Advanced
Tai Chi Chuan
Wind & Fire
Wheels

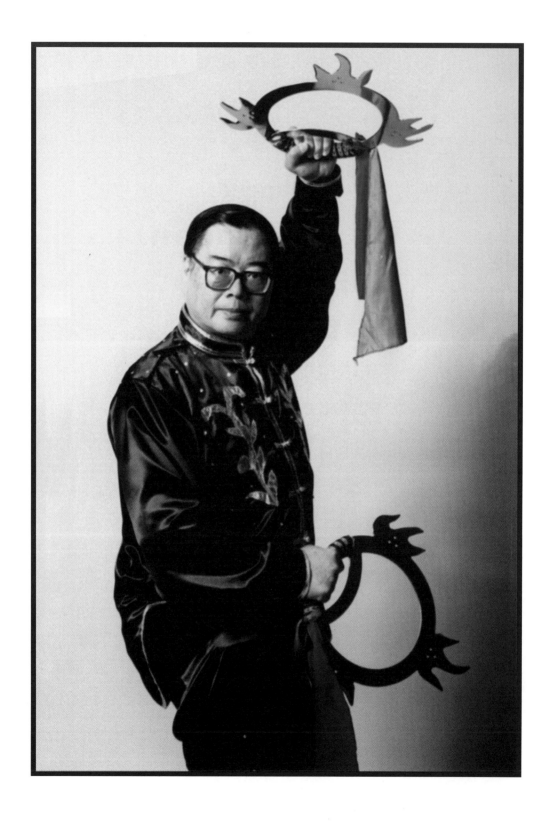

高 級
太極拳
風火輪

Advanced
Tai Chi Chuan
Wind & Fire
Wheels

by

Dr. Steve L. Sun, Ph.D.
9th Degree Black Belt

孫樹霖(釋德樹)著

Disclaimer

The author and publish of this material are **NOT RESPONSIBLE** in any manner whatsoever for any injury which may occur through reading or following the instructions in this book.

The activities, physical and otherwise, describe in this material may be too strenuous or dangerous for some people, and the reader should consult a physician before engaging in them.

First Printing
5

Library of Congress No: 99-093945

ISBN: 0-9671182-1-2

Printed in Canada

SLS Publication Center
A division of Siu Lum Studio, Inc.
27-29 East Eagle Road
Havertown, Pa.19083 USA
*Tel: (610) 789-1119 ** (610) 789-8771*
Fax: (610) 789-8771

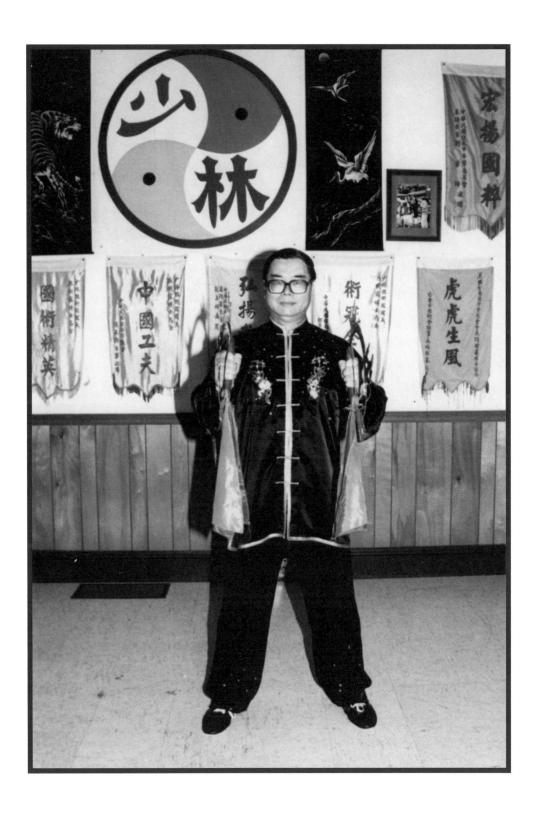

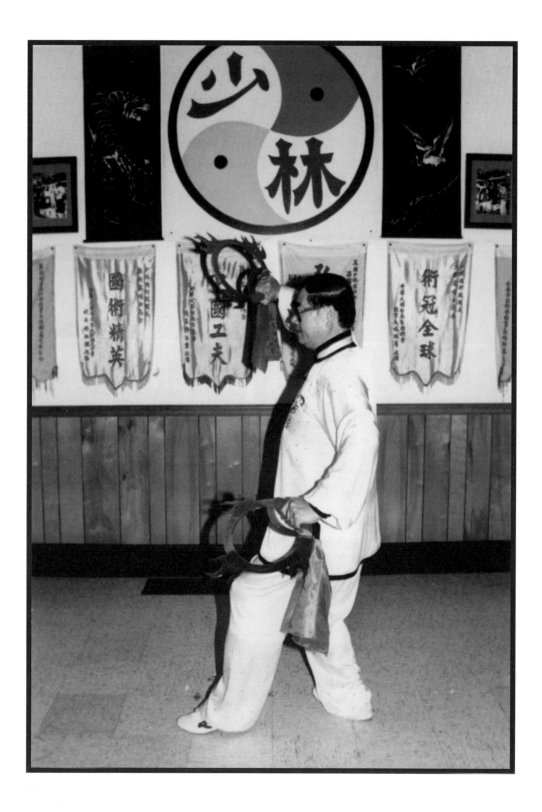

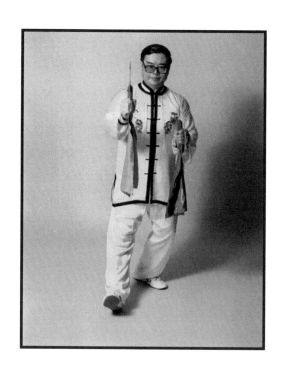

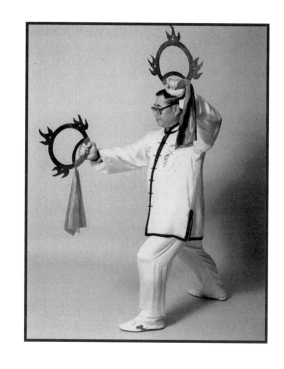

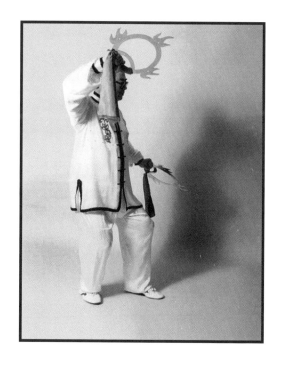

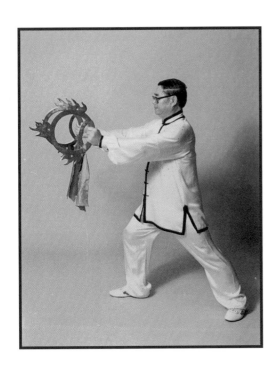

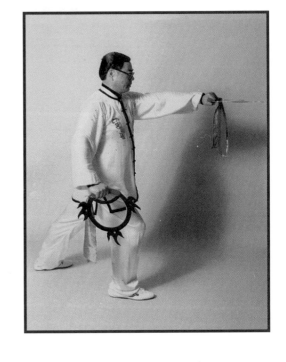

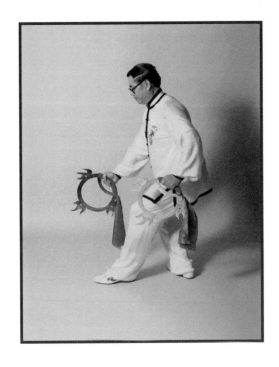

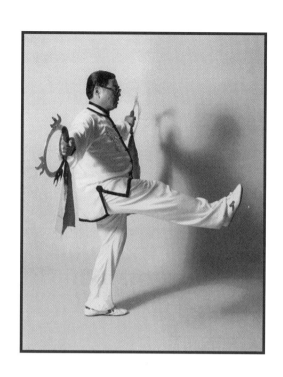

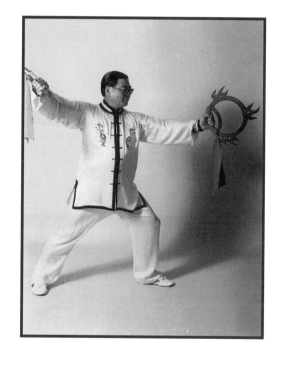

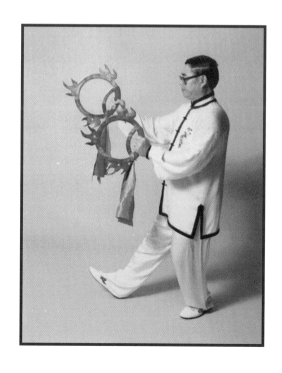

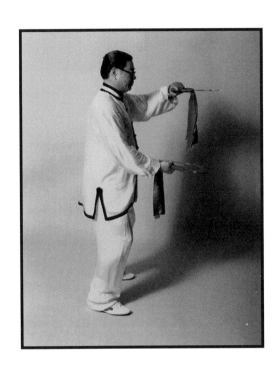

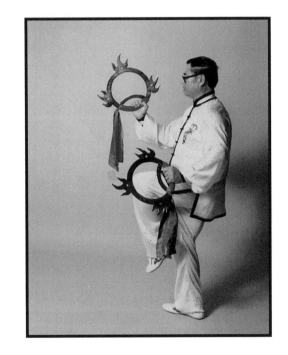

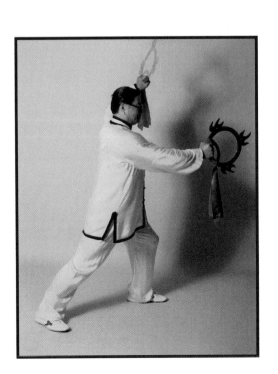

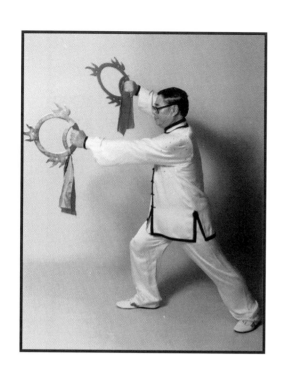

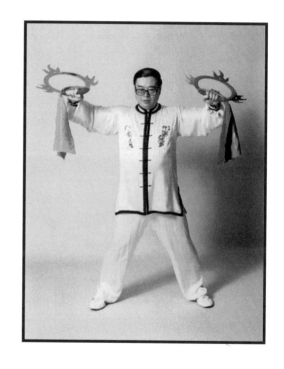

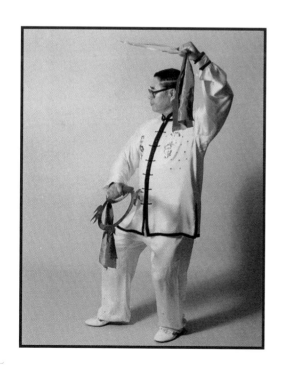

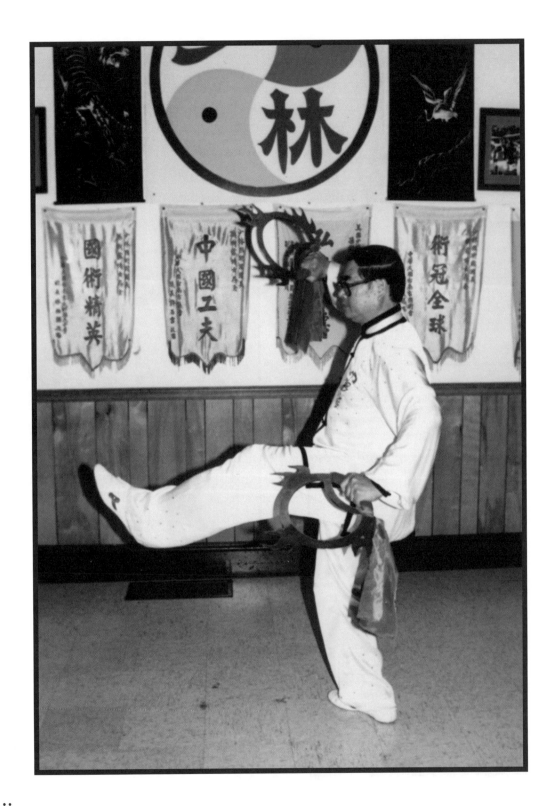

TABLE OF CONTENTS

DEDICATION TO
GRANDMASTER JOU TSUNG HWA

> *Every move of Tai-Chi Chuan is the movement of the universe. The awareness of the environment being engaged in a gigantic cosmic dance will suddenly dawn on you. You and the universe will become identical. You are then the Tai-Chi and the Tai-Chi is you and everything the universe reveals is you. This total identification is the foundation of universal harmony and peace. (Jou Tsung Hwa. The Tao of Tai-Chi Chuan)*

This eloquent quote from the heart of one of Tai-Chi's greatest grand masters conveys the spirit that Jou Tsung Hwa shared with us all. It is with the greatest humility that I dedicate this book to his memory.

In writing this book I have continually tried to make Jou Tsung Hwa's spirit central to every part of this book. We all knew him as a man who was dedicated to, **"Passing It On!"** His enthusiasm was partly based on his personal experience with the awesome benefits of Tai-Chi Chuan on his health as well as the growth in peace and harmony he saw in his students. While I personally have not been rescued from death's door by Tai-Chi as was Grand Master Jou, I have verified its life uplifting power in those I love and care for. What better expression could I find for who I am then to join Grand Master Jou in passing on the unique knowledge my family has given me of Tai Chi Wind-Fire Wheels.

The bedrock of Grand Master Jou's life was Taoism. As his students and friends knew, he was dedicated to cooperating in the flow of universal forces. **"Let it go!"** was his constant message whether the "it" be anger, pride, or intellectualization of the transcendent essence of Chi. Central to his cooperation in the connectedness of all was Grand Master Jou's emphasis on identifying with something other than self. As he would have said about the subject of this book, 'let go of any weapon as having singular power or uniqueness and become open to the wholeness that is the union of you, form, and weapon.' Realizing Grand Master Jou's vision of wholeness in Tai-Chi Chuan doesn't just happen. Players need a respectful grasp of correct technique, a firm base of internal strength, diligent practice, and wise guidance from a knowledgeable master. The purpose of this book is to help you achieve the first of these pre-requisites. The rest is up to you!

Readers of any advanced book in Tai-Chi Chuan must be careful to guard against pride in their accomplishments. In other words, I strongly advise students of Tai-Chi Wind Fire Wheels to absorb the wisdom of Grand Master Jou Tsung Hwa's book **The Tao of Tai Chi Chuan.** It is there that students will find a stress on simplicity and lightness of motion that is central to mastering the Wind Fire Wheels. As Grand Master Jou continually stressed, Tai-Chi is the natural movement of all parts of the body as one. The Wind-Fire Wheel is an awesome weapon whose appearance was meant to instill fear in opponents, but its power lies not in its appearance, or the sharpness of its blades, or in acrobatic and difficult movements, but in smooth and coordinated motion of wheels and body as a united whole.

My good friends, Pat Rice and Dr. John Painter, wrote moving testimonials to Grand Master Jou in a special issue of **Tai-Chi** magazine. Each stressed a central point from the grand master's teaching that is central to mastering the techniques and forms of this book. Pat Rice put the point as follows, "He constantly tested himself, created new theories, and tested again." Picking up the stress, John Painter reminded us that Grand Master Jou loved to say, "You just have to tell yourself 'I will do it!' then try to improve each day." Taken to heart, this wisdom is central to mastering the Wind Fire Wheels.

At the time of his death in August of 1998, Grand Master Jou Tsung Hwa was widely revered as a spiritual father to us all. While he is unable to write a foreword to this book as he did to its successor **(Tai-Chi Chuan Wind & Fire Wheels)**, his personal regard for me and that book remain one of the most heartfelt compliments I shall ever receive. Penned shortly before his death, Grand Master wrote to me in Chinese: "I received your book old brother [and] it is extraordinarily excellent." Thank you, brother, for those kind words and thank you for sharing your life with us.

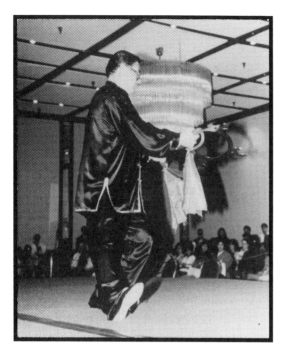

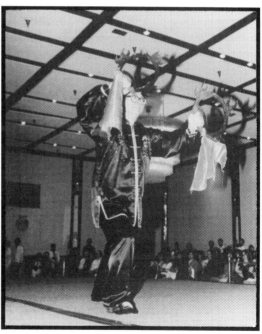

The author demonstrating the Tai-Chi Wind-Fire Wheels at Kuo-Shu Championship Tournament held in Hunt Valley, Maryland, July, 1995.

DEDICATION

This book is dedicated to my father, the late Grandmaster Sun Chun, who by his example, inspired me to study Chinese Martial Arts. My father was my hero, as many fathers are their sons heroes; it was he who first set my feet on the path I have followed all the days of my life. The techniques of Wind-Fire Wheels have been passed down from generation to generation in our family; and I thank my father for having entrusted me with this knowledge.

This book is further dedicated to Professor Wang Da-Sen, who instructed me in Tai-Chi Chuan and provided further instruction of Wind-Fire Wheel Techniques.

My father and Professor Wang Da-Sen provided my basic instruction of the Wind Fire Wheels. Through the years, my lovely wife, Emilia, has stood at my side, always providing the support and encouragement in my endeavors in the martial arts: my sons, David and Paul and their wives Toni and Suzanne, have also been strong supporters for me. It is therefore appropriate, that I dedicate this book to them, as well, for without them, I might have never chosen to write this book.

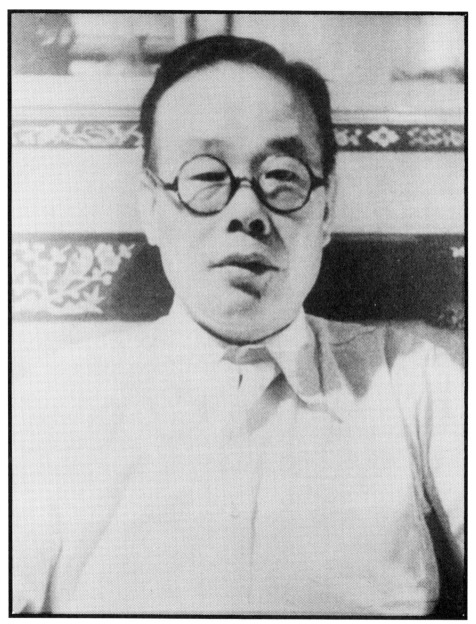

Great Grandmaster Sun Chun (孫郡), the author's father, who inspired the author to study Chinese Martial Arts and provided some of the basic Wind-Fire Wheels techniques.

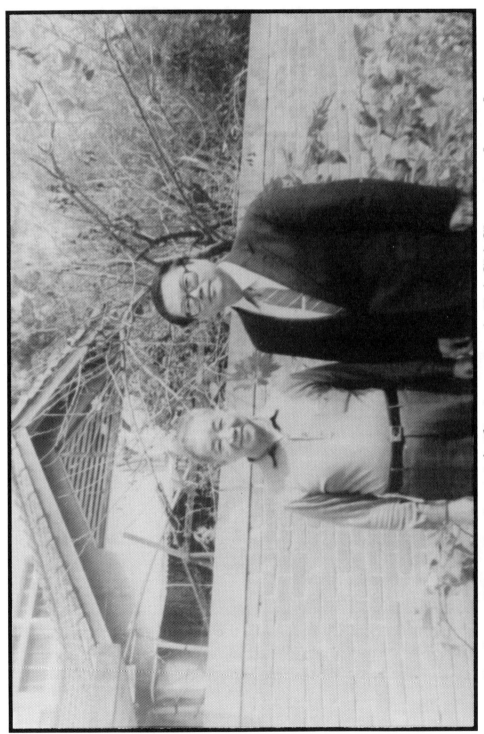

Professor Wang Da-Sen(王大琛), the author's Tai-Chi Chuan teacher, who provided some of the basic Wind-Fire Wheels techniques. Picture is taken in Tainan, Taiwan, 1985.

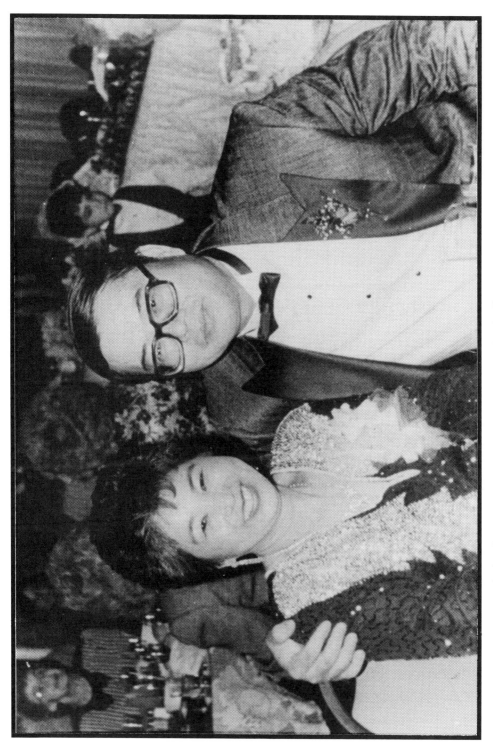

The author (孫樹霖) and his wife, Emilia (吳碧霞), celebrating 25th Wedding Anniversary (Silver Wedding) at their son's (David) Wedding Party, 1989.

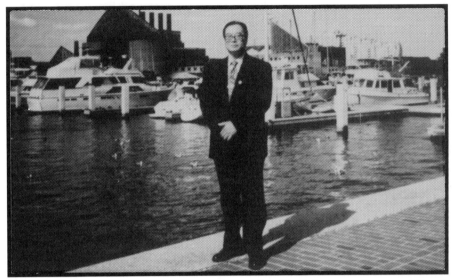

The author posing for a photo at the Baltimore Inner Harbor, Maryland, 1997.

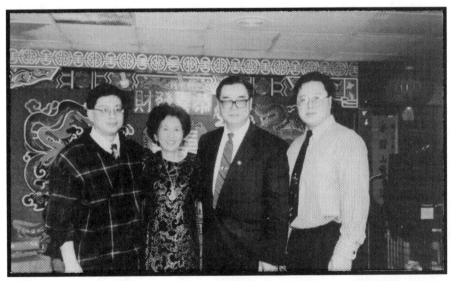

The author (second from right) posing for a family picture with his wife, Emilia and their sons, David(孫郁文, first right) and Paul(孫博文, first left). Picture is taken in Philadelphia, Pennsylvania, 1998.

ACKNOWLEDGMENTS

I would like to thank Mr. Andrew D. Schmith for taking all the photographs. I would also like to thank Maryann Leonard, Dr. Shahab Minassian and Professor Frank Wolek for helping me in writing this book. I would like to thank Toni Sun for helping me compile, edit and do most of the typing for this book. Thank you to Steve Barndt for posing in the Applications photos. A special thanks to Walter Bey for the inspiration and encouragement he gave me while writing this book. I would like to thank Ralph Wellington II for the computer graphic work done on this book. I would like to express my sincere gratitude to the following individuals for writing the foreword for this book: **Grandmaster Jou Tsung-Hwa, Grandmaster Wang Ju-Rong, Dr. Yang Jwing-Ming, Dr. John P. Painter, Director Pat Rice and Master Nick Gracenin.**

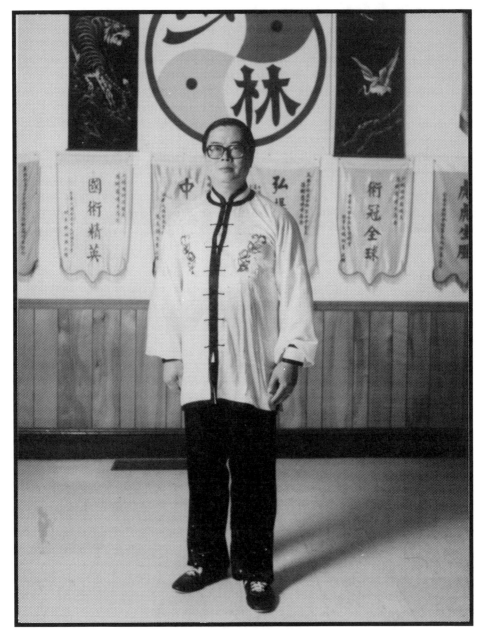

**Grand Master
Dr. Steve L. Sun**

ABOUT THE AUTHOR
GRANDMASTER DR. STEVE L. SUN

Grandmaster Dr. Steve L. Sun, certified Ninth Degree Black Belt, and founder of the Siu Lum Martial Arts Academy, has over forty-five years of experience in the martial arts. He is widely known for his wide array of knowledge of the martial arts, both internal and external, and also for his healing skills through acupressure. He has been featured in both _Inside Kung Fu_ and _Wu Shu Kung Fu_ in the United States and _Tai Chi & Alternative Health_ in Europe.

Grandmaster Sun was born on October 7, 1939 in Tainan, Taiwan, China. His father, a martial artist renowned for his skills, permitted his son to begin serious study of the martial arts when he was ten years of age. Grandmaster Sun's early training in the Northern and Southern Shaolin styles was conducted under the watchful guidance of his father and several well-known masters.

When Grandmaster Sun was eighteen years old, he entered National Cheng-Kung University in Tainan to study Civil Engineering. In college, he began the study of traditional Yang style Tai- Chi Chuan under Professor Da-Sen Wang and subsequently trained in Xing-Yi Quan under Master Kuo-Zong Chang. During this time, he continued to study, practice, and perfect his external martial art skills as well.

In 1962, he completed his B.S. degree in Civil Engineering and joined in ROTC training and then served in the Chinese Army Artillery Company stationed in Kin Moey Island. It was during the early 1960's when he met, courted, and finally married a beautiful and intelligent young woman- Emilia. While in the service, Dr. Sun taught Kung-Fu, Chin-Na, Shui Chiao and Knife and Gun Defense. After being honorably discharged in 1963, he returned to Cheng-Kung University to teach Civil Engineering courses as a teaching assistant.

In 1967, Dr. Sun came to the United States to study Civil and Environmental Engineering at the University of Pennsylvania in Philadelphia, Pennsylvania. At the request of a few graduate students, Grandmaster Sun began to teach Kung-Fu. In May of 1969, he was awarded a M.S. degree in Civil Engineering. Consequently, he continued his Ph.D. program in Water Resources and Environmental Engineering.

In 1973, Grandmaster Sun began working as an Environmental Engineering Consultant for United Engineers & Constructors, Inc. In May of 1975, Grandmaster Sun received a Ph.D. in Environmental Engineering from the University of Pennsylvania. In March 1977, Grandmaster Sun passed the Professional Engineer Certification, which is the most comprehensive examination for career Engineers.

While working full-time, Grandmaster Sun founded Sun's Siu Lum Kung-Fu Club. In 1983, Dr. Sun founded Siu Lum Martial Arts Academy in Havertown, Pennsylvania. Two years later, in 1985, he was received as a closed-door-31st generation disciple by the Shaolin Temple in the Henan province of China, and was instructed by the Abbot De-Chan in the ancient methods of internal Qigong, and in advanced Chin-Na techniques.

In 1986, Dr. Sun accepted a consultant position with Stone & Webster Engineering Corporation, in Cherry Hill, New Jersey. During this time, the Chinese Martial Arts Academy continued a steady growth, matching the growth of Grandmaster Sun's reputation of excellence. In 1990, Grandmaster Sun was named a recipient of the <u>Most Outstanding Martial Arts Gold Medal Award</u> from the World Martial Arts Federation of Taipei, Taiwan.

After 15 years as a Consulting Environmental Engineer, in the summer of 1991, Grandmaster Sun gave up his Engineering career to vigorously pursue his life dream of teaching martial arts full-time at the Chinese Martial Arts Academy he founded.

Numerous awards and recognition followed. In 1992, Grandmaster Sun completed an appointment as the 1992 Team Leader for the United States Kuo-Shu Team which competed successfully at the Seventh World Cup Chinese Kuo-Shu Tournament in Taiwan. In 1993, Grandmaster Sun was a recipient of the Top Ten Martial Arts Gold Medal Award. Additionally, Grandmaster Sun was appointed as the 1993 U.S. Team Leader for the Third "Overseas Chinese Cup" and 1993 Fourth "World Cup" International Martial Arts Championships. Under his leadership, the team garnered numerous gold medal awards and achieved Group Division Champion status in traditional forms.

Grandmaster Sun received the 1995 <u>The Martial Arts " Living Legends"</u> <u>Award</u> from Everhart's Nippon Kenpo Karate Do, of Washington, District of

Columbia. Current appointments include: United States Chairman of the Tainan Kung Fu Association; National Advisor of the United States of America Wushu Kung Fu Federation; United States East Coast President and Chairman of the International Kung-Fu Federation. In 1996, the United International KungFu Federation designated Grandmaster Sun "Sifu of the Year" and inducted Grandmaster into the "Hall of Fame". In 1997, Grandmaster Sun received the 6th World Cup International Martial Arts Championship "World Top One Hundred Exceptional Martial Artist Gold Medal Award" from International Martial Arts/Kung-fu Federation, U.S.A. In 1998, Grandmaster Sun was inducted into the "World Karate Union Hall of Fame", in which Dr. Sun received "Golden Lifetime Achievement Award of Honor".

In October, 1998, Grandmaster Sun published his first book entitled "Tai Chi Chuan Wind & Fire Wheels" which won the regard of six world well-known Martial Arts individuals who wrote a foreword for the book. On November 28, 1998, Dr. Sun was presented with Seven Most Outstanding Golden Awards by the World Chinese Medicine and Herbs United Association (W.C.M.H.U.A.) at "The Third World And Asian Traditional Medicine Conference" held in L.A., California, U.S.A.

On August 1, 1999, Dr. Sun participated in International Wushu Festival held at Union Square in San Francisco, California. Grandmaster Sun was recognized as one the most Outstanding Martial Artists by the World Traditional Chinese Sports Federation. On August 8, 1999, Dr. Sun was inducted into the "USA WKF Hall of Fame", in Baltimore, Maryland, in which Grandmaster Sun was honored and received "Outstanding Master Award".

Grandmaster Sun takes a strong pro-active role in tournament judging; and is certified as a National and International Kung Fu and Tai Chi Chuan Judge. He is also a Certified Senior Instructor of the United States Chinese Kuo-shu Federation. In addition to his extensive work in the martial arts, Grandmaster Sun is a skilled practitioner of the healing arts. In April of 1996, Grandmaster Sun opened the Chinese Chi-Kung Acupressure Center directly across from Siu Lum Studio to benefit the local community and increase public awareness of alternative Eastern medical techniques.

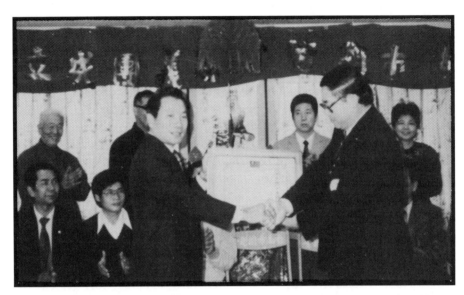

**The author receiving Eighth Degree Black Belt certificate from Grandmaster
Jui-Feng Yang (楊瑞峰), Chairman of the Tainan Kung-Fu Federation,
Tainan, Taiwan,1990.**

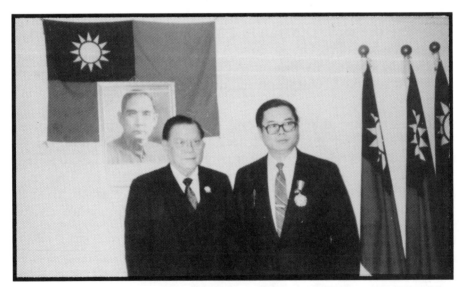

**The author receiving the Most Outstanding Martial Arts Gold Medal
Award from Dr. Shan-De Huang (黃善德), President of the world
Martial Arts Federation of Taipei, Taiwan, 1990.**

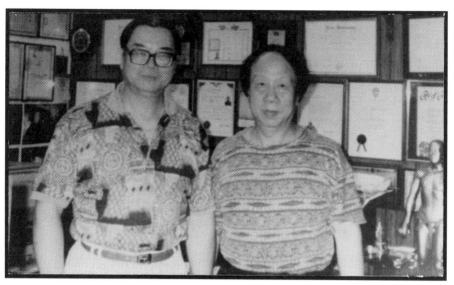

The author receiving Ninth Degree Black Belt from Dr. Che-Cheng Chiang(江志成), President of International Kung-Fu Federation, L.A.,U.S.A.,1995.

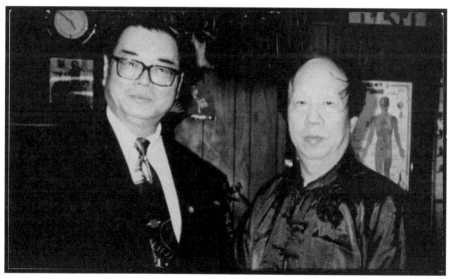

The author receiving Gold Cup Achievement Award from Dr. Che-Cheng Chiang, President of International Kung-Fu Federation, L.A., U.S.A., 1997.

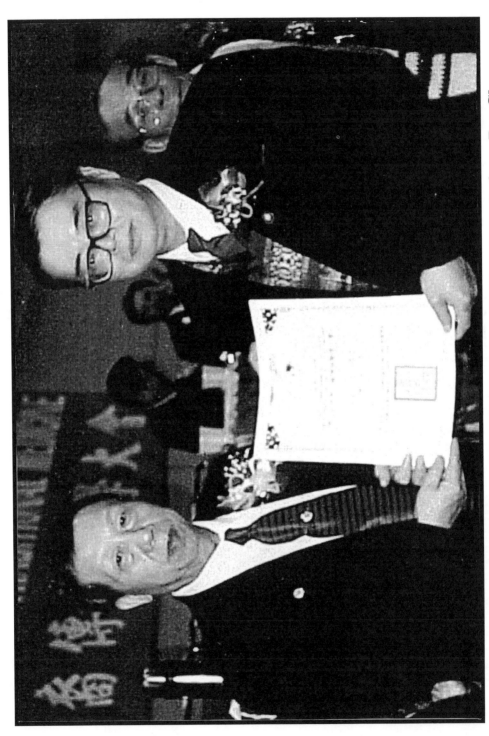

The author receiving Seven Most Outstanding Golden Awards from Dr. Che-Cheng Chiang, President of American Asian Federation, L.A., U.S.A., 1998.

FOREWORD

GRANDMASTER JOU TSUNG-HWA

When I began teaching Tai Chi Chuan in the United States in 1971, I had two mutually supportive objectives:

* to help Americans benefit in both internal and spiritual strength by following the Tai Chi principles developed by the Great Masters and

* to help people use these principles as I had to recover and to enhance their health.

From the first, I realized that these objectives would require cooperation with others who share my values. In my travels, I was constantly on the lookout for masters who Tai Chi was strong and true. One such person, indeed an exemplar of the kind of person I sought, was Dr. Steve L. Sun of the Siu Lum Studio. Here was a truly great practitioner of Tai Chi whose every move demonstrated internal power and respectful adherence to ancestral principle. Here also was a man of immense heart who had dedicated himself to encouraging others and to curing the physical weaknesses and impediments that limited their full enjoyment of life. In short, here was a man I wanted as a friend and comrade in my life's work.

Through the years, I have interacted with Dr. Sun often at Tai Chi seminars and at events around the country. I have seen how his expertise influences others I respect and how his unselfish warmth shines as a model to new masters here and abroad. I have also watched Dr. Sun emerge as a famous practitioner of Chi-Kung Acupressure. The point being that it is rare to find someone who combines internal power with an intellectual understanding of traditional medicine. Only those like Dr. Sun who have long years in Tai Chi and Chi-Kung have the internal power and sophisticated knowledge to treat the root causes of illness and physical weakness.

It came as no surprise when I saw a copy of this wonderful book *Tai Chi Chuan Wind Fire Wheels*. As I would have expected from Dr. Sun, his forms are not only respectful applications of Yang's Tai Chi to weapon use but are also intelligent and creative applications. How else can you describe the use of movements such as Brush Knee or Snake Creeps Down in ways that are both martial in intent and safe for the weapons user. As someone who is also dedicated to building on ancestral traditions, I have nothing but the greatest admiration for Dr. Sun's skill and accomplishment.

How wonderful it was too see how Dr. Sun used his knowledge of medicine and the human body to illuminate and enrich the forms he teaches here. His sophisticated presentation of content and performance is no accident. The book is exceptional in its attention to the medical implications of using this ancestral weapon. In providing a unique focus on the strength and coordination of the upper body. Dr. Sun has significantly enhanced the value of Tai Chi in developing internal strength. Here then are skills that will test and extend the internal power of any player regardless of prior accomplishments. I heartily recommend your close attention to and your serious practice of Dr. Sun's expertly designed forms.

Jou Tsung Hwa
Grandmaster
Founder of the Tai Chi Farm
Author of *The Tao of Tai Chi Chuan,*
The Tao of the I-Ching, and
The Tao of Meditation

FOREWORD

GRANDMASTER WANG JU-RONG

In 1989, soon after I moved to Houston, Texas, from Shanghai, I attended the United States Martial Arts Council wushu competition held in north Houston. There I met Dr. Steve L. Sun for the first time. Even at that first meeting, I noticed his enthusiasm for promoting wushu. He subsequently demonstrated his dedication to the art when in 1991, he gave up a lucrative career in engineering to teach a kung fu school - the American Chinese Kung Fu/Martial Arts Academy of Philadelphia, which he founded. I deeply respect this decision on his part. He indicated to me that he had two reasons for this move. First, he desired to make his own contribution to developing Chinese culture. In addition, having been taught wushu from childhood by his father, he wished to pass on the skills he had learned.

Now, Dr. Sun has invited me to write a foreword to this book, ***Taiji Wind Fire Wheel.*** Naturally I agreed, and I am glad to have this opportunity to congratulate him on the completion of this project and to wish him every success.

Since ancient times, many weapons have been used in traditional Chinese kung fu training. The most commonly quoted figure is eighteen different varieties of weapons. Actually, this figure is just half the story. It only takes into account the most commonly known weapons. To this list should be added a number of unusual weapons which were developed for specialized uses. The most accurate figure I have seen recognizes eighteen large weapons and eighteen small weapons, for a total of thirty-six. One of the most extraordinary and complex weapons is called "Feng Huo Lun" - the "Wind Fire Wheel". The name is also sometimes abbreviated to "Lun". In ancient China this "lun" was merely a solid metal ring or circular band. In its modern form, the ring has been flattened and a pattern of sharp curved points added to the outer edge, producing a lighter and more maneuverable weapon. These modifications give the "lun" the important ability to be used for blocking and defense, not just for attacking. It can be used as a single weapon or as a double weapon, according to the skill of the wielder.

The title of Dr. Sun's book is ***Taiji Wind Fire Wheel.*** The name immediately reveals the purpose - that is, combining traditional taijiquan with a traditional double weapon to develop a new wushu form that still retains the traditional flavor.

This book is divided into three parts. The first section introduces basic taiji movements using the "wind fire wheel." The movements retain the names of many familiar taiji postures, such as "Part Wild Horse's Mane," "Single Whip," "Wave Hands in Clouds," and so on. The basics shown in this section serve as the foundation for the intermediate and advanced routines presented in Sections 2 and 3 of the book, respectively. The movements are easy to learn and easy to memorize. The postures are performed using taiji techniques, and the "lun" is used to finish each movement. This form also has extra benefits that will enhance your practice. The routine uses three times the punching and kicking movements of the traditional form. It also emphasizes using both left and right sides in Bow Stances, Crouch Stances and One Legged Stances to give equal training to both legs. The stretching, balance and turning movements provide the health benefits inherent in all taiji forms. Practicing the double weapon form also increases arm and wrist power. It is not even necessary to begin by buying an expensive set of weapons. The beginner can fashion a lightweight practice wheel out of wood or cane. Later, if he wishes, he can switch to metal weapons and increase his power. Men, women, old and young, can all practice these easy to learn taiji style routines to improve their physical constitutions and general health.

Madame Wang Ju-Rong
Professor of Wushu
National Wushu Judge of China

FOREWORD

DR. YANG JWING-MING

It is well known that Japanese Karate was imported to America around 1950 by American soldiers who were serving in Japan and Okinawa. These Oriental martial arts captured the attention of Western society, and soon Karate spread throughout the world.

In the 1960's, Master Cheng, Man-Ching introduced Tai Chi Chuan, an internal Chinese martial art, to the Western world, and it caught the attention of Western society. Many people became fascinated with Tai Chi Chuan, which is very different from Japanese Karate.

The excitement over Chinese martial arts, both internal and external, reached its peak in the late 1960's, when Bruce Lee's motion pictures came to the West. Westerners finally began to realize the scope of Chinese martial arts, which have been developing for five thousand years.

President Nixon's visit to China in 1973 generated great interest in the study and understanding of Chinese culture. This is especially true of Chinese medicine, including acupuncture and Qigong for health and longevity. In addition, the arrival of many Chinese martial arts masters in the United States helped Western society gain a better understanding of real Chinese martial arts.

Today, Tai Chi Chuan is commonly recognized as one of the most effective methods of preventing sickness, calming the mind, building a sense of inner peace, lowering blood pressure, and many other health benefits.

Because of the open communication between China and the United States, many Tai Chi styles have become popular, including Yang, Chen, Wu, Sun, Hao, and Cheng. In addition to barehand Tai Chi Chuan sequences, many Tai Chi weapons are also taught. The most popular weapons are: Tai Chi saber, Tai Chi sword, Tai Chi staff, and Tai Chi spear. The practice of other Tai Chi weapons is seldom seen.

This book, written by Dr. Steve Sun, introduces to the West the usage of the Wind-Fire Rings in Tai Chi Chuan. Dr. Sun is a well-known martial artist, and he also has a doctorate in engineering. Therefore, the writing in his book is profound, logical, and scientific. I believe this book gives Tai Chi practitioners an opportunity to understand the applications of these extraordinary weapons.

Dr. Yang Jwing-Ming, Ph.D.
President, YMAA International

FOREWORD

DR. JOHN P. PAINTER

" And now Dr. Sun will demonstrate the Wind and Fire Wheels" as the announcer introduced my good friend Dr. Sun during the 1995 A Taste of China Masters demonstrations the thought crossed my mind. "Please not another gymnastic toy weapon demonstration." Peaking through the curtains I was presently surprised at what I saw. Dr. Sun holding two esoteric looking disc shaped knives with tongues of steel flame shooting from their rims was moving through a T'ai Chi Ch'uan routine. Instead of his hands performing the defensive tactics of deflect, neutralize and strike he was making all of his actions with these strange looking circular swords.

Being a lover of edged weapons, a law enforcement trainer and former bodyguard like my late teacher Li, Longdao I am seldom impressed by seeing the countless demonstrations with Chinese style tinfoil weapons, flips and other gymnastic tricks touted as real martial arts. Dr. Sun's demonstration was another matter entirely. Watching his actions even in slow motion it was obvious that not only did Dr. Sun know that what he was doing but that he also was a highly skilled martial arts practitioner. There were no huge long stances, no wasted motions and no actions appeared to be "just because they looked good."

I was witnessing what I so often long to see, in these demonstrations, practical yet beautiful martial arts. This was not a form Dr. Sun was demonstrating it was more than that. It was the way my teacher said forms should be,

" **Form can be empty or alive. The true form is not copied and then stamped out. A martial form is a receptacle that holds essential martial and physical principles arranged in a true pantomime of a combat with one or numerous invisible opponent. Without these things form is just dance.**"

Li, Longdao 1959

Now that Dr. Sun has released this book on Wind & Fire wheels I am very honored to help him promote it to the T'ai Chi Ch'uan martial arts community. This is an important work for it preserves a rare and interesting page of Chinese martial arts culture. Wind & Fire wheels can also be a fine way to get a little extra exercise and spice in our T'ai Chi Ch'uan routines. The book contains sound practical knowledge, history, and realistic applications all in one volume. It is also a way of proving the old maxim that, "if you truly know the hands you can know the weapon."

Unlike other eastern methods of self-defense that have separate hand and weapons techniques Chinese methods rely on making their weapons extensions of the hand. A real Chinese martial arts teacher who truly understands his arts principle, not just form can pick up almost any weapon from sword to firearm and in a few moments use it as if he had practiced with it for a long time. This is the mark of a true martial artist and I certainly can clearly see this mark on Dr. Steve Sun. I recommend his work to all interested in Chinese martial arts.

Dr. John P. Painter ND
Capt. American Rangers Law Enforcement Training
Jiulong Baguazhang Association, USA Representative
Arlington, TX.

FOREWORD

DIRECTOR PAT RICE

We who practice taijiquan in its various styles have learned many things about ourselves. As we increase our knowledge of self, we develop a great appreciation for the means of our growth. This is why many of us renew our dedication to the practice of taijiquan, recognizing that it has been the nest path to our higher self. Most of our insights come from our practice of barehand routines, and when we turn to the practice of weapons, we have additional opportunities to expand our journey inward.

Dr. Steve Sun has been both a student along this way, and also a leader for us to follow. His own thorough training and substantial credentials have brought him to a position of authority and trust. Like others who find themselves in such a place, he has turned his attention to service toward his community. With the publication of two books on the Wind-Fire Wheels, he enables many students to reach further in their studies and into themselves.

His publication of the first volume of Wind-Fire Wheels made an admirable presentation of this unusual weapon, and those attracted by this work and by the weapons themselves have eagerly anticipated this publication of further information. His work is both scholarly and readable, and truly honors his family traditional teachings.

Dr. Sun is not only a well-regarded teacher who is devoted to his own students and his own programs, he is an ardent supporter of others and their efforts. As Director of A Taste of China, an organization which since 1983 has promoted Chinese martial arts in general and presented annual seminars and tournaments, I feel fortunate to count Dr. Sun among our most valuable participants.

Pat Rice
Technical Committee Member, International Wushu Federation
Executive Board Member, United States Wushu Kungfu Federation
Director, A Taste of China
Winchester, Virginia

FOREWORD

MASTER NICK GRACENIN

I have been honored to write a foreword to Dr. Steve L. Sun's book TAI CHI CHUAN WIND AND FIRE WHEELS. Now I am happy to join other readers in welcoming a sequel. This advanced text will provide Tai Chi Chuan practitioners with even more insight concerning a truly rare weapon. Wushu of all styles and systems must be studied deeply to produce real benefits, and the availability of books by masters such as Dr. Sun facilitates that depth.

In my foreword to the author's initial publication I quoted the popular Tai Chi saying *"Xing ling yun shui"* - In appearance similar to floating clouds and flowing streams. The flow of time has now brought us to an inevitable and saddening loss.

It is with great sadness that I write to commemorate the passing of Master Jou Tsung-Hwa. For many years I have been honored to call Master Jou an advisor, a source of inspiration and most importantly, a true friend. Master Jou was in every sense of the word, a Teacher. Not only a Master of Chinese martial arts and academics, but a shining example of all that is good in humankind. Unfailing in generosity, perseverance and humility, Jou Tsung-Hwa was what many aspire to be - a true warrior poet. He has distinguished himself forever in the Chinese martial arts community through his many contributions, most notably his creation of the Tai Chi Farm. The dedication of this textbook to his memory is one of countless ways that "Mister Jou" will always remain with us.

I will always remember him for his gentle kindness to my wife and children, for his encouragement to always pursue higher levels of thought and ability, and for his wonderful smile. We have lost a leader, a teacher and friend, but his legacy remains with us forever. In years to come, we must never forget his example, to constantly reach for perfection, knowing that the process of doing so is the goal we seek.

Nick Gracenin

Executive Committee Member, International Wushu Federation
Founding Member, United States Wushu Kungfu Federation

PREFACE

I wrote this book as humble step in my continuing effort to pass on the inheritance of Chinese Great Masters. The book stems from over 50 years of research and experience in the Chinese Martial Arts, experience that resulted in three sets of Advanced Wind-Fire Wheels forms for Tai-Chi enthusiasts. I designed each forms to apply traditional Tai-Chi Chuan postures and movements to this ancient and powerful weapon. Tai-Chi players who are interested in weapon-based forms may now grow in their understanding and ability through careful study and patient and well structured practice of the book's contents.

Advanced Tai Chi Chuan Wind & Fire Wheels has been requested by experienced Tai-Chi players and masters throughout the world. I began writing and compiling the research that led to this book and its predecessor **(Tai Chi Chuan Wind & Fire Wheels)** following a demonstration of the Advanced Form in 1995 at a national Tai-Chi tournament - A Taste of China. I was further encouraged by my students and friends who wished to deepen their understanding of Tai-Chi Chuan. In short, I wrote the book as a learning tool for people who are enthusiastic about the role of Tai-Chi in developing their physical, mental, and spiritual well being.

I need to stress the significant qualifications for success in learning to do Tai-Chi with the Wind-Fire Wheels. Basic experience in barehanded Tai-Chi Chuan is absolutely essential. The physical strength and internal power, that comes from good form and teaching in Tai-Chi Chuan are also fundamental.

Finally, players need competent instruction from a Tai-Chi master. Learning the Wind-Fire Wheels is also unlikely without such guidance and false training will cause both external and internal injury. Readers with a solid base in Tai-Chi, a good teacher, and perseverance in the forms described here will surely acquire a sound command of this rare weapon.

I have also designed this book to be valuable for masters and advanced students dedicated to research on Tai Chi weapons. Every Wind-Fire Wheels posture is explained in simple and familiar terms and illustrated with photographs. Basic theory, methods, order of practice, and principles of weapon handling are presented in detail. My aim was to provide not only teaching but also depth in theory and training requirements. I will be very happy and honored if this book succeeds in advancing the research in Tai-Chi Chuan that is so essential in our revered and ever growing art.

This book is anchored on interaction with many masters and players throughout the world to whom I owe a great deal. Hopefully, the book will provide a return in enthusiasm for and advanced capability in Tai-Chi Chuan by both those who have helped me and those who they train and encourage. In this way, I will have given something back to the art of Tai-Chi Chuan, that is, to an art that continues to advance the longevity and happiness of its enthusiasts and the peaceful welfare of all people.

CHAPTER 1

INTRODUCTION TO ADVANCED TAI-CHI WIND-FIRE WHEELS

The Wind-Fire Wheels is a weapon that is close to my heart. Much of my early training in the Wheels came from my father who had been charged to pass on the training to future generations. So too had my grandfather trained my father and so on back through the generations of the Sun family. In other words, the knowledge and skill covered in this book continue both a great tradition and a great obligation. I sincerely pray that responsible readers also assume a similar obligation to seriously develop the knowledge and skill needed for passing the tradition on to new generations throughout the world.

Today we believe that what was once restricted and hidden knowledge be made public. We come to believe that it is not sufficient for beneficiaries of tradition to restrict themselves to passing it on to their own children. Instead, we believe there are now many talented and responsible people in the martial arts

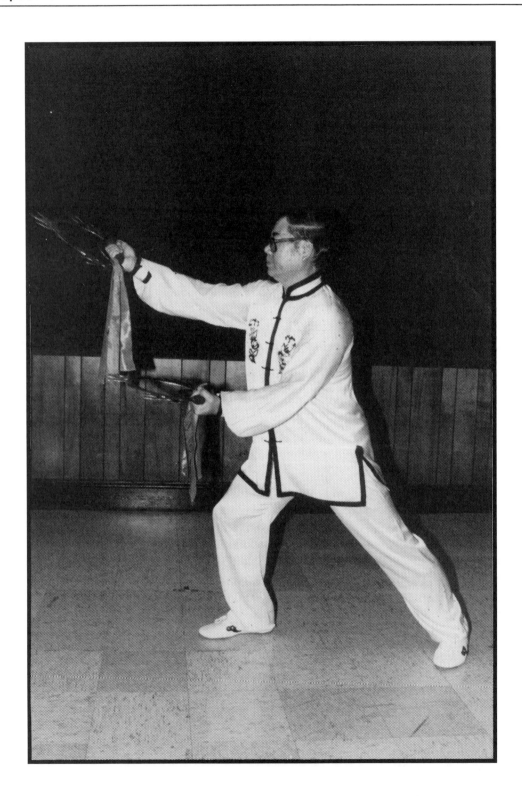

community who will respectfully learn that which was developed so carefully by our ancestors. Therefore, in July of 1995, I gave the first public performance of Tai-Chi Wind-Fire Wheels outside China. The occasion was the 1995 A Taste of China Master's Demonstration in Winchester, Virginia. The response was emphatically positive and quite overwhelming. Requests for further demonstrations, seminars, and teaching materials poured in as they also did after a second and third demonstration at the 1995 International Kuo-Shu Championships in Hunt Valley, Maryland and then at the 1995 World Wushu Championships in Baltimore, Maryland.

I soon saw that my personal demonstrations and seminars could not satisfy the Tai-Chi community's demand for knowledge of this wonderful weapon. Therefore, in 1998, I published the book **Tai-Chi Chuan Wind & Fire Wheels** through the **SLS Publication Center**. Where I might have once felt that one book would discharge my responsibility, the overwhelming response again indicated that I had opened a door I could never close. Therefore, I have accepted the further responsibility to organize and pass on not only the knowledge I gained from my ancestors but also that which I personally developed through 50 years of practice and reflection. This first step in that expanded effort, an advanced book on the theory and practice of Wind-Fire Wheels, will hopefully continue my life-long program of teaching and learning from others.

History of Wind-Fire Wheels

The origin of the Tai-Chi Wind-Fire Wheels is shrouded in the mysteries of China's past. While the weapon has an illustrious history in oral legend, it is not specifically mentioned in the ancient literature of Tai Chi. Weapons in the class of Wind-Fire Wheels are, however, encountered in literature from the latter part of the Ching dynasty (1644-1892) authored first by Yang Lu Chang (1799-1872) and then by Yang Ban-Hou (1837-1892). Even there, however, the literature is as sparse as we would expect given that the skill required could not have been common.

From a metallurgical point of view, the Wind-Fire Wheels share much of the same history as the Tai-Chi Jen which is a decidedly more common weapon dating back hundreds of years. This common history may be traced to the fact that production of swords and other cutting weapons from steel alloys reached high levels of craftsmanship during the Ching Dynasty. While several localities achieved renown in such weapons, three are held in especially high regard. Two of these esteemed areas, Lung Chuan and Wu Kan, are in eastern China in the

Zurgian Province. As students of Tai Chi might guess, the third location was at the Shaolin Temple-Chin Ying in Henan Province.

The Wind-Fire Wheels were hand-wrought by master metal smiths with long experience in crafting edged weapons. A smith would start with a flat piece of the special high-carbon steels reserved for bladed weapons. Patient heating was needed to make the steel ductile while maintaining its ability to take and hold a durable edge. Following such care, smiths forged the bar into a wheel. The smiths then drew the sides of the bright orange wheel into evenly tapered edges. The next step was to close the circle by forming a hand guard. The most critical steps centered on the three, three-pronged tongues of fire that are the slicing edges of each Wind-Fire Wheel. Each set of tongues was carefully forged as a unit from the best of cutting steel. Each was then forge-welded onto its wheel. Hand finishing with abrasive sand removed impurities such as metal scale and prepared the wheels for hand rubbing with oils and bee's wax that would give it lasting protection from rust. Finally, patient grinding and delicate hand filing brought each and every surface (save the area of the hand-hold) to an incorruptibly sharp cutting edge. Polishing and personally fitting a leather hand-hold completed a weapon that was fit only for the elite few with the patience, skill, and status to transform it into an awe-inspiring weapon.

The Significance of Wind-Fire Wheels in Tai-Chi Chuan

At times I wonder why so many accomplished martial artists are unaware of the Wind-Fire Wheels that my family has venerated for generations. One line of reflection on this question has led me to undertake this book. I noted that, until my publication of this book's predecessor *Tai-Chi Chuan Wind & Fire Wheels*, knowledge of the weapon was restricted to oral tradition. Knowledge of such value to the martial arts community was, in other words, hidden in time and in teaching conveyed from father to child. In some families, the knowledge died when there was no heir to learn it. In other cases, it was lost because there was no one within a family's circle ready or worthy of receiving it. I realized also that my family and others responsibly transmitted the skill outside the circle of their own bloodlines when they recognized a capability and dedication to learning. In other words, some families were open to sharing with outside orientals who had proven themselves by achieving Master status.

As liberating as this openness was, the knowledge continued to die just as tragically when some family circles failed to extend themselves to new masters. Indeed, the tragedy deepened as the knowledge was being lost to an increasingly world-wide community in the martial arts. It was thus that I came to see that it was time to extend my family's knowledge to a global community in which I have found numerous deserving people. In other words, it was time to use the more public means of publishing multiple books and giving seminars at all levels in order to preserve a body of knowledge that could no longer be allowed to disappear in the whims of family history.

Why do Tai-Chi Wind-Fire Wheels have so much significance for me? One response focuses on their uniqueness in expressing the traditional essence of Tai-Chi Chuan. This is one of very few double-handed weapons available in Tai-Chi Chuan. As such, the weapon emphasizes the coordination of body movements at the heart of Tai-Chi. Both arms and both legs must work in harmony with the torso to achieve a flowing and powerful movement in Wind-Fire Wheel forms.

While traditional practice develops the total body, I have found that the practice of western students favors development of the lower body. In other words, I recognized the value of training that would restore the balanced development of the total body emphasized in traditional teaching. Tai-Chi Wind-Fire Wheels satisfy that need through the coordinated strength they require in the arms and upper torso. The longer forms at the core of this book are impossible for someone unused to handling weights in extended positions from the body. So important is this issue of balanced use of the body that I have devoted a special chapter to its coverage.

The significance of Tai-Chi Wind-Fire Wheels extends further to its compatibility with traditional barehanded Tai-Chi Chuan. Forms for working with some treasured weapons such as the cudgel encourage adaptations to capture the weapon's physical length and flexibility. Tai-Chi movements and forms with Wind-Fire Wheels, on the other hand, are easily anchored on the same principles of barehanded Tai-Chi. Save for minor adaptations to protect the player from self-injury, readers will recognize the same fluid, slow, and graceful action found in Yang's Tai-Chi.

The final point about the significance of Wind-Fire Wheels concerns the central role of intent and spirit in Tai-Chi Chuan. Weapons in general have played a major role in developing advanced skills precisely because they require significant concentration and sense of martial purpose for correct use. Yet, for too many generations, weapons fell into disfavor when firearms rose to martial prominence. Weapons such as Wind-Fire Wheels, Tai-Chi Jen, and Broad Sword declined to purely symbolic significance in dances, ceremonies, and rituals.

Throughout the world, Masters are recognizing the value of weapons to develop their students' concentration, appreciation of intent, and spirit. It is in this sense that I believe that the Tai-Chi Wind-Fire Wheels have a special role. The heart of using Wind-Fire Wheels lies in the value of the tongues of fire for slicing. While each set of tongues was awesomely sharp, the key to the their effectiveness was a user's smooth and powerful rotation. In other words, the most critical Wind-Fire skill is the same coordinated fluidity of circular motion at the heart of Tai-Chi Chuan. So too does the curvature of each tongue reflect the circular motion in the player's body and as the tongues are thrust in circular piercing motions towards an opponent.

The circularity of the weapon and its use reflects the balance of Yin and Yang that tradition teaches us is central to Tai-Chi Chuan as well as all life. In other words, the value of the tongues in slicing and thrusting is balanced by using the edges between each set of fire for blocking. However, just as tradition teaches us that Ying and Yang are infinitely embedded in each other, so is the sharpness of these blocking edges useful in destroying an opponent's weapon.

Tradition also teaches us the importance of being perpetually prepared to respond to an opponent's energy. Players who use the Wind-Fire Wheels learn that such preparedness is critical as their personal safety requires them to never drop their sense of the wheels' position. Preparedness is more than control of position, however, it is also an ability to sense the energy of those around you in relation to your own. It is here that the fine metal composition of two metal wheels acts like an energy sensing dowsing rod.

The Critical Importance of Safety

Readers are cautioned that working with the Wind-Fire Wheels requires a great deal of coordination and care. Indeed, those who would take up the wheels should have already acquired proficiency in a prior weapon such as the straight or broad sword. Even though the weapons used in modern Tai-Chi Chuan are not sharp, handling the Wind-Fire Wheels requires players to be fully aware of the position of the weapon in relation to their own and others' bodies. This is especially true of the orientation and proximity of the three sets of fire tongues that remain dangerously pointed. Turning the Wind-Fire Wheels too close to one's body is a problem that reality will quickly correct.

There is an especially distinct risk of serious injury to inexperienced players who would play with the wheels on a dare or lark. Untutored people lacking the strength, balance, coordination, and inner sense of positioning that comes from serious study of barehanded forms of Tai-Chi run significant risk of falling on points, cutting themselves on edges, or otherwise injuring themselves and others. With experience and the mutual respect for and awareness of others that characterizes a well functioning studio, players will possess the base they need for safe enjoyment of this potent weapon.

A Look Ahead

This book builds on the foundation of basic moves and forms covered in the author's earlier book, *Tai-Chi Chuan Wind & Fire Wheels*. That book presented a set of twenty-one (21) basic movements; three forms designed for novice, intermediate, and advanced players, and twenty-two (22) martial art applications of basic movements. The current book opens with a deeper discussion of the health and internal benefits players obtain from working with the wheels. The book then presents eight (8) additional movements for advanced level players. These movements and the applications of them presented in a later chapter are entirely of my own design. Each is, however, firmly anchored on traditional Tai-Chi Chuan principles and developed from barehanded movements used in advanced forms of Tai-Chi Chuan.

Consistent with the inspiration of this book in the life and teaching of Grand Master Jou Tsung Hwa, I begin the integration of basic movements with a presentation on their use in Chi-Kung. That base for an advanced treatment of internal energy states leads to three, complete forms each of which requires and will reward advanced skill and concentration.

Conclusion

I was initially introduced to this beautiful and potent weapon in the extensive training in martial arts I received in Taiwan from my father, Grandmaster Sun Chun. The foundation I received from my father was extended in training under several renowned teachers beginning first with training in external Kung Fu systems and expanding to internal forms. Professor Wang Da-Sen, an outstanding teacher of Tai-Chi Chuan, played an integral part in developing my expertise with Wind-Fire Wheels.

Soul-Searching reflection on the global state of the martial arts today has led me to follow Grand Master Jou Tsung Hwa in using my humble talents to write a series of books on the use of weapons in Tai-Chi Chuan. This second book in that commitment is an outgrowth of a two-pronged effort to educate the martial arts community about this personally significant weapon. In other words, the books themselves are coupled with demonstrations, seminar leadership, and training programs I have conducted regularly since 1995. The first step in this outreach program was the selection of a special group of my own students to learn and make group demonstrations with the Wind-Fire Wheels. My students and I have followed that beginning with repeated demonstrations and seminars. We are proud to say that, judging from the enthusiastic response, this part of our work will continue for a long time to come.

CHAPTER 2

FUNDAMENTAL TRAINING AND BASIC EXERCISES

2.1 Introduction

As with all new techniques, it is advisable to begin the learning process through a variety of warm-up exercises. This is applicable to both the beginner and the experienced player. So too, when beginning to learn to use the Wind-Fire Wheels, there are a series of movements which allows the player to learn and develop an expertise in using the Wind-Fire Wheels. As the Wheels are approximately 2 - 3 pounds each, heavier than most weapons, it is necessary to build up to their use in the form. Without this, it is difficult to complete the form without tiredness or injury. Only those who have trained extensively can perform the form immediately, without the introductory movements. There are additional reasons for performing the movements in the beginning of training. They are as follows:

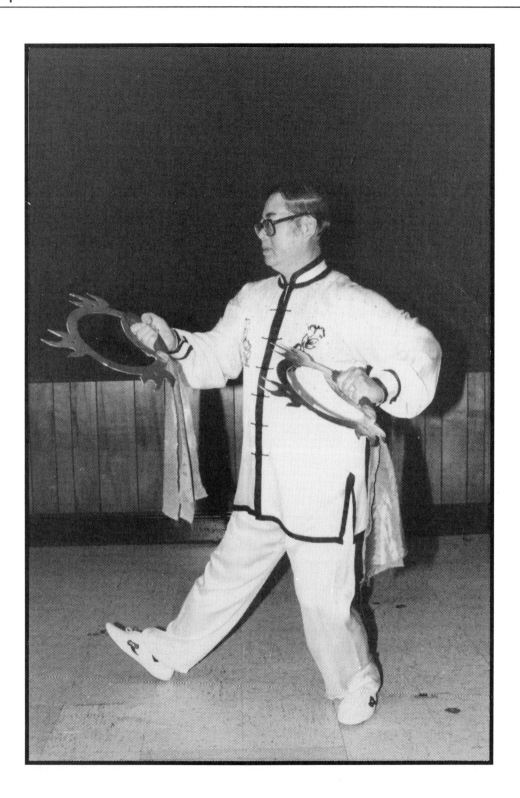

1. Learning the Basic Techniques
2. Training the arm strength and improving the stance of the feet
3. Coordinating the body with the weapon
4. Power and endurance training
5. Familiarize the player with the techniques used in the performance of the form

Because of the size, shape and sharpness of the weapon, it is important to know how to move while holding these weapons and to increase an awareness of their position in relation to the body in order to prevent injury. The weapon is quite broad when compared to other types of weapons, such as the straight or broad sword. In addition, there are flame-like appendages which extend an additional inch to an inch and a half beyond the edge. When completing some moves, such as Brush Knee, there is an increased possibility of gouging or scraping the body or limbs, particularly the leg and head, while performing the movement. Practicing the movements repeatedly before going into the form allows the player to develop the body-weapon position awareness needed to prevent injury.

The weight of the weapons puts an added stress on the arms and upper body. Over time, with increased practice, the body builds endurance and strength. Many of the players, particularly the females, who have practiced the movements have noticed an increase in the definition and tightening of the muscles of the upper arm. This strengthening is needed, again, to prevent stress related injuries, particularly to the elbow region. So too, the player must learn to position the feet and lower body correctly in order to maintain the balance and proper alignment when performing the movements. The balance improves, especially when performing the kicks, as the practicing time increases. By practicing the movements, the player can become familiar with the weight of the weapon, the shifting of the weight which occurs due to the change in the location of the weapon, gradually increasing the amount of time which the movements can be performed without becoming tired, causing strain or losing one's balance.

Just as identified earlier, the weapons substantial weight adds an additional factor when performing the form. Any form which is performed over an extended period of time therefore will require greater endurance, strength and power in order to complete it with the fluidity expected. The gradual introduction of more complex movements allows for the power to build, the Chi to develop, as well as the physical strength of the body to increase. The movements are the building blocks to the form. It is upon these blocks or foundation that the player builds.

By practicing the basic movements, the player becomes aware of the position of the weapon in relation to the body and learns to move with greater coordination and ease. The moves can become synchronized, smoother, performed as is the barehand movements. Though this may be a weapon, it is still Tai-Chi and requires that the player adhere to the basic concepts as explained in the literature and taught by the various Masters. The hand, leg and body must reach the various "end-point" of the movements at the same time. This takes practice and focus.

By practicing the individual movements, the player learns how each is performed without having to worry about the sequence of the form. Once the player is practiced in the individual techniques and feels confident in the balance and strength, he or she may move on to the full form. This familiarity and comfort with the individual movements enables the player to learn the form faster without having to focus totally on individual factors, such as balance, position, coordination, etc. There are different levels in the forms as well, each building on the other. This allows the player to learn the forms at different levels of achievement helping to decrease loss of interest and injury. As the player becomes proficient in each form, the challenge of more complex form to "sink the teeth into" waits.

It should be noted, that the learning and practice of weapons in Tai-Chi improves the player's performance in the barehand forms. Weapons improves the root and the development of the internal energy, the Chi. In addition, the player becomes more conscious of the movement of the waist, the balance, and the position of the body, feet and arms during the practice. This awareness subsequently carries over into the performance of the barehand forms. The body becomes sensitized to the position, the movement flow, the balance and the energy flow during the performance of the moves.

Now that the purpose for practicing the movements is understood, it is time to begin learning the individual movements. Once the player has begun the form, the movements will take on greater meaning and should be returned to even while learning the form. This practices helps the player to perfect the form, and to continue improving the body strength, endurance, coordination and fluidity.

2.2 BASIC TECHNIQUES

1. Vertical Striking
2. Wind-Fire Turning Wheels
3. Part Wild Horse's Mane
4. Ward Off
5. Roll Back
6. Roll Back And Press
7. Push
8. Single Whip
9. Lifting Hand
10. White Crane Spreads Its Wings And Heel Kick
11. Brush Knee And Step Forward
12. Playing The Lute
13. Wind-Fire Protecting The Head And Heel Kick
14. Front Striking, Open Blocking And Forward Striking With Bow Stance
15. Reverse Reeling Forearm
16. Wave Hands Like Clouds
17. High Pat On Horse
18. Heel Kick And Strike To Ears
19. Lower Body And Stand On One Leg
20. Fair Lady Shuttles Back And Forth
21. Needle At Sea Bottom And Fan Through Back
22. Embrace The Tiger And Return To The Mountain
23. Fist Under The Elbow
24. Brush Knee And Punch Down
25. Diagonal Flying
26. Strike The Tiger
27. White Snake Spits The Poison
28. Step Forward And Strike Down
29. Step Back And Ride The Tiger

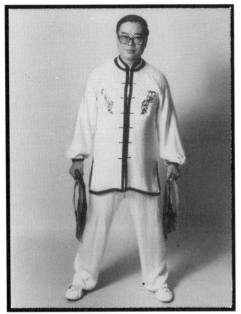

Figure 2-1

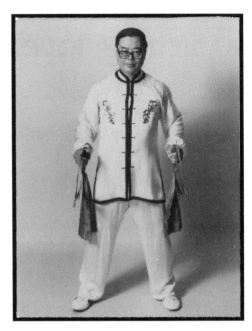

Figure 2-2

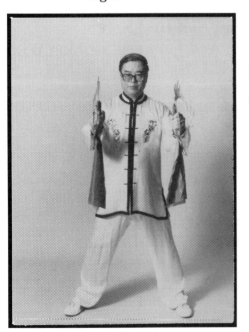

Figure 2-3

1. BASIC TECHNIQUES - Vertical Striking (Figures 2-1 to 2-3)

Stand with the feet shoulder width apart, arms at the sides with the weapon grasped in the hand parallel to the body (one weapon in each hand)

Slowly raise the arms to shoulder height, keeping the weapon in a vertical position, arms slightly bent (about 90 degrees)

Extend the weapon forward slightly, keeping the arms slightly bent (about 20 degrees)

Slowly lower the weapon to about hip level

Bring the weapon in closer to the body until the arm is again bent about

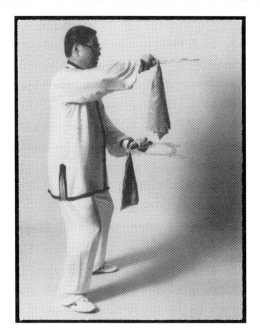

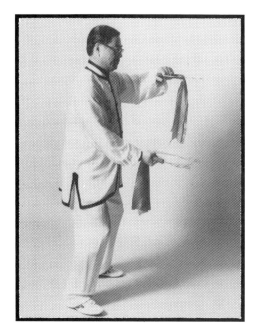

Figure 2-4   **Figure 2-5**

90 degrees

Raise the weapon slowly to shoulder height

Repeat this circular movement for a total of three times

On the last circle, bring the weapons all the way down to the sides of the body as in the start of the movement

Repeat the entire movement for a total of five times (15 circles)

2. BASIC TECHNIQUES - Wind-Fire Turning Wheels (Figures 2-4 to 2-7)

Stand with the feet shoulder width apart, arms at the sides with the weapon grasped in the hand parallel to the body (one weapon in each hand)

Slowly raise the arms keeping the weapon in a vertical position to mid-chest height, arms slightly bent (about 45 degrees)

Slowly rotate the hands in a circular motion bringing the left hand downward on the outside of the ball to waist level and the right hand upward on the outside of the ball to shoulder height (Keep the hands parallel)

Rotate the weapons again keeping the hands parallel until the right hand is at waist level and the left hand is at shoulder height

15

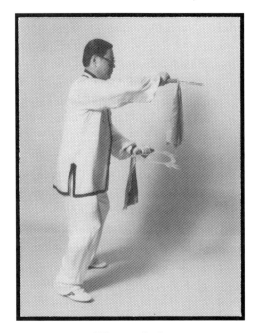

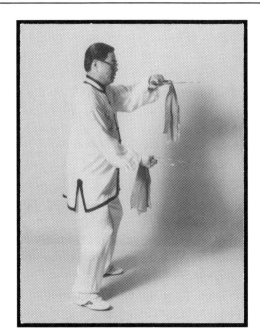

| **Figure 2-6** | **Figure 2-7** |

Repeat this circular movement for a total of ten times

Rotate the weapons until they are in the original position with the weapon in a vertical position at mid-chest height at the sides of the body, arms slightly bent (90 degrees)

Lower the weapons to the sides

Repeat the movement 3 times

3.   BASIC TECHNIQUES - Part Wild Horse's Mane (Figures 2-8 to 2-11)

Stand with the feet shoulder width apart, arms at the sides with the weapon grasped in the hand parallel to the body (one weapon in each hand)

Slowly raise the arms keeping the weapon in a vertical position to mid-chest height, arms slightly bent (about 90 degrees)

Shift the weight of the body to the left, turn the right foot 45 degrees in or to the center, shift the body weight to the right

Bring the left foot into the right instep, touch the toe to the floor

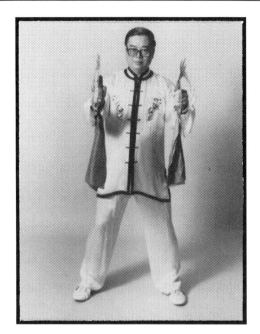

Figure 2-8

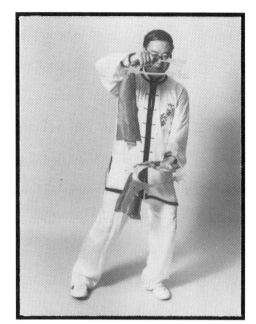

Figure 2-9

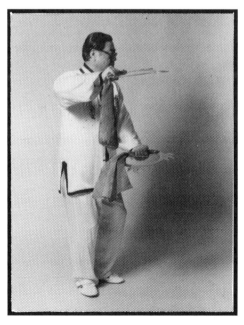

Figure 2-10

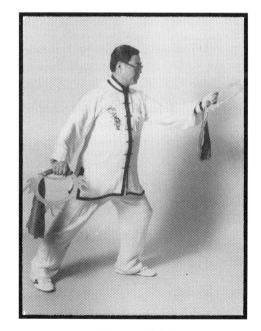

Figure 2-11

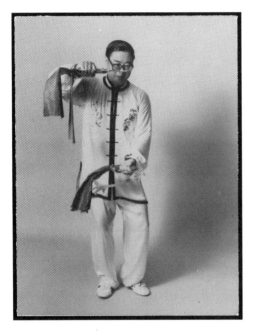 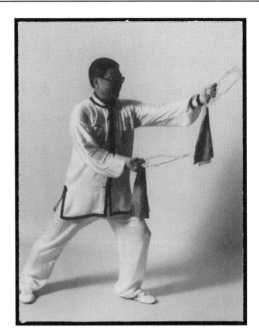

| Figure 2-12 | Figure 2-13 |

Rotate the left arm across the front of the body to the right side, palm up about hip height and the right hand palm down about shoulder height, to make the ball (Weapons should parallel each other)

Slowly step out to the front with the left foot into Bow Stance

Bring the left hand in an upward arc to approximately mid-chest, left palm facing up, weapon parallel to the floor

Simultaneously, bring the right hand down the back the ball and, in a scooping action, up the bottom of the ball to the front about abdomen height, weapon parallel to the ground, palm up

Return to the starting position

Repeat the movement 4 more times

Repeat the movement to the right 5 times.

4. BASIC TECHNIQUES - Ward Off (Figures 2-12 to 2-15)

Stand with the feet shoulder width apart, arms at the sides with the weapon grasped in the hand parallel to the body (one weapon in each hand)

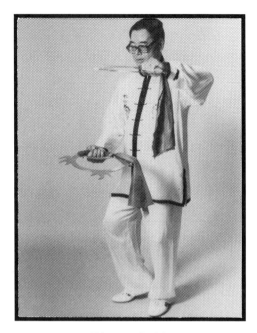

Figure 2-14

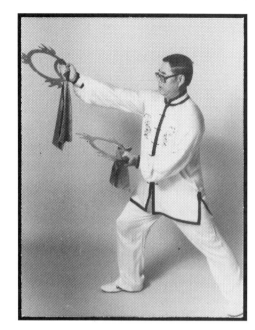

Figure 2-15

Slowly raise the arms keeping the weapon in a vertical position to mid-chest height, arms slightly bent (about 90 degrees)

Shift the weight of the body to the left, turn the right foot 45 degrees in or to the center, shift the body weight to the right

Bring the left foot into the right instep, touch the toe to the floor

Rotate the left arm across the front of the body to the right side, palm up about hip height and the right hand palm down about shoulder height, to make the ball (Weapons should parallel each other)

Slowly step out to the front with the left foot into Bow Stance

Bring the left hand in an upward arc to approximately mid-chest, left palm facing up, weapon parallel to the floor

Allow the right hand to drop in a downward arc to just below hip height, palm towards the body, with the weapon at approximately 25 degrees angle toward the floor

Return to the original position

Repeat the movement 4 more times

Repeat the movement to the right 5 times.

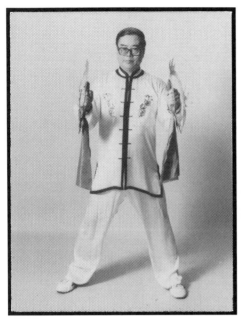

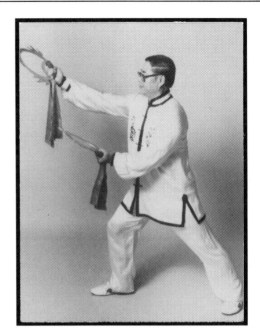

Figure 2-16   **Figure 2-17**

5. BASIC TECHNIQUES - Roll Back (Figures 2-16 to 2-18)

Stand with the feet shoulder width apart, arms at the sides with the weapon grasped in the hand parallel to the body (one weapon in each hand)

Slowly raise the arms keeping the weapon in a vertical position to mid-chest height, arms slightly bent (about 90 degrees)

Step out with the left foot to the front, into Bow Stance

Raise both weapons simultaneously to about waist height, arms bent at 90 degrees

Push out in a double strike to the front, keeping the weapons parallel to each other and perpendicular to the floor

Shift the weight to the right foot, allowing the toes of the left foot to rise, heel remaining on the floor

Rotate both weapons simultaneously up and out in a circular motion (imagine two circle on the outside of the body)

Bring the weapons back to the waist with the weapons toward the

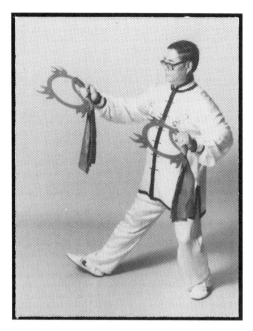

Figure 2-18

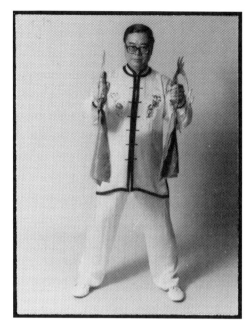

Figure 2-19

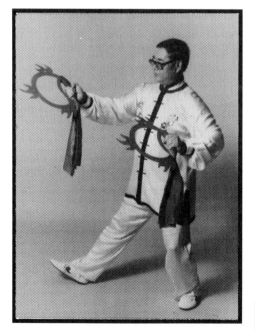

Figure 2-20

front

Shift the weight on to the left foot into Bow Stance

Push out in a double strike to the front, keeping the weapons parallel to each other and perpendicular to the floor

Return to the starting position

Repeat the movement 4 more times

Complete the movement on the right side

6. BASIC TECHNIQUES – Roll Back And Press (Figures 2-19 to 2-21)

Stand with the feet shoulder width apart, arms at the sides with the weapon grasped in the hand parallel to the body (one weapon in each hand)

Slowly raise the arms keeping the weapon in a vertical position to mid-chest height, arms slightly bent (about 45 degrees)

Shift the weight of the body to the left, turn the right foot 45 degrees to the right, shift the body weight to the right

Bring the left foot into the right instep, touch the toe to the floor

Rotate the left arm down and the right hand up to make the ball

Slowly step out with the left foot into Bow Stance

Bring the right hand up to shoulder height, right palm facing up, weapon parallel to the floor

Bring the left hand down to hip height, palm face down weapon at approximately 45 degree angle perpendicular to the floor

Shift the weight of the body back to the right foot, slowly draw back the arms in downward slicing motion palms facing each other parallel to the floor

Shift the weight forward onto the left foot (Bow Stance) rotate the right hand in an upward arc (up the front side of the ball) to just above forehead height turning the weapon so it is at a 45 degree angle perpendicular to the floor, palm facing out, thumb toward the floor, bring the left hand forward under the bottom of the ball in a vertical strike, the weapon perpendicular to the floor, palm facing to the mid line

Turn the left foot as far as possible to the right, shift the weight to the left foot, bring the right foot in to the instep, touch the floor with the toe

Bring the left hand up along the back of the ball until the palm is facing down parallel to the floor making the top of the ball, pull the right hand so the palm is facing up, parallel to the floor making the bottom of the ball

Slowly step out with the right foot into Bow Stance

Bring the left hand up to shoulder height, left palm facing up, weapon parallel to the floor

Bring the left hand down to hip height, palm face down weapon at approximately 45 degree angle perpendicular to the floor

Shift the weight of the body back to the left foot, slowly draw back the arms in downward slicing motion palms facing each other parallel to the floor

Return to the starting position

Complete the movements four more times

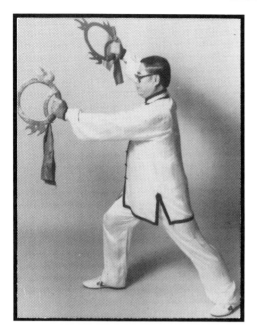

Figure 2-21

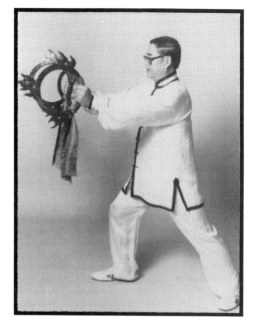

Figure 2-22

7. BASIC TECHNIQUES - Push (Figures 2-22 to 2-25)

Stand with the feet shoulder width apart, arms at the sides with the weapon grasped in the hand parallel to the body (one weapon in each hand)

Slowly raise the arms keeping the weapon in a vertical position to mid-chest height, arms slightly bent (about 45 degrees)

Shift the weight of the body to the left, turn the right foot in towards the center of the body, shift the weight to the right

Step out with the left foot into Bow Stance

As the weight shifts to the front foot, extend both hands, palms facing each other to the front to about mid-chest height

Roll the weight onto the back foot, allowing the front foot to rise off the ground

Bring the arms up and back, turn the palms face down, weapons angled slightly upward, approximately 10 or 15 degrees to approximately shoulder height

Slowly turn the palms until they are once more facing each other as the

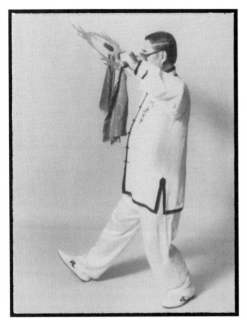 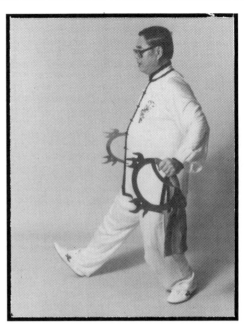

Figure 2-23   **Figure 2-24**

arms continue in the circular motion down the sides to waist height

As the body weight is shifted forward into Bow Stance, extend the arms forward, palms facing each other, weapons perpendicular to the floor to about mid-chest

Shift the weight to the left foot, turn the right foot toward the center, shift the weight to the right foot

Bring the elbows back into the waist area

Bring the left foot into the instep of the right foot

Step out into left Bow stance

As the weight shifts to the front foot, extend both hands, palms facing each other to the front to about mid-chest height

Return to the original starting position

Repeat the move for a total of 4 moves

Complete the movement 5 times on the right side

8. BASIC TECHNIQUES - Single Whip (Figures 2-26 to 2-28)

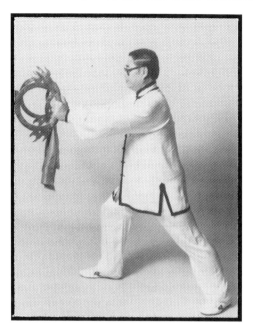

Figure 2-25

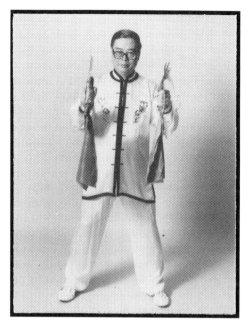

Figure 2-26

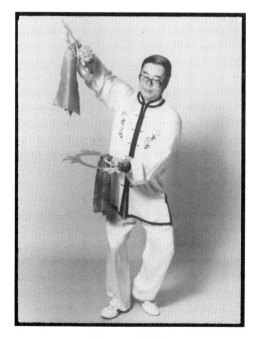

Figure 2-27

Stand with the feet shoulder width apart, arms at the sides with the weapon grasped in the hand parallel to the body (one weapon in each hand)

Slowly raise the arms keeping the weapon in a vertical position to mid-chest height, arms slightly bent (about 45 degrees)

Shift the weight of the body to the left, turn the right foot 45 degrees to the right, shift the body weight to the right

Bring the left foot into the right instep, touch the toe to the floor

Bring the left hand, palm up, to about the height of the bottom rib

Extend the right arm out to the side, palm down, to about ear height, the weapon should be angled to approximately 45 degrees downward

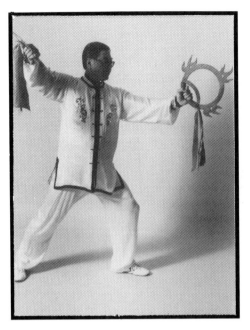

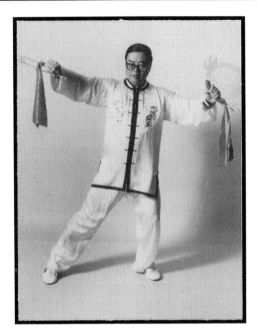

| Figure 2-28 | Figure 2-29 |

(thumb side down) toward the floor

As the left leg moves out into Bow stance position, turn the left hand to palm down, the weapon parallel to the floor

Bring the left hand laterally across the waist region, with the palm down

Once the body and weapon are facing front, turn the weapon so it is perpendicular to the floor (a chest strike), the palm facing to the right

Return to the starting position

Repeat the movement 4 times

Complete the movement 5 times to the right

9. BASIC TECHNIQUES - Lifting Hand (Figures 2-29 to 2-31)

Stand with the feet shoulder width apart, arms at the sides with the weapon grasped in the hand parallel to the body (one weapon in each hand)

Slowly raise the arms keeping the weapon in a vertical position to mid-chest height, arms slightly bent (about 90 degrees)

Raise both hands outward to the sides palms forward, weapons

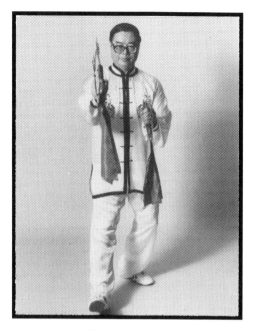

Figure 2-30

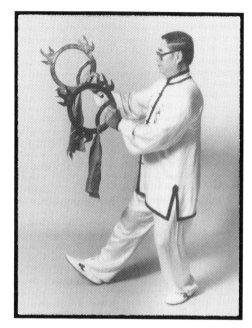

Figure 2-31

perpendicular to the floor (The body is in the shape of a "T" with a downward sloping top)

Shift the weight to the right foot

Lift the right foot to complete a low front kick with the heel being placed on the floor, the weight remains on the left foot

Bring both hands/weapons to the front, weapons are now perpendicular to both the floor and the body, the right weapon is about shoulder height, arm bent about 120 degrees, left hand is about mid-chest height bent about 90 degrees

Complete a circular forward strike with first the right weapon, then the left weapon (the strike with the left weapon should be initiated 2 -3 seconds after the right strike is initiated)

Return to the starting position

Repeat the movement 4 more times

Complete the movement 5 times on the other side

10. BASIC TECHNIQUES - White Crane Spreads Its Wings And Heel Kick (Figures 2-32 to 2-35)

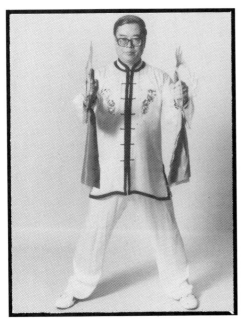

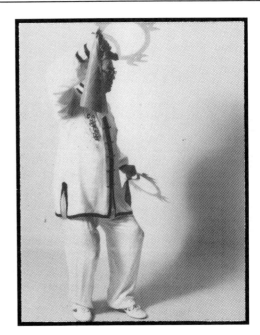

Figure 2-32   **Figure 2-33**

Stand with the feet shoulder width apart, arms at the sides with the weapon grasped in the hand parallel to the body (one weapon in each hand)

Slowly raise the arms keeping the weapon in a vertical position to mid-chest height, arms slightly bent (about 90 degrees)

Shift the weight of the body to the left, turn the right foot in toward the center 45 degrees to the right, shift the body weight to the right

Bring the left foot into the right instep, touch the toe to the floor

Rotate the right arm down and the left hand up to make the ball

Slowly raise the left leg until the thigh is parallel to the floor, knee bent, foot parallel to the floor

Swing the left hand across the front of the body with the left leg, palm down, to rest at the left side at a 45 degree angle from the body

Bring the right hand up the back of the ball to forehead height (the thumb of the hand should still be visible at the edge of the peripheral vision while looking forward), the palm should be facing the forehead, the weapon angled slightly up

Extend the lower left leg out, toe towards the ceiling, into a heel kick position

Bend the leg at the knee, place the foot to the front on the floor

Return to the starting position

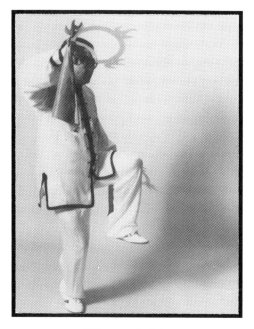

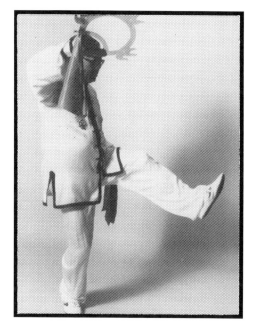

Figure 2-34   **Figure 2-35**

Repeat the movement 4 more times

Complete the movement 5 times on the other side

11. BASIC TECHNIQUES - Brush Knee And Step Forward (Figures 2-36 to 2-38)

Stand with the feet shoulder width apart, arms at the sides with the weapon grasped in the hand parallel to the body (one weapon in each hand)

Slowly raise the arms keeping the weapon in a vertical position to mid-chest height, arms slightly bent (about 90 degrees)

Shift the weight of the body to the left, turn the right foot 45 degrees in towards the center, shift the body weight to the right

Bring the left foot into the right instep, touch the toe to the floor

Rotate the right arm down and the left hand up to make the ball

Slowly step out with the left foot into Bow Stance

Swing the left hand across the front of the body in a downward slanted arc, left to right, with the left leg, palm down, to rest at the left side at a 45

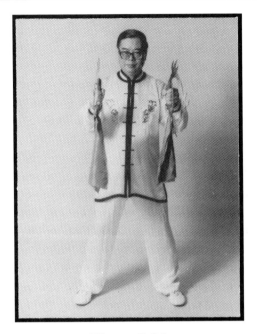

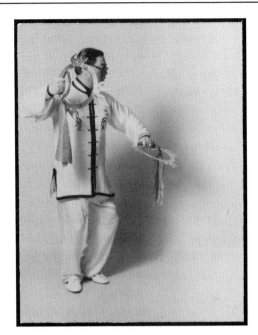

Figure 2-36   **Figure 2-37**

degree angle from the body

Bring the right hand up the back of the ball to slightly above mid-chest height, palm toward the body, weapon perpendicular to the floor

As the waist turns, bring the right hand to the front, holding the weapon perpendicular to the floor

After the weapon passes the body, (while looking forward you should see the fist holding the weapon) turn the weapon palm down to a mid chest strike position

Return to the starting position

Repeat the movements 4 times to the left

Complete the movement 5 times to the right

12. BASIC TECHNIQUES - Playing The Lute (Figures 2-39 to 2-43)

Stand with the feet shoulder width apart, arms at the sides with the weapon grasped in the hand parallel to the body (one weapon in each hand)

Slowly raise the arms keeping the weapon in a vertical position to mid-chest height, arms slightly bent (about 90 degrees)

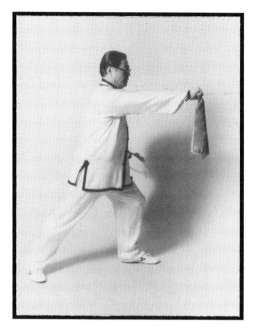

Figure 2-38

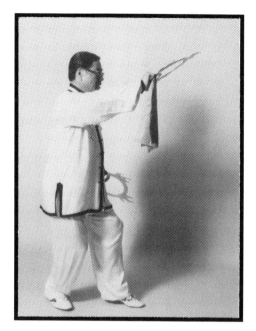

Figure 2-39

Shift the weight of the body to the left, turn the right foot 45 degrees in towards the center, shift the body weight to the right

Stand equally weighted on both feet

Swing the right weapon, palm down to the right dropping down the right side, then across the front of the body to the left palm down at about hip height, then up the left side of the body to about shoulder or mid-chest height, in a circular motion across the front of the body

Turn the left hand, so the palm is facing up (the arm will need to go out to the left slightly to avoid contact with the body)

The weapons should be parallel, palms facing each other (left hand on the bottom, palm facing up, right hand on the top, palm facing down)

Move the weapons across the front of the body from left to right to mid body

Shift the weight to the right foot

Step out with the left foot, placing the heel on the floor the toe up

Draw the left hand up and the right hand down in a pulling motion, still with the left palm up and the right palm down the (left palm should be just to the left of the center of the body)

Bring the right hand to hip height, weapon angled at about 45 degrees out from the body

The left hand should be brought up to shoulder height, palm face angled

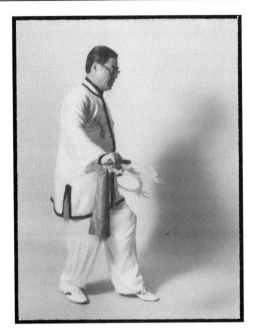

Figure 2-40

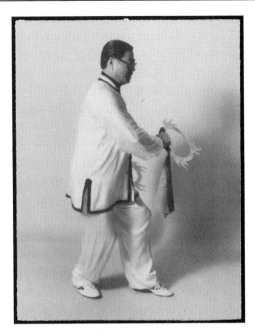

Figure 2-41

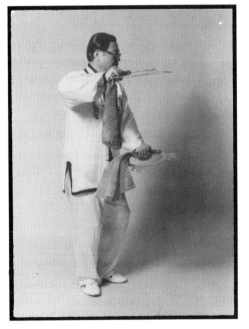

Figure 2-42

at about 45 degrees towards the body

Return to the starting position

Repeat the movement 4 times on the left

Complete the movement 5 times to the right

13. BASIC TECHNIQUES — Wind-Fire Protecting The Head And Heel Kick (Figures 2-44 to 2-47)

Stand with the feet shoulder width apart, arms at the sides with the weapon grasped in the hand parallel to the body (one weapon in each hand)

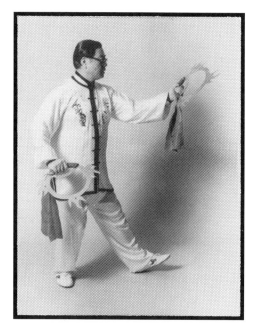

Figure 2-43

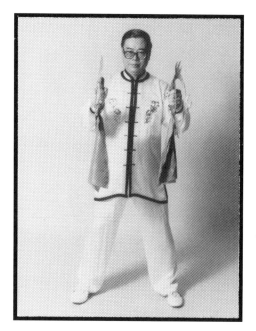

Figure 2-44

Slowly raise the arms keeping the weapon in a vertical position to mid-chest height, arms slightly bent (about 90 degrees)

Shift the weight of the body to the left, turn the right foot 45 degrees in towards the center, shift the body weight to the right

Bring the left foot into the right instep, touch the toe to the floor

Rotate the right arm down and the left hand up to make the ball

Slowly raise the right leg until the thigh is parallel to the floor, knee bent, foot parallel to the floor

Swing the left hand up from the bottom of the ball until it is just above the head, palm down, weapon parallel with the floor facing forward

Drop the right hand downward in an arc to the right side

Extend the lower left leg out, toe towards the ceiling, into a heel kick position

Bring the right hand up and across the body about waist height, continue in a horizontal motion slowly raising the arm until it is about shoulder height when the it reaches the right side

Bend the leg at the knee, place the foot on the floor

Bring the right hand down to the waist, palm towards the body, weapon perpendicular to the floor

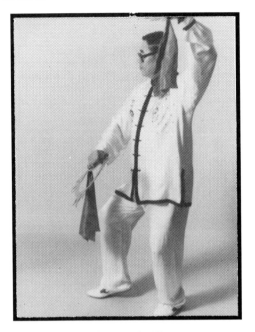

Figure 2-45

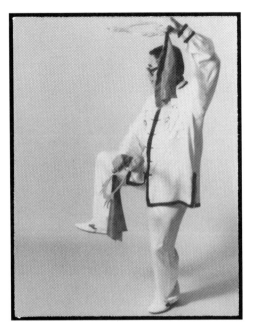

Figure 2-46

Return to starting position

Repeat the movement 4 more times

Complete the movement 5 times on the right

14. BASIC TECHNIQUES - Front Striking, Open Blocking And Forward Striking With Bow Stance (Figures 2-48 to 2-51)

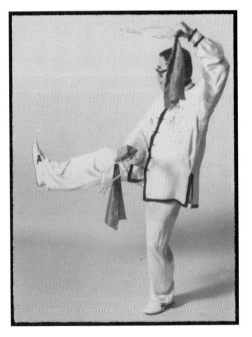

Figure 2-47

Stand with the feet shoulder width apart, arms at the sides with the weapon grasped in the hand parallel to the body (one weapon in each hand)

34

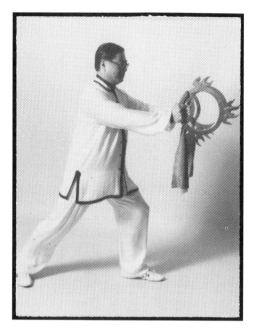

Figure 2-48

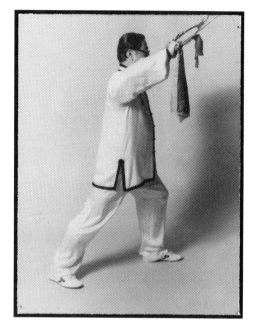

Figure 2-49

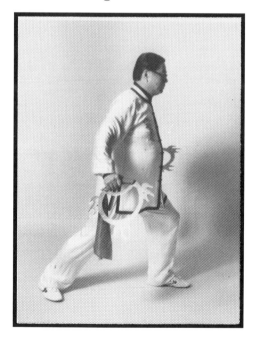

Figure 2-50

Slowly raise the arms keeping the weapon in a vertical position to mid-chest height, arms slightly bent (about 90 degrees)

Step out with left foot into Bow Stance with both hands extended forward at mid-chest height

Slowly raise the hands to forehead height rotating the weapons until they are in a slight "V" shape, the inner portion of the weapons slanted towards the floor, palm to the outside

Bring the weapons back in a circular motion to the side of the body at shoulder height

Continue in the circular motion down to waist level, moving around the ball in a circular movement (Imagine two circles on either side of the body)

Turn the hands parallel palms facing

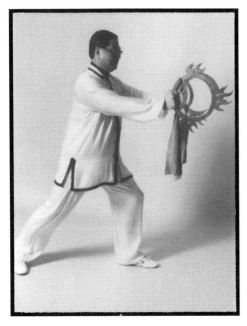
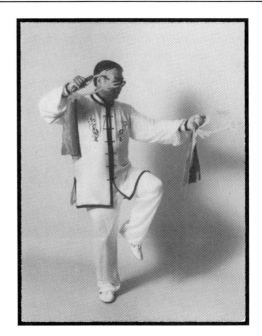

Figure 2-51   **Figure 2-52**

Extend the hands out forward from the body

Repeat the movement for a total of 5 rotations

Bring the weapons all the way down to the sides of the body as in the start of the movement, bringing the left foot back to the original position

Repeat the movement in right arrow stance

15. BASIC TECHNIQUES - Reverse Reeling Forearm (Figures 2-52 to 2-56)

Stand with the feet shoulder width apart, arms at the sides with the weapon grasped in the hand parallel to the body (one weapon in each hand)

Slowly raise the arms keeping the weapon in a vertical position to mid-chest height, arms slightly bent (about 90 degrees)

Shift the weight of the body to the left, turn the right foot 45 degrees in towards the center, shift the body weight to the right

Bring the left foot into the right instep, touch the toe to the floor

Rotate the right arm down and the left hand up to make the ball

Extend the left arm to the front, palm up, weapon at a slight downward angle to the floor

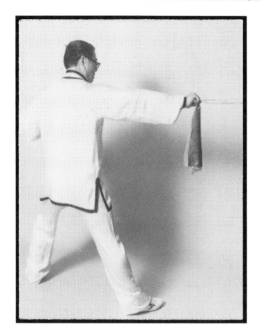

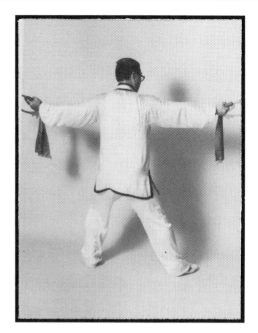

Figure 2-53   **Figure 2-54**

Lift the left leg, toe pointed downward

Bring the right hand towards the front, passing parallel to the left hand about an inch above the left hand, weapons parallel to each other and the floor

Step backwards with the left foot slightly to the left side, shift the weight to the left leg

Draw the left arm back towards the body, while the right arm remains extended to the front

Continue drawing the left arm to the back until it is extended to the rear keeping the weapon pointed away from the body

Turn the body with the movement

Turn the right foot to the center of the body, shift the weight to the right foot

Lift the left leg with the tow pointed downward

Bring the right hand towards the front, passing parallel to the left hand about an inch above the left hand, weapons parallel to each other and the floor

Step backwards with the left foot slightly to the left side, shift the weight to the left leg

Draw the left arm back towards the body, while the right arm remains extended to the front

Continue drawing the left arm to the back until it is extended to the rear

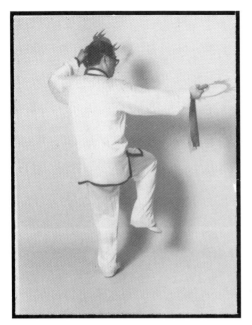

Figure 2-55

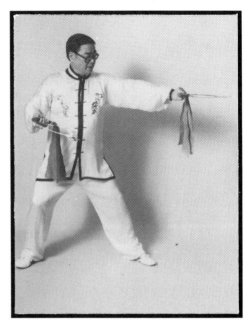

Figure 2-56

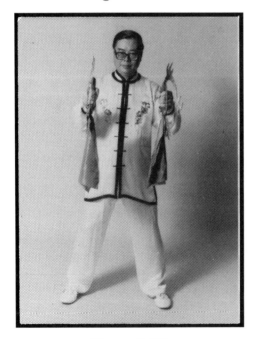

Figure 2-57

Return to the starting position

Repeat the move for a total of 4 more times

Complete the move 5 times to the right

16. BASIC TECHNIQUES - Wave Hands Like Clouds (Figures 2-57 to 2-60)

Stand with the feet shoulder width apart, arms at the sides with the weapon grasped in the hand parallel to the body (one weapon in each hand)

Slowly raise the arms keeping the weapon in a vertical position to mid-chest height, arms slightly bent (about 90 degrees)

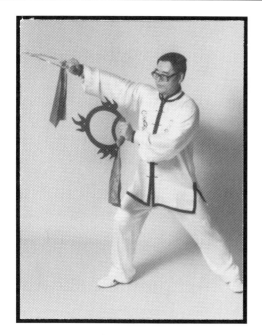

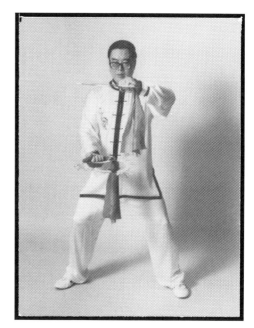

Figure 2-58   **Figure 2-59**

Turn the hands over in a circular form bringing the right hand to the top about shoulder height and the left hand to the bottom about waist height

Turn the hands and the waist to the right as far as the waist can turn comfortably

Rotate the hands in a circular motion (around the ball) keeping the hands palms facing each other equal distance apart

Step out with the left foot to the left side, keeping the weight on the right foot

Turn the hands and the waist slowly to the left, keeping the hands parallel, palms facing, until the waist has turned as far as it can be comfortably

Shift the weight from the right foot to the left foot in symphony with the movement of the hands until the weight is on the left

Turn the hands over in a circular form bringing the right hand to the top about shoulder height and the left hand to the bottom about waist height

Bring the feet together, about a fist distance apart, weight on the left foot

Turn the hands and the waist to the right as far as the waist can turn comfortably

Shift the weight from the left foot to the right foot in symphony with the movement of the hands until the weight is on the right

Rotate the hands in a circular motion (around the ball) keeping the hands palms facing each other equal distance apart

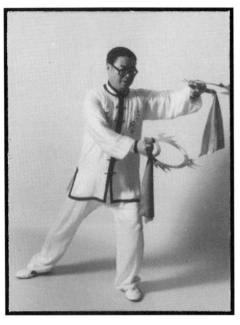

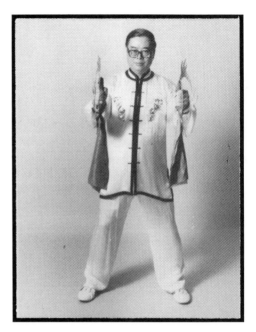

Figure 2-60   **Figure 2-61**

Repeat the move for a total of 4 more movements to the left
Then repeat the movement to the right for 5 movements

17. BASIC TECHNIQUES - High Pat On Horse (Figures 2-61 and 2-62)

Stand with the feet shoulder width apart, arms at the sides with the weapon grasped in the hand parallel to the body (one weapon in each hand)

Slowly raise the arms keeping the weapon in a vertical position to mid-chest height, arms slightly bent (about 90 degrees)

Shift the weight of the body to the left, turn the right foot 45 degrees in towards the center, shift the body weight to the right

Bring the left foot into the right instep, touch the toe to the floor

Rotate the right arm up and the left hand down to make the ball to the center of the body

Step out and touch the floor with the left toe in Cat Stance

Extend the right hand towards the front, passing parallel to the left hand about an inch above the left hand, weapons parallel to each other and the floor,

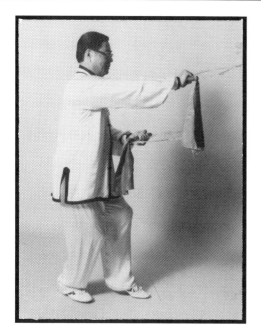

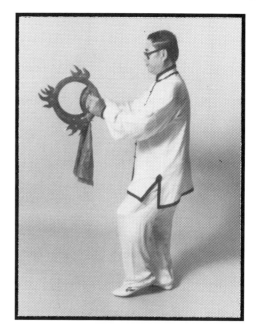

Figure 2-62   Figure 2-63

palms facing

Retract the left hand until the weapon is about one inch from the body, palm up, weapon parallel to the floor, keep the weapon angles away from the body slightly

Extend the right hand forward, palm down, weapon parallel to the floor until the hand is about shoulder height and is extended comfortably away from the body, to the front

Return to starting position

Repeat the movement 4 times

Complete the movement 5 times to the right

18. BASIC TECHNIQUES - Heel Kick And Strike To Ears (Figures 2-63 to 2-69)

Stand with the feet shoulder width apart, arms at the sides with the weapon grasped in the hand parallel to the body (one weapon in each hand)

Slowly raise the arms keeping the weapon in a vertical position to mid-chest height, arms slightly bent (about 90 degrees)

Shift the weight of the body to the left, turn the right foot 45 degrees in

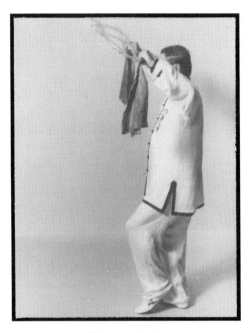

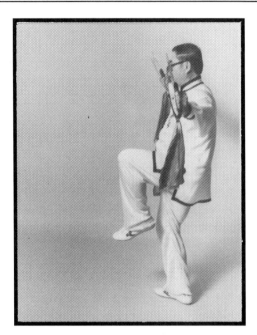

Figure 2-64   **Figure 2-65**

towards the center, shift the body weight to the right

Bring the left foot into the right instep, touch the toe to the floor

Maintain the hands at about mid-chest height, perpendicular to the floor

Raise the left leg until the thigh is parallel to the floor, the knee is bent and the foot is parallel to the floor

Raise the hands in outward circular arc to either side of the body, the hands should be palm forward at about shoulder height, weapons perpendicular to the body and perpendicular to the floor

Raise the lower leg until it is extended outward with the heel out, the toe pointed up

Bend the leg at the knee and place the foot flat on the floor into Bow Stance position Bring the hands in an upward circular arc and forward to about ear height. The palm should be down angles slightly towards each other, the weapons each at an upward 45 degree angle towards the center

Shift the weight to the right foot

Allow the palms to rotate slowly toward each other until the palms are facing and dropping toward the floor in an downward arc

Allow the front foot to rise off the floor, the heel remains in contact with the floor

Shift the weight back onto the forward foot

Allow the arms to continue their circular motion back towards the front

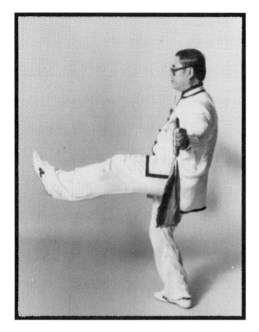

Figure 2-66

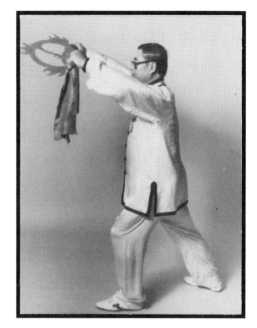

Figure 2-67

and upward to the head area once more until they reach about ear height, the palms facing downward and slightly toward the center, the weapons angled 45 degrees toward the center

Shift the weight to the back leg turn the left foot toward the center, shift the weight to the left foot

Bring the right foot into the left instep, touch the toe to the floor

Maintain the hands at about mid-chest height, perpendicular to the floor

Raise the left leg until the thigh is parallel to the floor, the knee is bent and the foot is parallel to the floor

Raise the hands in outward circular arc to either side of the body, the hands should be palm forward at about shoulder height, weapons parallel to the body and parallel to the floor

Raise the lower leg until it is extended outward to the front with the heel out, the toe pointed up

Bend the leg at the knee and place the foot flat on the floor into Bow Stance position.

Bring the hands in an upward circular arc and forward to about ear height. The palms should be down angles slightly towards each other, the weapons each at an upward 45 degree angle towards the center

Shift the weight to the left foot

Allow the palms to rotate slowly toward each other until the palms are

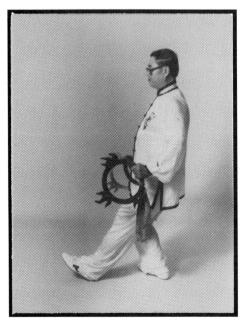
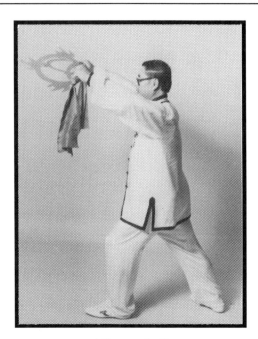

Figure 2-68   **Figure 2-69**

facing and dropping toward the floor in an downward arc

Allow the front foot to rise off the floor, the heel remains in contact with the floor

Shift the weight back onto the forward foot

Allow the arms to continue their circular motion back towards the front and upward to the head area once more until they reach about ear height, the palms facing downward and slightly toward the center, the weapons angled 45 degrees toward the center

Shift the weight to the back leg turn the right foot toward the center, shift the weight to the right foot

Return to the starting position

Repeat the move 4 more times

Complete the movement 5 times on the right

19. BASIC TECHNIQUES - Lower Body And Stand On One Leg (Figures 2-70 to 2-73)

Stand with the feet shoulder width apart, arms at the sides with the weapon grasped in the hand parallel to the body (one weapon in each hand)

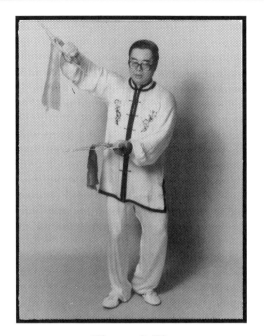
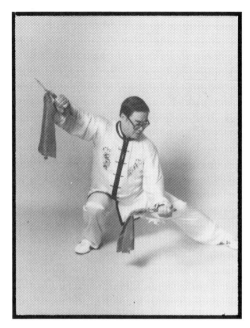

Figure 2-70   **Figure 2-71**

Slowly raise the arms keeping the weapon in a vertical position to mid-chest height, arms slightly bent (about 90 degrees)

Shift the weight of the body to the left, turn the right foot 45 degrees in towards the center, shift the body weight to the right

Bring the left foot into the right instep, touch the toe to the floor

Bring the left hand, palm up, to about the height of the bottom rib on the right side

Extend the right arm out to the side, palm down, to about ear height, the weapon should be angled to approximately 45 degrees downward (thumb side down) toward the floor

Extend the left leg out as far as possible comfortably to the side

Lower the body down on the right leg, the left leg extended to the side

Slowly shift the body weight onto to the extended left foot, moving from the right leg, into Horse Stance, then shift the full weight on to the left leg

Allow the left hand to move in a horizontal motion, palm up, the weapon parallel to the floor, the back of the hand should remain close to the extended leg

As the balance is established on the left leg, the body should straighten and the right leg should be raised until the thigh is parallel with the floor, the knee bent and the foot parallel to the floor

The right hand swings in a small arc on the right coming up with elbow bent at 90 degrees, palm toward the center, weapon parallel to the body at about

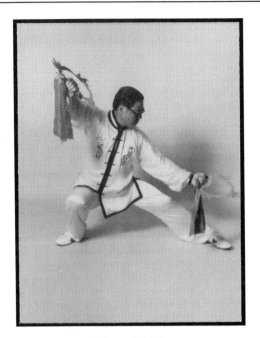

Figure 2-72

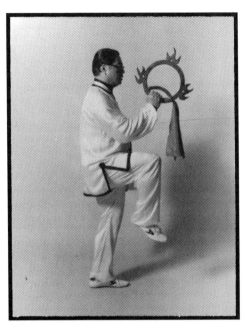

Figure 2-73

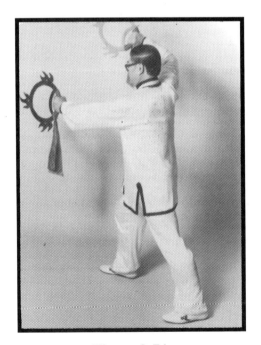

Figure 2-74

shoulder height

The left hand swings to the left side, palm toward the body at a 45 degree angle

Return to starting position

Repeat the movements 4 more times

Complete the movement 5 times on the right

20. BASIC TECHNIQUES - Fair Lady Shuttles Back And Forth (Figures 2-74 to 2-77)

Stand with the feet shoulder width apart, arms at the sides with the weapon grasped in the hand parallel to

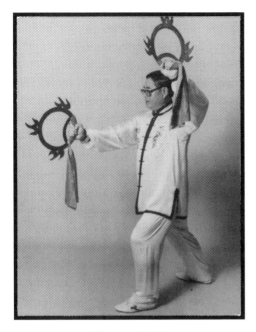
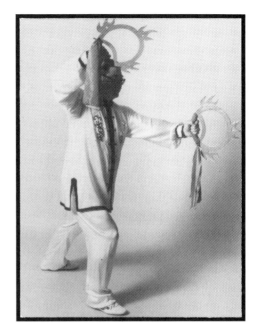

Figure 2-75   **Figure 2-76**

the body (one weapon in each hand)

Slowly raise the arms keeping the weapon in a vertical position to mid-chest height, arms slightly bent (about 90 degrees)

Shift the weight of the body to the left, turn the right foot 45 degrees in towards the center, shift the body weight to the right

Bring the left foot into the right instep, touch the toe to the floor

Rotate the left hand down and the right hand up to make the ball

Slowly step out with the left foot into Bow Stance

Bring the left hand up the front of the ball, slowly turning the palm out and forward until it is about forehead height (the thumb should be down and visible on the edge of the peripheral vision when looking forward)

Bring the right hand around the back of the ball to waist level

As the waist turns, bring the right hand out from the waist to a forward strike about mid-chest, the palm should be toward the center, the weapon perpendicular to the body

Shift the weight to the right foot, turn the left foot to the center, shift the weight to the left leg

Bring the right foot into the right instep, touch the toe to the floor

Rotate the right hand down and the left hand up to make the ball

Slowly step out with the right foot into Bow Stance

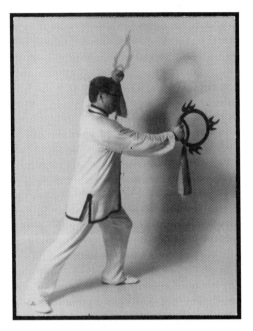

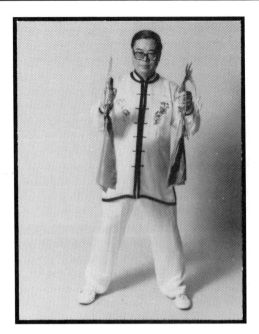

Figure 2-77   Figure 2-78

Bring the right hand up the front of the ball, slowly turning the palm out and forward until it is about forehead height (the thumb should be down and visible on the edge of the peripheral vision when looking forward)

Bring the left hand around the back of the ball to waist level

As the waist turns, bring the left hand out from the waist to a forward strike about mid-chest, the palm should be toward the center, the weapon perpendicular to the body

Return to the starting position

Repeat the movement 4 more times

Complete the movement 5 times to the right

21. BASIC TECHNIQUES - Needle At Sea Bottom And Fan Through Back (Figures 2-78 to 2-80)

Stand with the feet shoulder width apart, arms at the sides with the weapon grasped in the hand parallel to the body (one weapon in each hand)

Slowly raise the arms keeping the weapon in a vertical position to mid-chest height, arms slightly bent (about 90 degrees)

Shift the weight of the body to the left, turn the right foot 45 degrees in towards the center, shift the body weight to the right

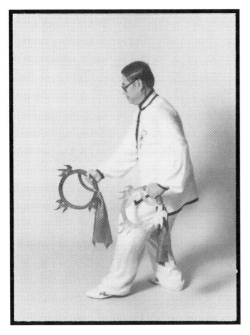

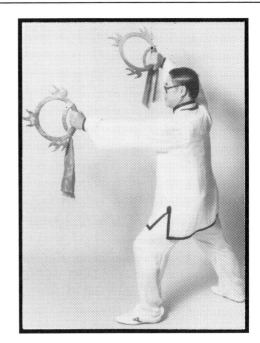

Figure 2-79   **Figure 2-80**

Bring the left foot into the right instep, touch the toe to the floor

Rotate the right arm down and the left hand up to make the ball

Swing the left hand down in an arc palm down, across the front of the body from right to left, simultaneously bring the left leg out to the front, to rest at the left side at a 45 degree angle from the body, in a Cat Stance (toe touching the floor, heel raised)

Bring the right hand up the back of the ball to strike down toward the floor, slightly in front of the knee, the palm should be toward the center, the weapon perpendicular to the floor

Step forward with the left foot into Bow Stance

Bring the right hand in an upward arc to about forehead height, turning the palm to the outside, the weapon angled at a 45 degree angle down toward the center

The left hand comes up from the side to about mid-chest height and then out and to the front in a chest strike, palm toward the center, the weapon perpendicular to the floor

Return to the starting position

Repeat the movements 4 more times

Complete 5 movements to the right

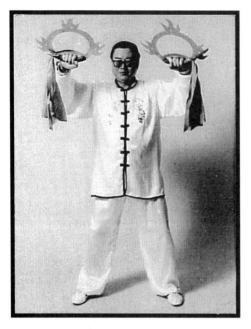

Figure 2-81

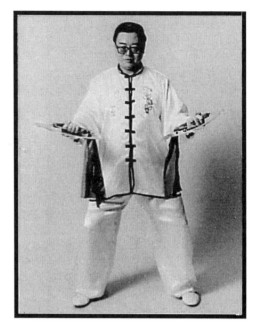

Figure 2-82

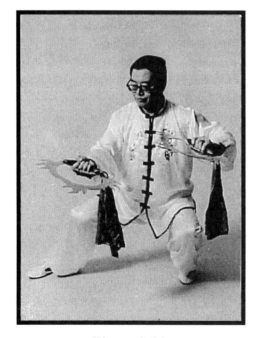

Figure 2-83

22. BASIC TECHNIQUES - Embrace The Tiger And Return To The Mountain (Figures 2-81 to 2-84)

Stand with feet shoulder width apart, hands with the Wind-Fire Wheels at the sides of the body

Step out to the left side into a high Horse Stance

Raise the hands arching out from the sides of the body until the weapons are about forehead height on either side of the head, palm down, the weapons should be angled at about 45 degree

Bring the weapons in an outward circular motion until the weapons are about the level of the diaphragm, palms

50

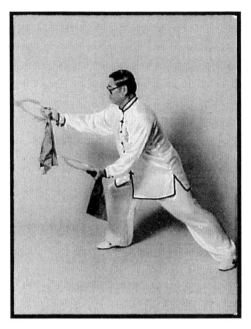

Figure 2-84

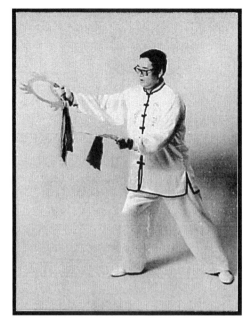

Figure 2-85

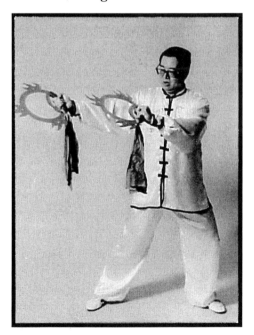

Figure 2-86

up, tipped at a slight angle (about 10 degrees) up to the outside

Drop down into a deep Horse Stance

Shift the weight to the left leg

Turn the left hand so it is palm down, the right hand is about waist height, the left hand about diaphragm height

Shift the weight to the right leg and rise to a normal Bow Stance

Swing the weapons to the right turning the right hand to palm out about upper diaphragm height, the left weapon in a forward punching motion at about groin height

Return to the starting position

Repeat 4 times to the right

Complete 5 times to the left

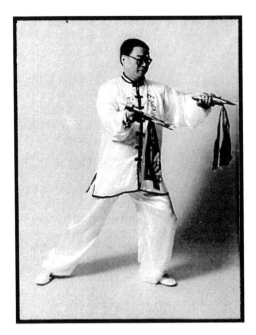

Figure 2-87

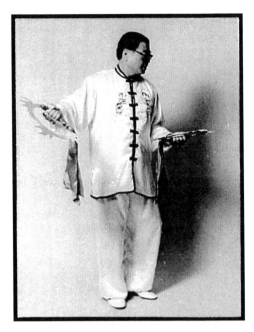

Figure 2-88

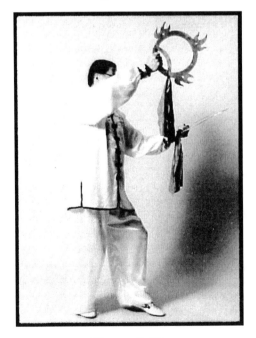

Figure 2-89

23. BASIC TECHNIQUES - Fist Under The Elbow (Figures 2-85 to 2-90)

Stand with feet shoulder width apart, weapons on either side of the body

Raise the weapons to shoulder height, bending the elbows

Shift the weight to the right foot and then shift the weight to the left foot

Step into left Bow Stance, weapons palm facing at waist height

Strike left weapon, palm up, to throat height

Strike with the right weapon, palm to center, in a vertical forward cutting motion, to mid abdomen

Return to starting position

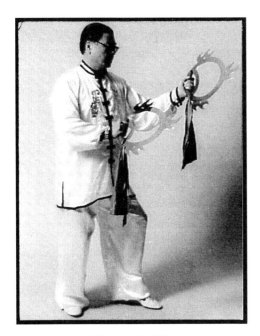

Figure 2-90

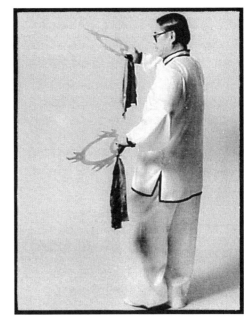

Figure 2-91

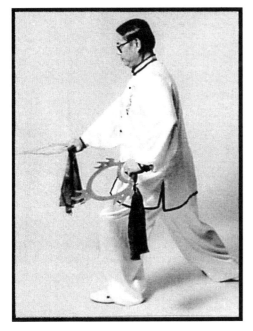

Figure 2-92

Repeat the movement 4 times

Complete the movement 5 times to the right

24. BASIC TECHNIQUES - Brush Knee And Punch Down (Figures 2-91 And 2-92)

Stand with the feet shoulder width apart, arms at the sides with the weapon grasped in the hand parallel to the body (one weapon in each hand)

Slowly raise the arms keeping the weapon in a vertical position to mid-chest height, arms slightly bent (about 90 degrees)

Shift the weight of the body to the left, turn the right foot 45 degrees in towards the center, shift the body weight to the right

Bring the left foot into the right instep, touch the toe to the floor

Rotate the right arm down and the left hand up to make the ball

Slowly step out with the left foot into Bow Stance

Swing the left hand across the front of the body in a downward slanted arc, right to left, with the left leg, palm down, to rest at the left side at a 45 degree angle from the body

Bring the right hand up the back of the ball to about shoulder height, the weapon should be perpendicular to the floor, parallel to the body

As the waist turns, bring the right hand in a downward punching motion until level with the knee

Return to the starting position

Repeat the movements 4 times to the left

Complete the movement 5 times to the right

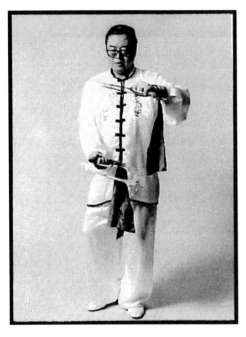

Figure 2-93

25. BASIC TECHNIQUES — Diagonal Flying (Figures 2-93 and 2-94)

Stand with the feet shoulder width apart, arms at the sides with the weapon grasped in the hand parallel to the body (one weapon in each hand)

Slowly raise the arms keeping the weapon in a vertical position to mid-chest height, arms slightly bent (about 90 degrees)

Turn the hands over in a circular form bringing the left hand to the top about shoulder height and the right hand to the bottom about waist height

Shift the weight to the left, step out to the right side in a sideways Bow Stance

The weight should be on the right foot, the body at an angle to the floor

Bring the right hand, palm up, in an arc type movement, until the right weapon is extended to the right of the body, to about slightly above of the head

Bring the left hand, palm down, in a downward arc, the weapon should be parallel to the leg, weapon pointing towards the floor

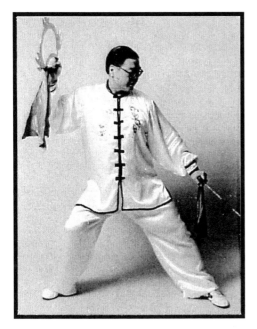

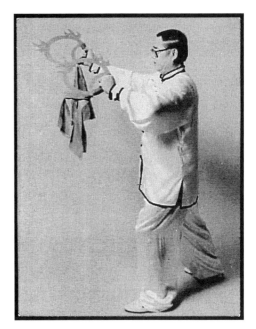

Figure 2-94 Figure 2-95

Repeat the move for a total of 4 more movements to the left
Then repeat the movement to the right for 5 movements

26. BASIC TECHNIQUES — Strike The Tiger (Figures 2-95 to 2-98)

Stand in left Bow Stance
Raise the weapons, parallel to each other, palms facing towards the center, right hand head height, left hand shoulder height
Turning with the waist, swing the weapons in a downward arc to the left
Turning with the waist, swing the weapons in a downward arc to the right
Turn with the waist to the left to Bow Stance
Bring the left weapon in an upward arc to the height of the head, the palm is down
Bring the right weapon in a horizontal arc to the center of the body, palm down
Return to the starting position

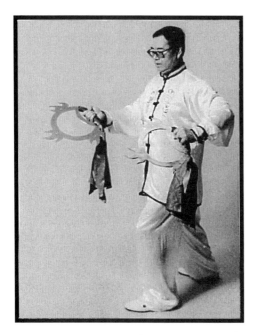

Figure 2-96

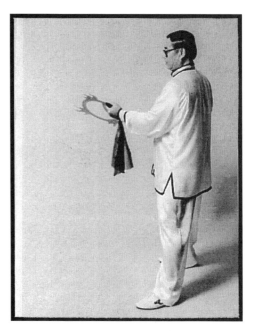

Figure 2-97

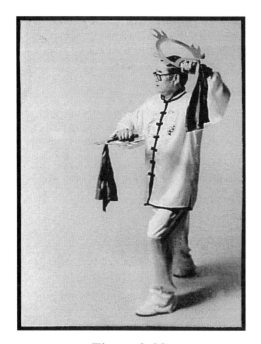

Figure 2-98

Repeat the movement 4 times

Complete the movement 5 times to the right

27. BASIC TECHNIQUES – White Snake Spites The Poison (Figures 2-99 and 2-100)

Stand in left Bow Stance

Raise the left weapon to mid chest height, parallel to the body

Turn the left weapon, palm up, to a 45 degree angle to the floor

Raise the right, palm up, in an upward thrusting motion across the top of the left weapon

Repeat the movement four times

Repeat the movement five times on the right

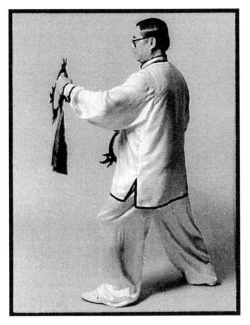

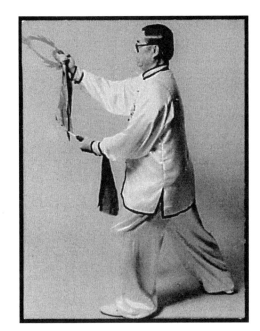

Figure 2-99   **Figure 2-100**

28. BASIC TECHNIQUES — Step Forward And Strike Down (Figures 2-101 and 2-102)

Stand with feet together, the weight on the right foot, the left foot next to the right

Step forward into Bow Stance

Raise the right hand to shoulder height, palm down, the weapon parallel to the floor at about a ten degree angle to the right

Bring the left hand to about hip height, palm down, parallel to the floor at about a 15 degree angle to the left

Bring the left hand to the side of the body in a downward arc, the weapon should be at a 45 degree angle away from the body

Bring the right hand in a circular motion, the outside of the body, and then in a forward thrusting motion, from the waist

The weapon should be perpendicular to the floor at about waist height

Repeat 4 times to the left

Complete 5 time to the right

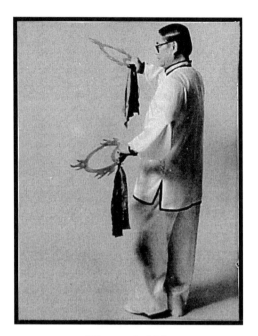

Figure 2-101

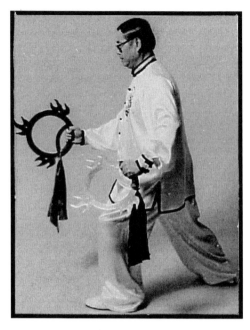

Figure 2-102

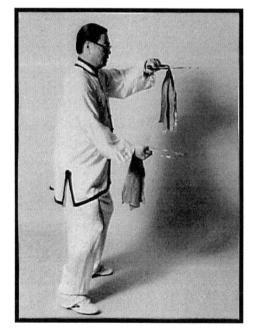

Figure 2-103

29. BASIC TECHNIQUES — Step Back and Ride The Tiger (Figures 2-103 to 2-106)

Stand with feet shoulder width apart, arms at the sides with the weapon grasped in the hand parallel to the body

Slowly raise the arms keeping the weapons in a vertical position to mid-chest height, arms slightly bent (about 90 degrees)

Turn the hands over in a circular form bringing the right hand to the top about shoulder height and the left hand to the bottom about waist height

Turn the hands and the waist to the right as far as the waist can turn

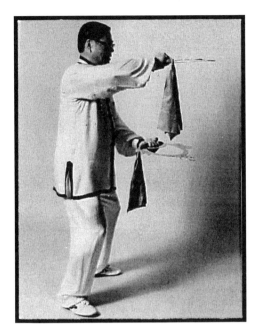

Figure 2-104

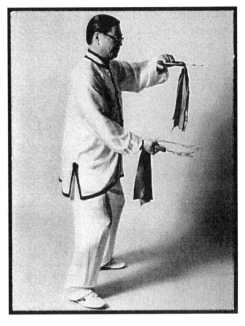

Figure 2-105

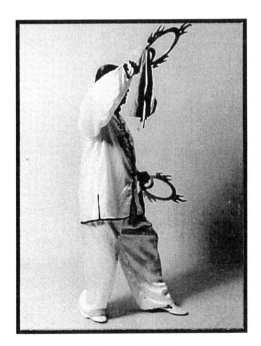

Figure 2-106

comfortably

Rotate the hands in a circular motion (around the ball) keeping the hands palm facing each other, equal distance apart

Shift the weight to the right leg and extend the left foot forward, toe first into Cat Stance

Bring the right weapon in an upward arcing motion to above the head, the weapon should be parallel to the floor, at about a 45 degree angle, pointing up

Bring the left weapon in a downward arcing motion to the left side of the body, at a 45 degree angle pointing toward the floor

Repeat the movement 4 times

Repeat the movement 5 times on the right

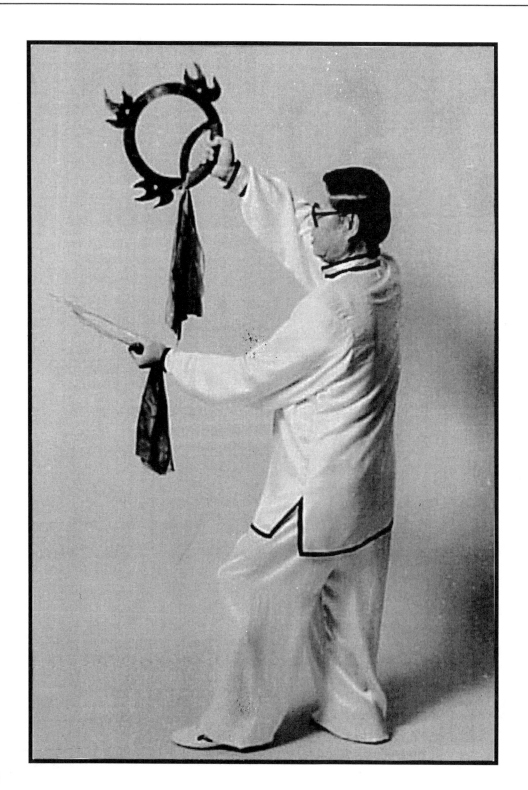

CHAPTER 3

SIMILARITIES BETWEEN THE WIND-FIRE WHEELS AND THE BAREHAND FORM

3.1 Introduction

The Wind-Fire Wheels are two handed weapons and as such are an ideal complement to the barehanded, traditional Yang form. Each Wind-Fire-Wheels movement has its counterpart in the traditional form. Since the Wind-Fire-Wheels are extensions of the hands, almost every Tai-Chi technique can be modified to the form. Thus, it is extremely important that the player acquire both good knowledge and training in the basic movements of the barehand technique. One should observe the basic principles of Tai-Chi while training in this elegant form. A solid background in the martial applications of the movements will be a plus, as they are too similar to the Wind-Fire Wheels form

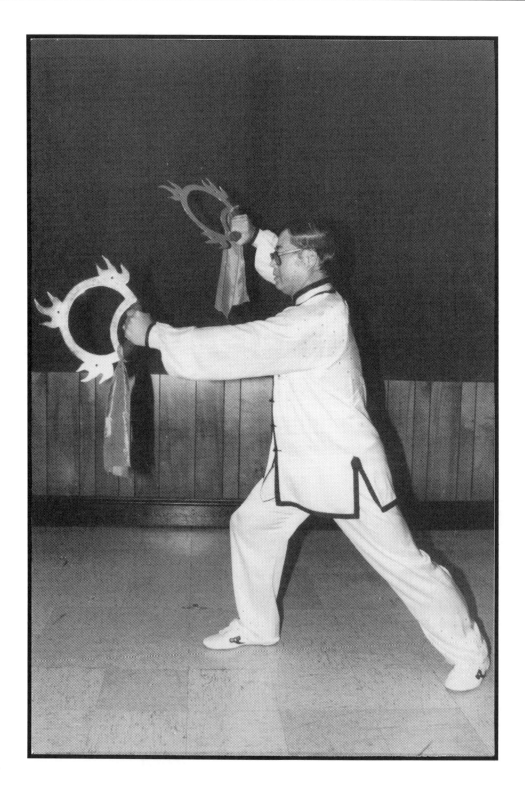

concepts. Indeed, the Yang form is a spectacular martial art as well as a health-maintaining art. The Wind-Fire-Wheels form takes full advantage of both aspects in very similar ways. Breathing sequences with each Wind-Fire-Wheels movement are quite similar to those used in barehand and should be adhered to.

Finally, the movement of internal energy during the barehand form, a level of achievement for more advanced students, should follow the same general patterns in the Wind-Fire-Wheels form. The player's knowledge and skill in Tai-Chi will parallel those of the Wind-Fire-Wheels and their refinement will help improve skills in this unique form. This chapter will demonstrate the similarities between the basic blocks and strikes that are used in both the Yang style of Tai-Chi Chuan and Wind-Fire-Wheels.

3.2 Wind-Fire Wheels Similarities

1. **Commencing**
2. **Roll Back**
3. **Push**
4. **Part Wild Horse's Mane**
5. **Single Whip**
6. **Lifting Hand**
7. **White Crane Spreads Its Wings**
8. **Brush Knee And Step Forward**
9. **Playing The Lute**
10. **Wave Hands Like Clouds**
11. **High Pat On Horse**
12. **Heel Kick And Strike To Ears**
13. **Reverse Reeling Forearm**
14. **Snake Creeps Down**
15. **Golden Rooster Stands By One Leg**

16. **Fair Lady Shuttles Back And Forth**
17. **Needle At Sea Bottom**
18. **Fan Through Back**
19. **Embrace The Tiger And Return To The Mountain**
20. **Fist Under The Elbow**
21. **Brush Knee And Punch Down**
22. **Diagonal Flying**
23. **Strike The Tiger**
24. **White Snake Spits The Poison**
25. **Step Forward And Strike Down**
26. **Step Back And Ride The Tiger**

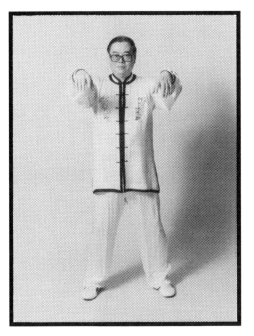

Figure 3-1

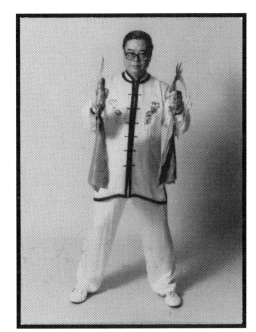

Figure 3-2

3.2.1. Commencing

The Yang form commences with the lifting of both hands. The Wind-Fire-Wheels are also raised together in a relaxed manner (Figures 3-1 and 3-2). As in the barehand technique, the breath is inhaled as the Wind-Fire-Wheels are lifted and exhaled as they are brought forward and down in a circle (three times). Note as per Yang principles that the head and back remain straight, the knees are slightly bent and the feet are shoulder-width apart. The eyes look forward. The lifting of hands is a blocking maneuver for self defense just as in barehand.

3.2.2. Roll Back

The roll back movement for Wind-Fire-Wheels is close in structure to barehand. Both require a relaxed, centered stance. Flexibility of the waist is

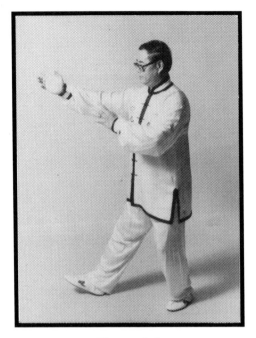

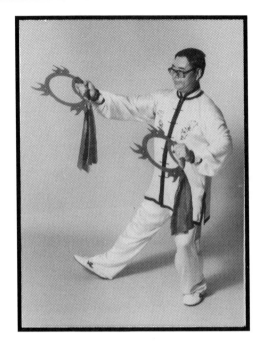

Figure 3-3   Figure 3-4

very important. As in barehand, the eyes must follow the movement of the hands (weapons). The breath is inhaled in both techniques. One must be sure to keep the arms level with the thorax. Note that the palm and toe positions are the same, and that one must be centered over the width of the stance rather than leaning back (Figures 3-3 and 3-4). The Roll Back movement uses the same blocking/deflecting technique as barehand.

3.2.3. Push

The Push movement is exceedingly similar in both forms. A rooted, centered approach is a key requirement. Both employ a circular look which is seen in Figures 3-5 to 3-12. Note that the elbows are not locked in either. The palm and toes placements are similar. Breathing during the movements is the same: inhale when rolling back, exhale when pushing. The arms move in the same circular motion to block and strike in similar manners. Both strikes end up at chest level with the eyes forward and the thorax straight. The self-defense applications are similar. Initially the weapons block/deflect an attack. A strike to the thorax completes the application.

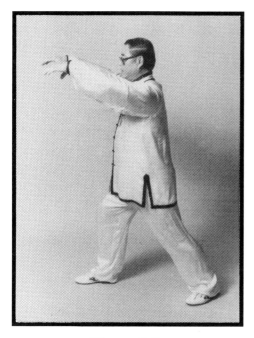

Figure 3-5

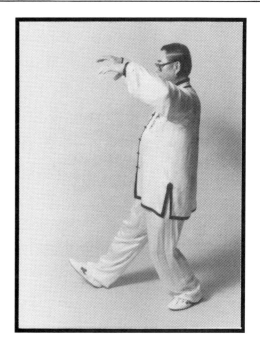

Figure 3-6

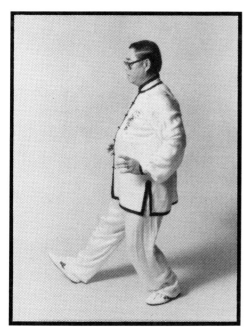
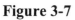

Figure 3-7

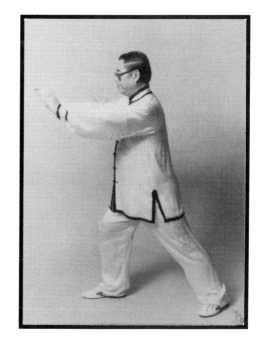

Figure 3-8

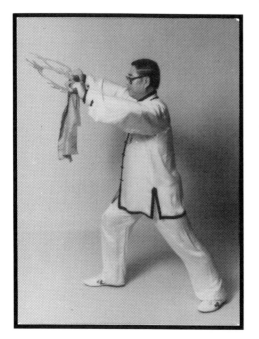

Figure 3-9

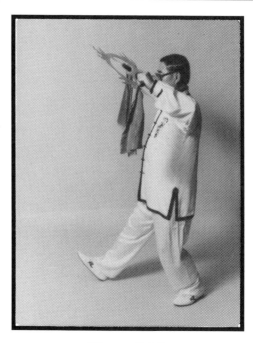

Figure 3-10

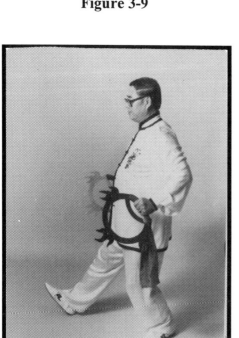

Figure 3-11

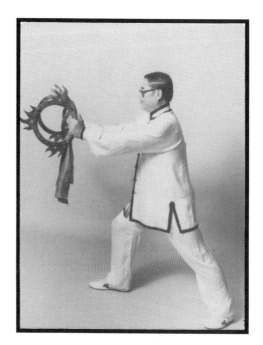

Figure 3-12

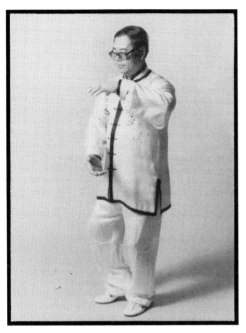

Figure 3-13

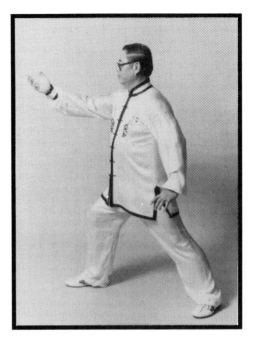

Figure 3-14

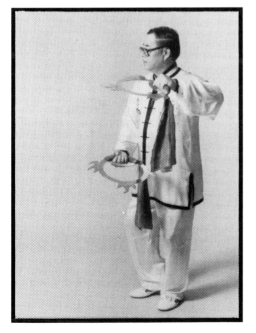

Figure 3-15

3.2.4. Part Wild Horse's Mane

Figures 3-13 to 3-16 demonstrate the sameness of movement for both techniques. Both employ the smooth use of the arms and waist, particularly during the strike. The palm positions and level of the hands must correlate with the barehand move. As in barehand the blocking hand is level with the waist and the striking hand is at upper thorax level. Once again, the breathing pattern must be the same. One inhales as the weapons (hands) are brought to face each other and exhales with the strike. The Bow Stance is identical. The initial portion of the movement blocks/deflects the incoming attack. A single hand strike to the upper body disables the

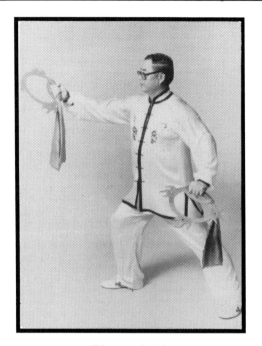

Figure 3-16

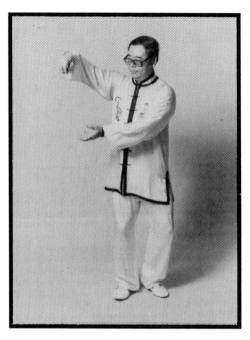

Figure 3-17

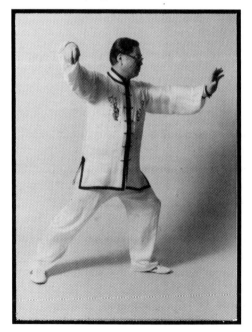

Figure 3-18

opponent. This is identical with the barehand application.

3.2.5. Single Whip

One of the most graceful yet most powerful movements in this form is the Single Whip. Note the same stances, start and finishing positions (Figures 3-17 to 3-20). The right hand is placed in the same manner as the barehand: raised and above the level of the left arm. The eyes follow the weapons early in the move, and eventually follow the left weapon as with barehand. The waist must be flexible and relaxed for easy completion of this portion of the move in either technique. The level of placement of the left hand during the strike is the same, at head level, but unlike barehand the left palm faces out and

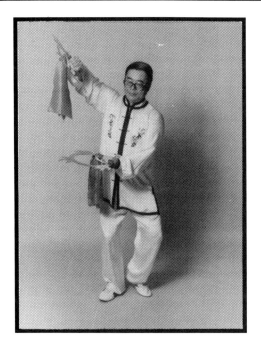

Figure 3-19

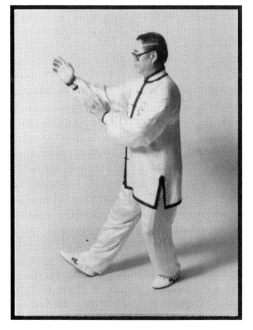

Figure 3-21

Figure 3-20

away from the chest. The weapon is turned at the beginning of the strike to allow for this (Figure 3-19). The strike is completed in the same sweeping motion. Breathing during the move is identical. One inhales while bringing the weapons towards the body initially, then exhales when the left hand sweeps out. Similarities with the barehand applications are seen here. An attack from either side can be locked/deflected. A right hand strike initially to a right-sided attacker, and a left-handed one later are possible just as in barehand.

3.2.6. Lifting Hand

The familiar Lifting Hands movement of the Yang style is identically performed with the Wind-Fire Wheels (Figures 3-21 and 3-22). The gentle turn of

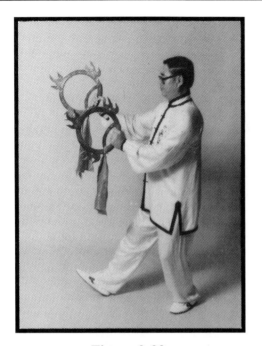

Figure 3-22

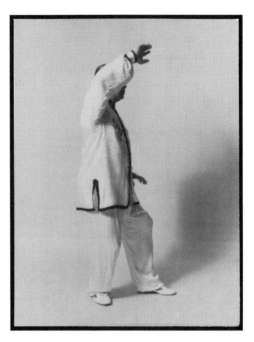

Figure 3-23

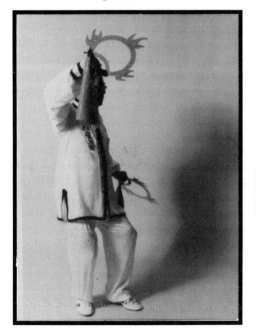

Figure 3-24

the waist to the right and the 90% - 10% weight difference for the left and right feet, respectively, are the same. The palms face each other. The blocking and striking applications are quite similar.

3.2.7. White Crane Spreads Its Wings

Once again, the Wind-Fire Wheels correspond to the traditional Yang move. The hands spread with the palms outward in the same manner, and a 90% - 10% Cat Stance finishes the move. The right hand weapon protects the head as in the barehand (Figures 3-23 and 3-24)

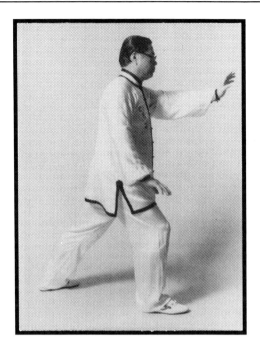 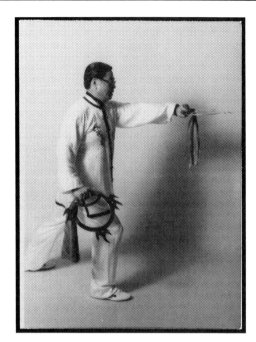

Figure 3-25   **Figure 3-26**

3.2.8. Brush Knee And Step Forward

The Brush Knee move for the Wind-Fire-Wheels is comparable to the traditional Yang move. Some similarities are shown in Figures 3-25 and 3-26. A balanced Bow Stance is important. The back is straight. The palm placements and hand levels coincide. As in the Yang style, one must take care to lift the toe to a 45 degree angle before turning the foot to avoid knee injuries. In contrast to the traditional move, the weapon is turned from its vertical position during the forward strike and struck palm down (Figure 3-26). The same barehand self-defense applications of blocking and striking are easily seen.

3.2.9. Playing The Lute

Almost identical to the Yang move, this technique contains the required circular block, 90% - 10% stance and forward strike. Note the same hand placement (Figures 3-27 and 3-28). In both techniques, the left foot turns 45 degrees as the right hand makes a circle. Applications for both techniques are comparable.

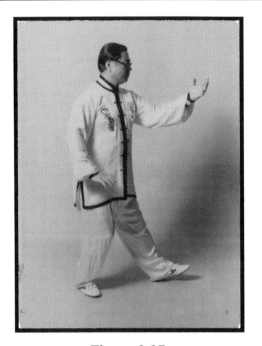

Figure 3-27

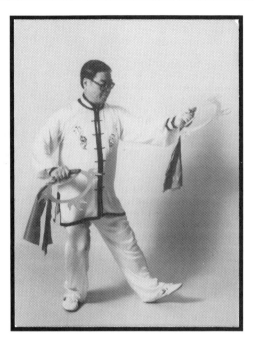

Figure 3-28

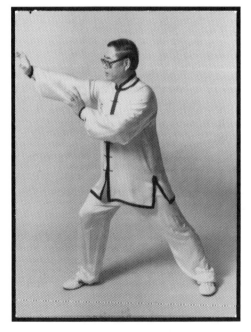

Figure 3-29

3.2.10. Wave Hands Like Clouds

The classic cloud-hands of Yang is followed in almost parallel fashion. The foot placements are identical. The hand placements are similar with the palms facing each other (Figures 3-29 to 3-34). As in the barehand, relaxed movements of the waist are required and very important. The outstanding blocking/deflecting applications of the barehand technique are nearly the same here.

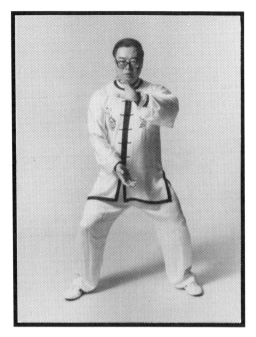

Figure 3-30

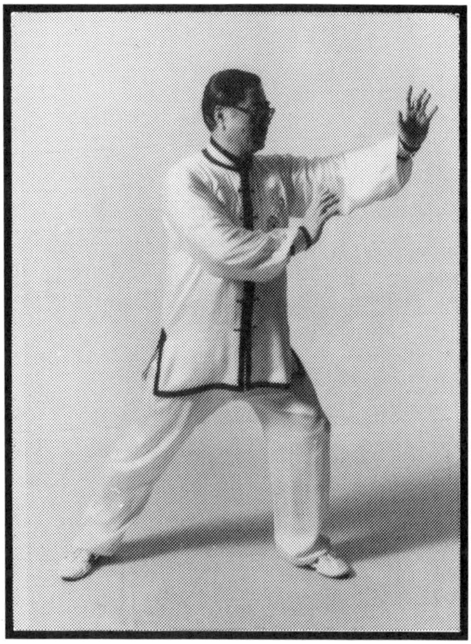

Figure 3-31

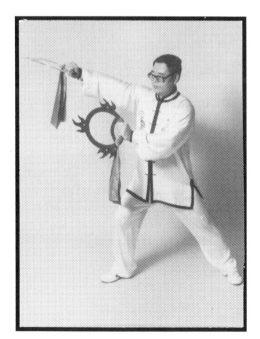

Figure 3-32

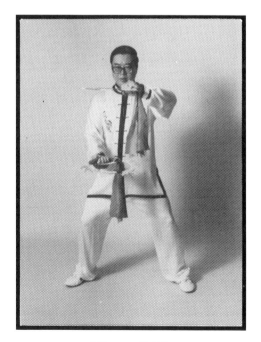

Figure 3-33

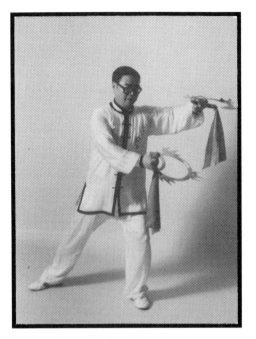

Figure 3-34

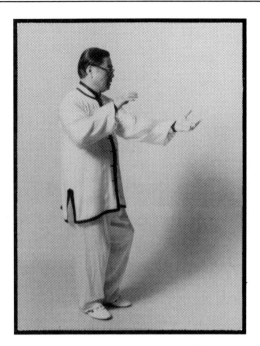

Figure 3-35

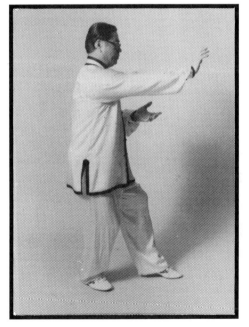

Figure 3-36

3.2.11. High Pat On Horse

High Pat On Horse is performed just as in barehand (Figures 3-35 to 3-38). The 90%-10% Cat Stance coincides with the same hand movements. Both palms face each other. The breath is exhaled with the forward strike as in barehand. The applications are similar for both techniques, such as the right hand strike to the arm, upper body or head.

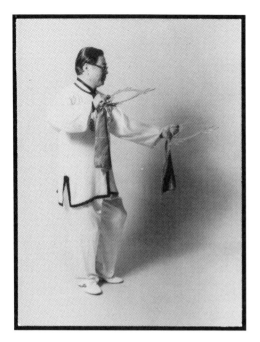

Figure 3-37

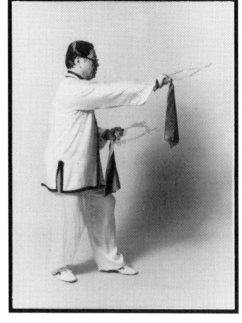

Figure 3-38

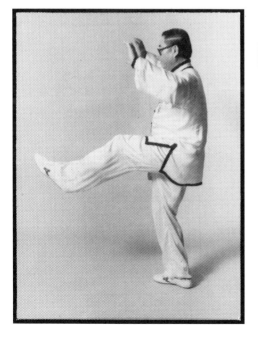

Figure 3-39

3.2.12. Heel Kick And Strike To Ears

The Heel Kick of the Wind-Fire Wheels form is the same as in the Yang style (Figures 3-39 to 3-46). Note, however, the lower hand placement of the weapons in Figure 3-43. Otherwise the step-down and strike, centered and balanced, is identical. The Bow Stance, hand placement of the ear strike and exhalation at the end are comparable. The Yang-like applications include bilateral blocks with the weapons and ear strikes.

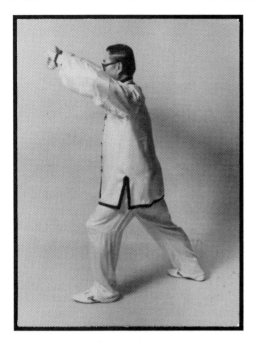

Figure 3-40

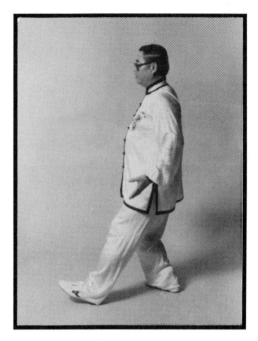

Figure 3-41

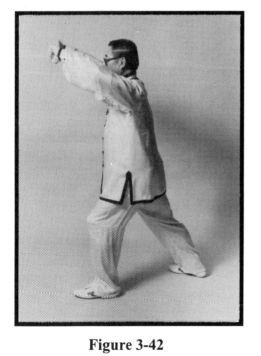

Figure 3-42

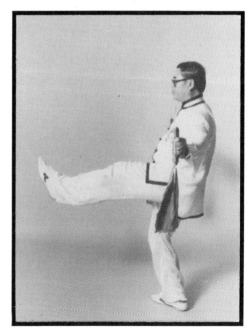

Figure 3-43

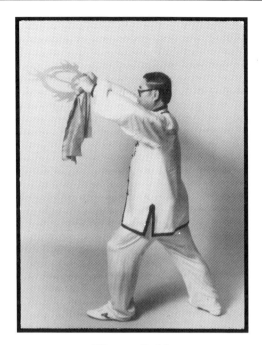

Figure 3-44

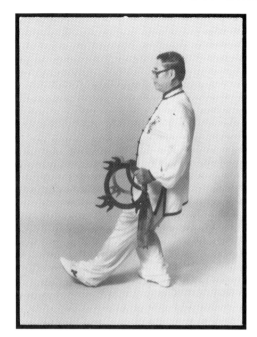

Figure 3-45

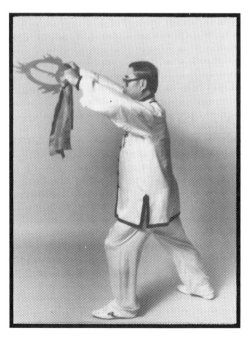

Figure 3-46

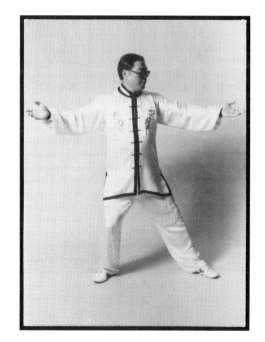

Figure 3-47

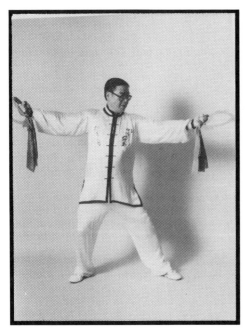

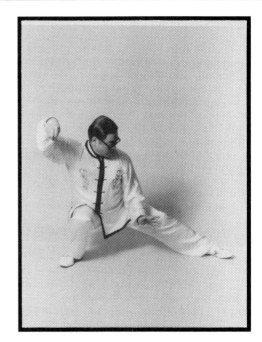

Figure 3-48   Figure 3-49

3.2.13. Reverse Reeling Forearm

The movement is identical for both forms. Note the head and hand positions (Figures 3-47 and 3-48). The centered stance is the same. The eyes follow the hands or weapons in both techniques, and the breathing techniques are similar.

3.2.14. Snake Creeps Down

One of the more advanced moves of the form is Snake Creeps Down. The same Single Whip beginning is followed by the low sweeping motion, similar to the hand strike of the barehand form (Figures 3-49 to 3-52). One must exhale with this latter move just as in barehand, and the body must be centered. The deflecting action of the right hand followed by the downward strike are the same.

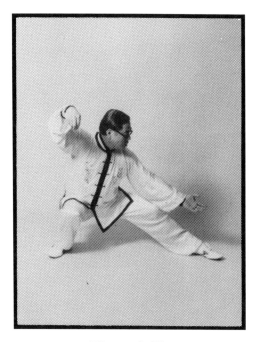

Figure 3-50

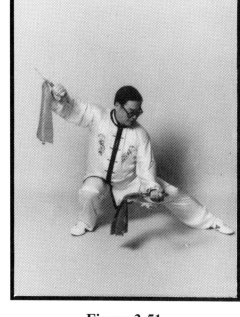

Figure 3-51

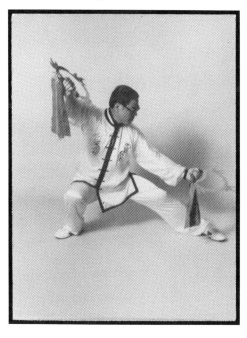

Figure 3-52

3.2.15. Golden Rooster Stands By One Leg

The Golden Rooster is performed identically in both forms. The raised vertical position of the right hand weapon follows tradition (Figures 3-53 and 3-54). Note the same level of placement of the left hand. The blocking application for this hand and the right hand upward strike are similar to the barehand. Exhalation of the breath when completing this movement is identical in both forms.

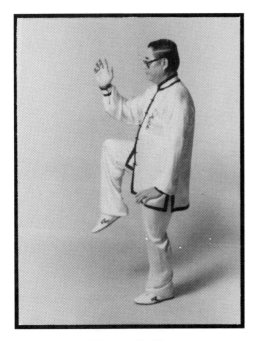

Figure 3-53

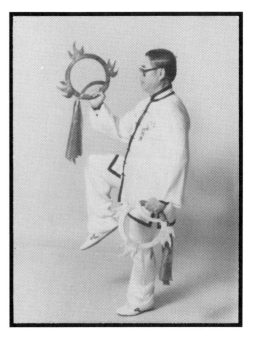

Figure 3-54

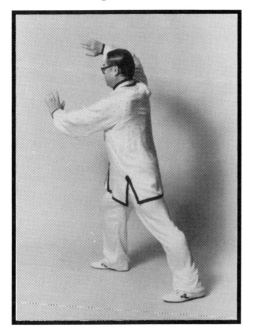

Figure 3-55

3.2.16. Fair Lady Shuttles Back And Forth

A beautiful analogy to the Yang movement, the Fair Lady is performed like the traditional move (Figures 3-55 to 3-62). As in Yang, the Bow Stance is off to the right at 45 degrees.

The upper hand is placed to the side of the forehead for protection. The forward strike requires a vertical weapon, just as the barehand form requires a more vertical striking hand.

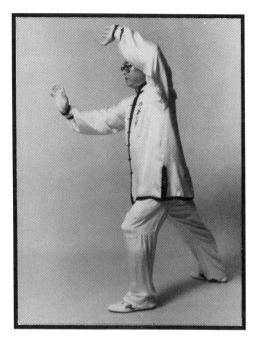

Figure 3-56

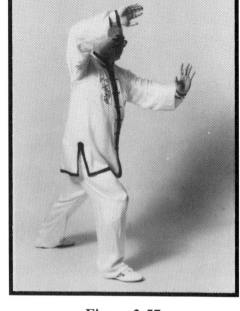

Figure 3-57

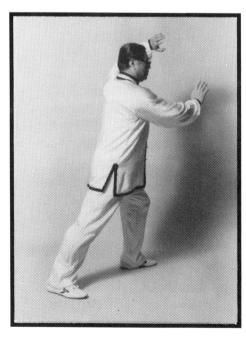

Figure 3-58

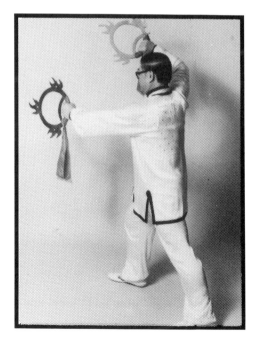

Figure 3-59

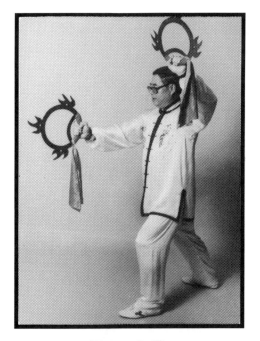

Figure 3-60

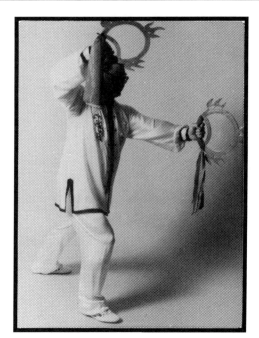

Figure 3-61

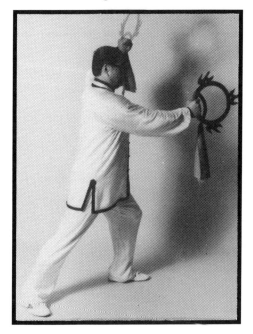

Figure 3-62

3.2.17. Needle At Sea Bottom

The Needle at Sea Bottom movement is similar to the barehand technique. Both demand a 90% - 10% foot stance and a downward strike. Note the same left hand placement (Figures 3-63 and 3-64). Exhalation is required in both with the strike.

3.2.18. Fan Through Back

The Fan Through Back is carried out the same for both forms. A sweeping upper hand provides a block for the head. Both demand a vertical strike starting from the side of the body (Figures 3-65 and 3-66). One must exhale during the strike as in barehand.

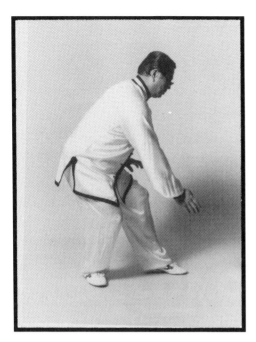

Figure 3-63

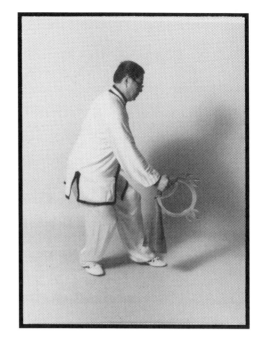

Figure 3-64

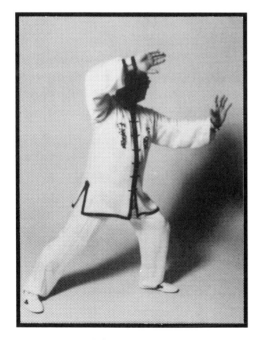

Figure 3-65

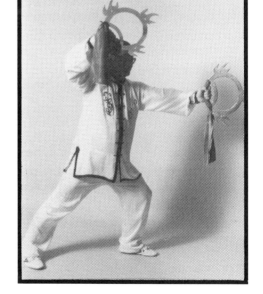

Figure 3-66

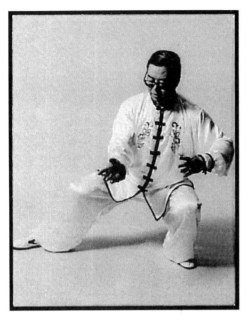 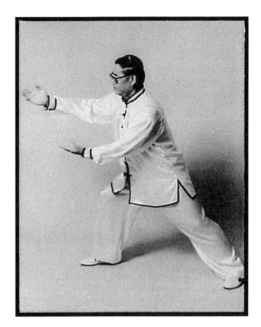

Figure 3-67   Figure 3-68

3.2.19. Embrace The Tiger And Return To The Mountain

Embrace Tiger and Return to Mountain is performed almost identically to the barehand movement. Note the low, centered stances for both (Figures 3-67 to 3-70). Gentle movements of the waist allow for a smooth, healthy sequence with or without the weapon. The breathing pattern is the same, with inhalation on the "Embrace" and exhalation on the "Return".

3.2.20. Fist Under The Elbow

The complex, lethal Fist Under the Elbow barehand movement is followed faithfully with the Wind-Fire Wheels (Figures 3-71 to 3-82). A wide, relaxed centered stance is required for both at the beginning. Notice the dragging movement in the barehand (Figure 3-72) being mirrored by the slicing of the wheels (Figure 3-78). Next, both techniques require right and left hand blocks followed by a left hand strike, the latter while exhaling. A right hand chop or slice is identical. The completion of the movement, as the name explains, ends in a similar left hand block. Modifications of the barehand move are required here to avoid self-injury.

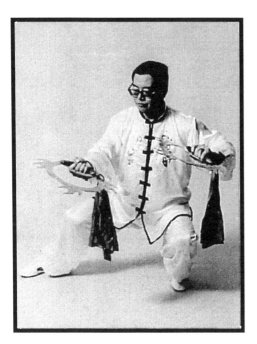

Figure 3-69

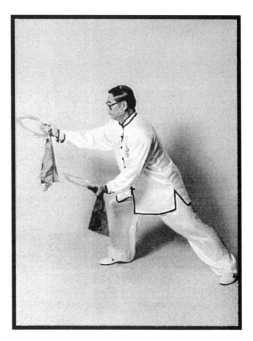

Figure 3-70

3.2.21. Brush Knee And Punch Down

This simple, elegant movement is identical to the barehand. A left hand block, while inhaling, is followed by a right hand strike while exhaling (Figures 3-83 to 3-86).

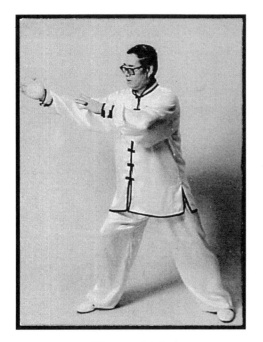

Figure 3-71

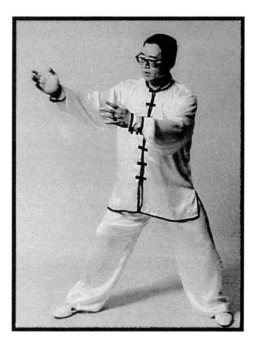

Figure 3-72

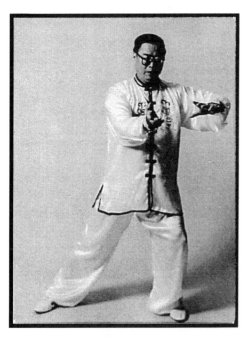

Figure 3-73

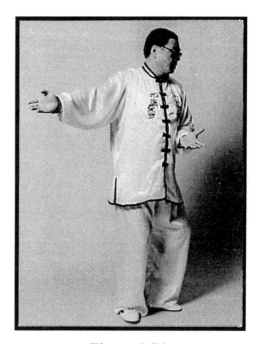

Figure 3-74

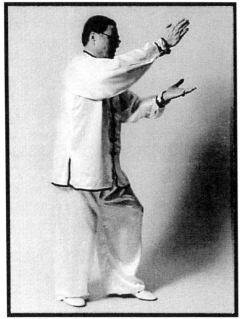
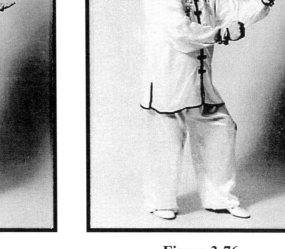

Figure 3-75   Figure 3-76

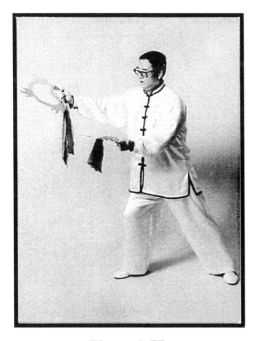
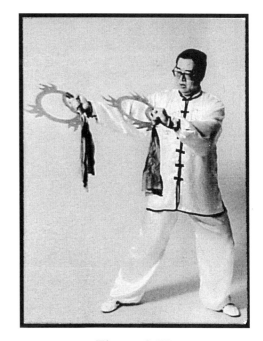

Figure 3-77   Figure 3-78

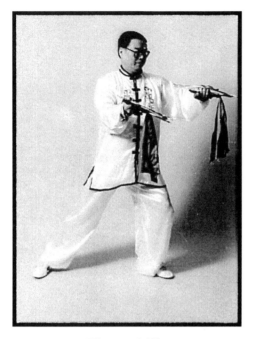

Figure 3-79

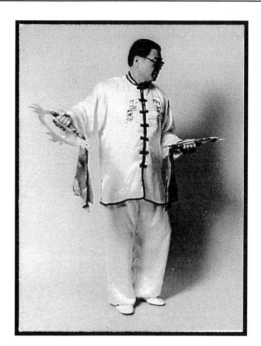

Figure 3-80

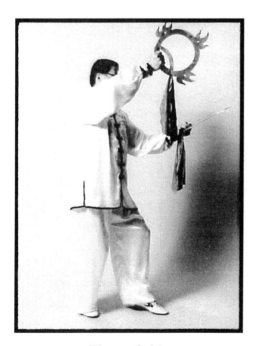

Figure 3-81

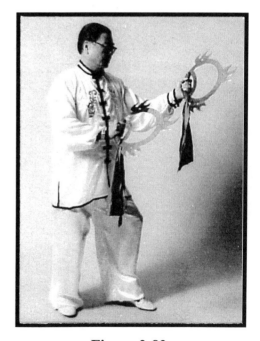

Figure 3-82

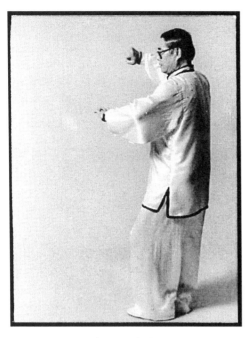

Figure 3-83

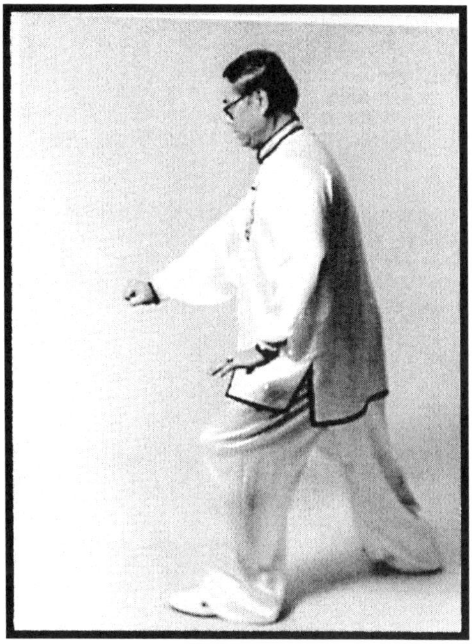

Figure 3-84

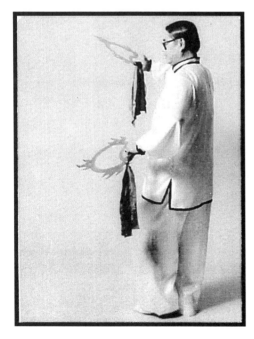

Figure 3-85

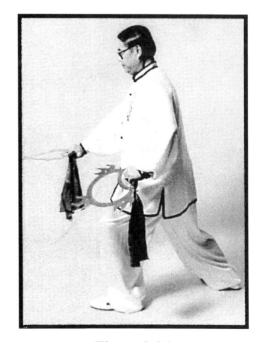

Figure 3-86

3.2.22. Diagonal Flying

In this movement the bare-hand form translates easily into the weapon form. In both (Figures 3-87 to 3-90) the sweeping motion of the lower hand, in concert with the waist and exhalation, is evident. The chi "ball" is made while inhaling in both techniques.

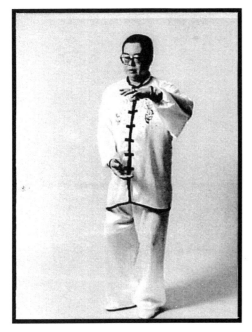

Figure 3-87

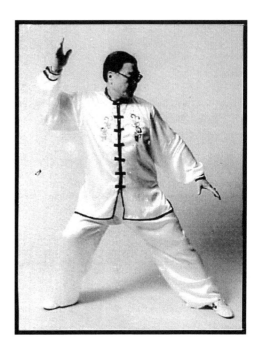

Figure 3-88

3.2.23. Strike The Tiger

The graceful Strike the Tiger movement is seen in its similarity to the barehand form in Figures 3-91 to 3-98. One can easily understand how the sweeping arm movements, Bow Stance and finishing strike are close in meaning to the barehand technique. Both techniques emphasize the gentle turning of the waist and adequate hand placements for optimal blocking for the head. Note how each technique demands that the body turns to a 45 degree finishing Bow Stance, with the head facing forward.

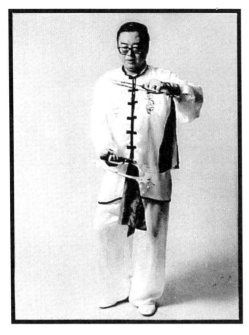

Figure 3-89

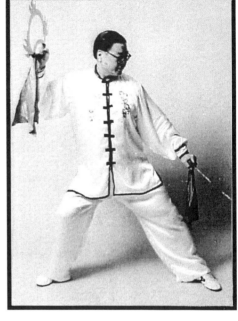

Figure 3-90

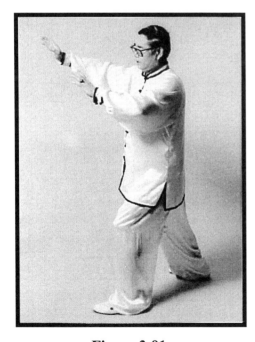

Figure 3-91

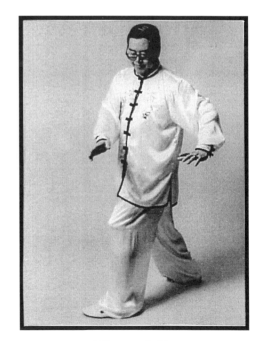

Figure 3-92

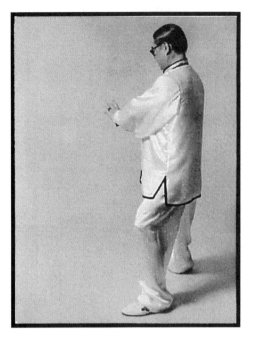

Figure 3-93

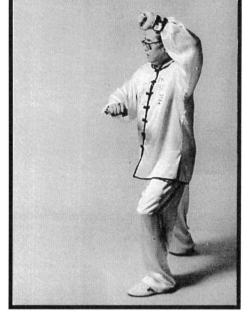

Figure 3-94

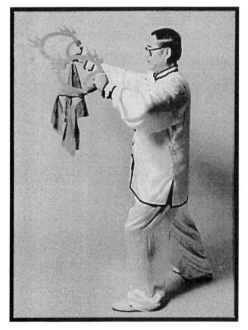

Figure 3-95

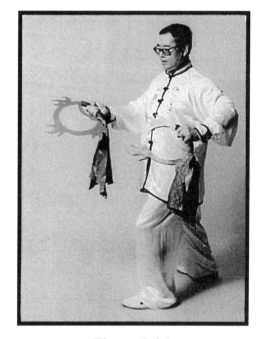

Figure 3-96

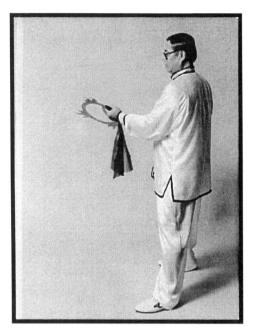

Figure 3-97

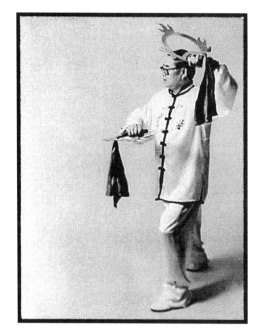

Figure 3-98

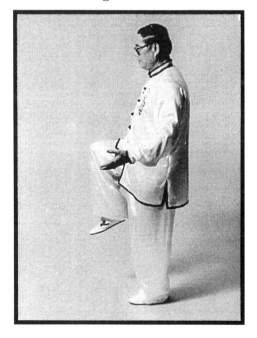

Figure 3-99

3.2.24. Strike To Ears With Both Fists

In Figures 3-99 to 3-102, the identical techniques for the Strike to Ears movement is easily noted. One inhales as the hands are brought down. Notice that the palm placement is similar. The Wind-Fire Wheels movement requires a centered stance at the end, as does the barehand. The applications are quite similar, with bilateral temple or ear strikes smashing into the unfortunate opponent.

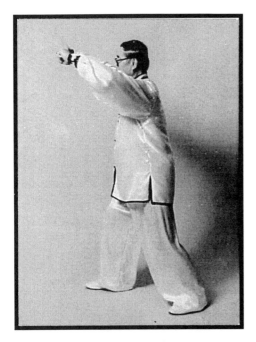

Figure 3-100

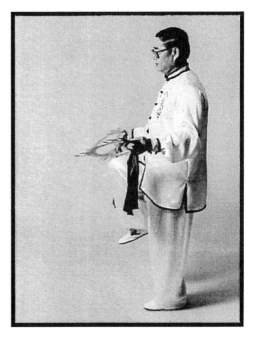

Figure 3-101

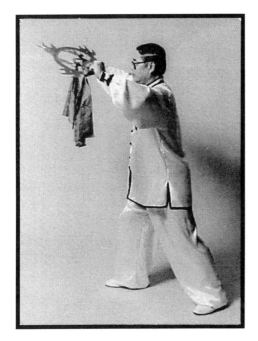

Figure 3-102

3.2.25. White Snake Spits The Poison

The White Snake movement (Figures 3-103 to 3-106) is similar to the barehand, and due to safety precautions not identical. The beginning of both techniques is a block with the left hand. Note the similar arm placement. The palm turns upward with the strike when using the weapon technique, downward with the barehand. Both techniques end with the upper weapon striking to the face. The weapon form actually allows the lower hand to take advantage of the tongues of fire, trapping an attacking weapon with the downward move.

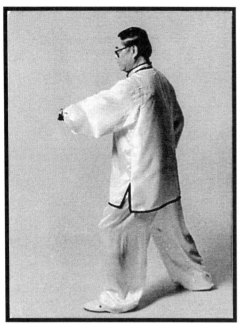

Figure 3-103

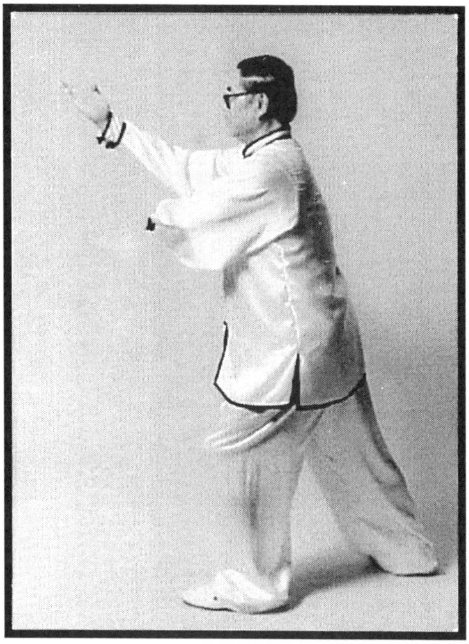

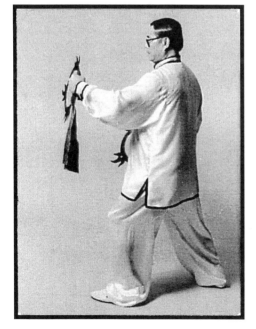

Figure 3-105

Figure 3-104

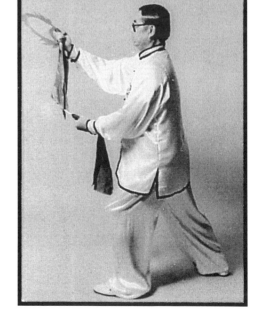

Figure 3-106

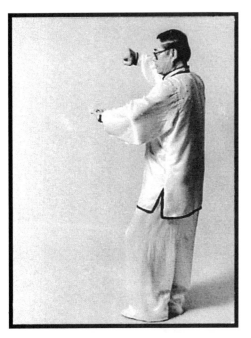

Figure 3-107

3.2.26. Step Forward And Strike Down

The barehand and Wind-Fire Wheel techniques for this movement, seen in Figures 3-107 to 3-110, are comparable. Blocking by the lower hand or weapon while inhaling, striking down with the upper fist or weapon while exhaling is easily seen. The waist, relaxing and flowing, turns with the strike, and the body ends in a Bow Stance in both.

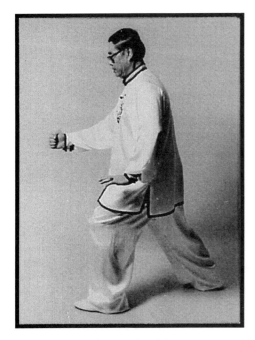

Figure 3-108

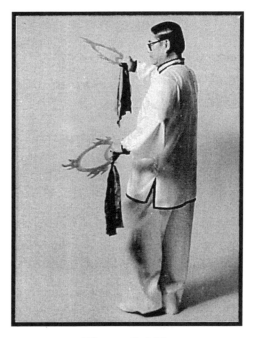

Figure 3-109

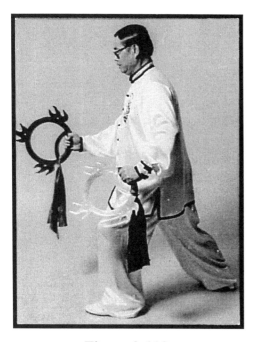

Figure 3-110

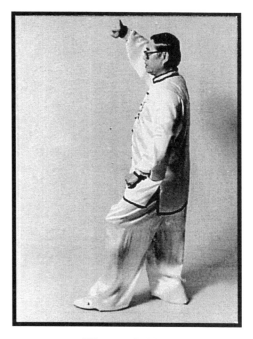

Figure 3-111

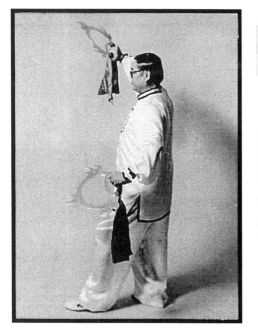

Figure 3-112

3.2.27. Step Back And Ride The Tiger

This classic movement is simply and gracefully demonstrated in Figures 3-111 to 3-112. The movements in both forms are almost indistinguishable. Blocking upward and down, both protect the head and body. Cat Stances and a gentle turn of the waist are important elements of both techniques.

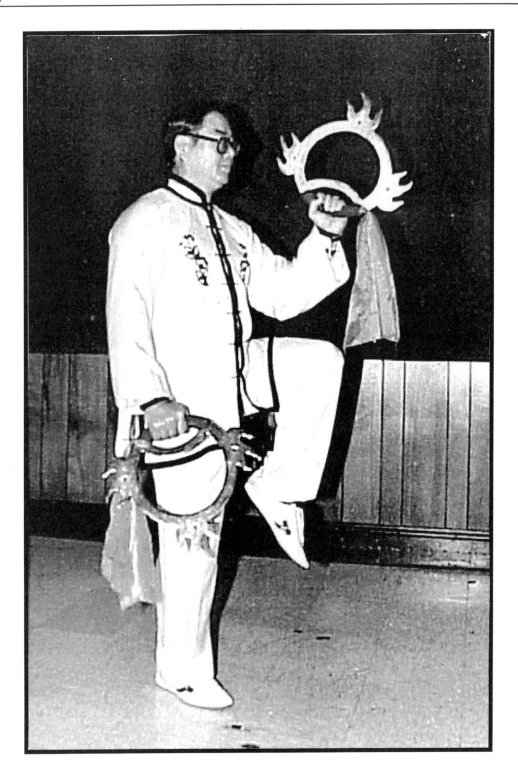

CHAPTER 4

THE VALUE OF THE WIND-FIRE WHEELS

4.1 Introduction

The learning process for Tai-Chi players, as in all types of education, requires a "give and take". This process involves not only the instructor but the core of the technique as well (the technique must reward the player for the time and effort extended). Knowledgeable players will ask themselves what benefits a certain technique or weapon will give them personally. The Wind-Fire Wheels offer many enhancements to a player's training. The health benefits are outstanding. The overall increased muscle tone and lung capacity are very noticeable even early in training. The increased circulation of internal energy, a marked enhancement with this weapon, may theoretically boost the body's immunologic processes. The self-defense benefits of this weapon are quite useful. Granted, the modern-day use of these ancient weapons are minimal. However, in the most basic sense, they offer excellent training for the very real circumstance of defending ones' self with objects in both hands. Finally, the Wheels reinforce the self-defense aspects of the traditional barehand technique.

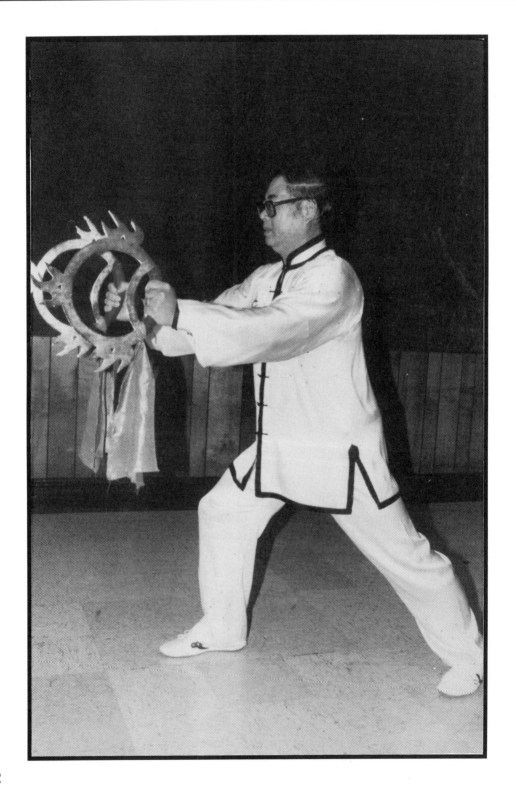

In this chapter the ultimate benefits of practicing this form are given.

4.2 The Value Of The Wind-Fire Wheels

4.2.1 For Strength And Power Training

The unique structure and bilaterality of the Wind-Fire Wheels confer likewise unique effects on the player's body, and eventually on the player's strength. Although its weight is greater than most weapons in the Tai-Chi arsenal, the wheel increases muscular tone without increasing bulk (which would decrease fluidity). It is light enough, conversely, to allow for adequate control of the weapon. The circular shape brings the structure of the weapon closer to the body than other weapons (e.g., straight sword), and the width is greater. These final two characteristics require more effort to balance the weapon laterally, on either side of the arm, rather than the weapon pointing entirely in the same direction as the arm. Finally, the tongues of fire protruding from the circle require care and balance, resulting in strength-building, to avoid injury during use.

The Wind-Fire Wheels provide excellent training for all areas of the body. One will especially notice these effects on the arms and thorax. During early training, the strength value is felt in the wrists, hands, and forearms. One may feel mild soreness at the start followed in short by a steady decrease as the form is learned. Later in training, the biceps and deltoid muscles feel stronger. As with all Tai-Chi forms, these weapons will provide for a great deal of lower body power. One will soon realize that the greatest and ultimate benefit will be in loosening the waist and strengthening the lower limbs. Indeed because of the unique shape and weight, coupled with the intent of the form itself, the effort required to remain centered is an excellent adjunct to rooting training.

4.2.2 For Endurance And Spiritual Training

One of the unique characteristics of this weapon and form is the endurance training it provides. As the days, weeks and months of training pass,

103

there is an increasing feeling of ease and confidence. The Wheels become lighter in the hands. For the intermediate player this should take only a matter of a few weeks to realize. Fatigue in the wrists, hands, arms and especially shoulders will occur. These symptoms will fade. Endurance training, however, is not limited to the upper body. The remarkable amount of centering and balance required to perform the movements will slowly build the endurance level of the lower body, making the form a superior method for overall training.

As the player learns and perfects the form, a growing level of confidence and well-being follows. This change is different than that felt with other weapons. Players in our school have remarked about the intense feeling of heat and energy while performing the movements. They notice a feeling of accomplishment and relaxation after the form. In its most fundamental aspect, training in the Wind-Fire Wheels form instills a remarkable amount of patience and dedication itself. This benefit will extend to the player's approach to daily life experiences.

4.2.3 For Internal Chi Circulation

The development of Tai-Chi Chuan is forever intertwined with the existence and circulation of Chi. This very real physical force pervades the human body. It reaches and exerts effects on all organs and tissues. Without this energy health and even life itself can not be maintained. The circulation of Chi can be linked to the nervous system, which conducts this energy. The specific pathways of conduction are termed meridians (14 total) and vessels (two total) which themselves are associated with an organ of the body. The smooth, unimpeded flow of Chi throughout the system promotes health.

Blockages or restrictions of Chi flow will result in illness. The type of illness will depend on which meridian (and therefore organ) is affected. Nerve injuries are an example of a restriction. In response to these phenomena, centuries of investigation and practice have led to the development of acupuncture/acupressure theory. Cavities, or acupuncture points, in specific locations on the meridians provide target areas for needle insertion (or external pressure) in an attempt to open or "re-adjust" the blocked or aberrant Chi circulation.

The practice of Tai-Chi Chuan activates and promotes the smooth circulation of Chi throughout the body. Chi not only flows more easily through the meridians and vessels but also into the tissues (especially the extremities). Blood flow to the tissues and internal organs also increase. Less stress throughout the body is noted. The slow movements and deep breathing are virtually linked to these events. Chi can be moved either through the "Small Circulation " within the abdomen, thorax and head or the "Grand Circulation " which additionally includes the extremities. What is just as important, however, is the elevation of martial techniques and understanding of them after years of training. Using these skills the Tai-Chi martial artist can more easily develop Chi circulation throughout the entire body and learn to control its movement for self-defense.

Wind-Fire Wheel training is an excellent method to develop Chi circulation. The path to achieving this is similar to the barehand form. Once the practitioner learns the sequence of movements and breathing, he/she will notice the signs of Chi circulation with continued practice (warmth, perspiration, increased blood flow to the skin, a sense of well being, etc). Intermediate and advanced players who are more knowledgeable in circulating Chi can incorporate this understanding by moving Chi through the Small and Grand Circulations. In time as the martial techniques are better understood the practitioner will be able to use this knowledge. The circulation of Chi will be controlled and be more easily delivered to the opponent through the weapons.

4.2.4 For Health Improvement

The health benefits provided by the Wind-Fire Wheels is delivered through two means: Tai-Chi Chuan and Chi-Kung. These vital entities are different in some aspects but so related in others. The Wind-Fire Wheels system takes advantage of both. The system combines firmness and gentleness, fullness and emptiness and peace and tranquility. There are harmony, continuity and softness in the movements. The form requires a fusion of will, vital force and spirit. The combination of tranquility and movement seen in both Tai-Chi Chuan and Chi-Kung results in an intense cultivation of inner health when the system is practiced.

Tai-Chi Chuan is well known (especially in China) for its therapeutic effect on many illnesses. It is not surprising that many of these illnesses are stress-related: gastritis, intestinal ulcer, cardiac disease, respiratory diseases, hypertension, arthritis and psychological disorders are examples. Stress reduction, increased endurance, improved cardiorespiratory function, improved balance and enhanced immunologic function are achieved. Various academic researchers in Western traditional medicine (including one of this book's contributing editors) are currently studying the beneficial effects of acupuncture, Tai-Chi and Chi-Kung on selected diseases and on immune function. There is preliminary evidence that acupuncture or Chi-Kung can be used successfully to treat some female endocrinologic disorders. New evidence will soon be published that confirms an enhancement in the functions of specific leukocytes (white blood cells) in the circulation, which provide disease resistance. Tai-Chi has been found to reduce the incidence of accidental falls in the elderly. The Tai-Chi Chuan system will lead the practitioner on a path towards mental, physical and spiritual health. Because the Wind-Fire Wheels system follows Tai-Chi principles, these outstanding health advantages are within reach of the practitioner.

Chi-Kung is a general term for many different forms of internal energy exercises devised for meditational and therapeutic purposes. It incorporates the meridian theory of traditional Chinese medicine, and uses both cerebral hemispheres for its purpose. Thus Chi-Kung is quite the same as Tai-Chi and, in fact, has been touted as the forerunner to all martial arts. Chi-Kung differs from Tai-Chi by its simpler forms. The practitioner can then concentrate all efforts on improving the ability to feel inside the body. Its benefits certainly include all those that Tai-Chi provides and more.

In the Wind-Fire Wheels system, Tai-Chi Chi-Kung sets have been developed to take advantage of both techniques. Some forms in the sets are actually simplified movements adopted from the Tai-Chi Chuan sequence. These simple exercises will give practitioners a feeling for their Chi and start them on the road to understanding how to work with their Chi. As Chi circulation improves, the practice of Tai-Chi Chuan becomes more successful. Health and martial arts skill will become enhanced.

The best way to improve health with the Wind-Fire Wheels form is to follow these important principles:

Breathing should be deep, long, slow, fine and even. This will facilitate the delivery of blood (and oxygen) into the peripheral tissues.

1. Coordinate the movements of the hands, feet, elbows, knees, shoulders and hips. Understand the basic techniques, theory, methods and function of all movements. Correct and harmonious movements are the requirements for advancing your skill in the weapon.

2. Emphasize the inner concentration when practicing Chi-Kung. Successful Chi-Kung practice is based on converting the external concentration

into the inner concentration. The term inner concentration is defined as the flow of thought that regulates and protects the cerebrum through either the transmission or guarding of the flow of thought, to manifest the function of Chi and set life itself into motion.

With long term and constant practice in the Wind-Fire Wheels system, the following specific organ systems will undergo improvements:

1. Cardiorespiratory: Increased cardiac output and lung capacity.

2. Gastrointestinal: Improved appetite and gastrointestinal absorption, improved hepatic and gall bladder function, decreased blood cholesterol.

3. Vascular: Reduction in arteriosclerosis.

4. Extremities: Enhanced, smoother joint mobility, increased tendon and bone strength.

5. Vertebral: Enhanced, smoother vertebral mobility, prevention of age-related vertebral changes.

6. Central nervous system: Enhanced sense of well-being and mood, improved vision and hand-eye coordination, faster reaction times, improved balance

7. Immunologic: Enhanced resistance to infectious disease.

4.2.5 For Self-Defense

The form incorporates many of the movements characteristic of the Yang Style. Thus, it reinforces the refinement of these movements and their applications. It helps train the player to use these applications with an object in their hands, therefore expanding the training they receive with barehand techniques. It is unlikely that one would specifically use these ancient weapons in self-defense should an attack occur (obviously the legality of carrying them on one's person is questionable at best). However, if the need arises players can use the basic principles of this form should they have heavy, compact objects in their hands. Because of the compact nature of the wheels, as opposed to longer weapons, the applications of the Yang movements are extended in quite a natural way. The blocking techniques, for example, are extremely practical in their applications. An attacker carrying a long weapon - a staff or cudgel for example - can be blocked in numerous ways including the angle between the tongues of fire and the wheel, and the trapping ability of the wheel's circle itself. The dual nature of the weapons offers several advantages. These include: 1) The unique use of both hands to block an oncoming attack, 2) the use of one hand to strike/slice after the other has blocked, 3) the ability to kick while blocking and striking with both hands, 4) better balance from the weight of the weapons when kicking and 5) the ability to block or strike multiple attackers with both hands armed. As in other Tai-Chi forms, the ultimate goal of extending internal energy through the weapon may be the key to successfully disabling an opponent.

CHAPTER 5

ADVANCED FORM I

5.1 Introduction

Previous chapters have undoubtedly sparked your interest in an advanced use of the Wind-Fire Wheels. You understand that the weapon is ancient in origin, that it has inspired awe and fear, and that it promises significant gains in your command of Tai-Chi and health. The previous chapter has shown you how your knowledge of barehanded Tai-Chi movements relates to using the Wind-Fire Wheels, and you are now able to grasp the power of the weapon. You may have even seen a demonstration of Wind-Fire Wheels and felt the internal power, rhythm, and grace that accompanies their use in Tai-Chi. Now you are ready for a personal test of whether this weapon makes sense for you and of how prepared you are to make use of it. In other words, you are ready to learn, practice, and perform a complete form of Wind-Fire movements.

This chapter describes and illustrates the first advanced form for using

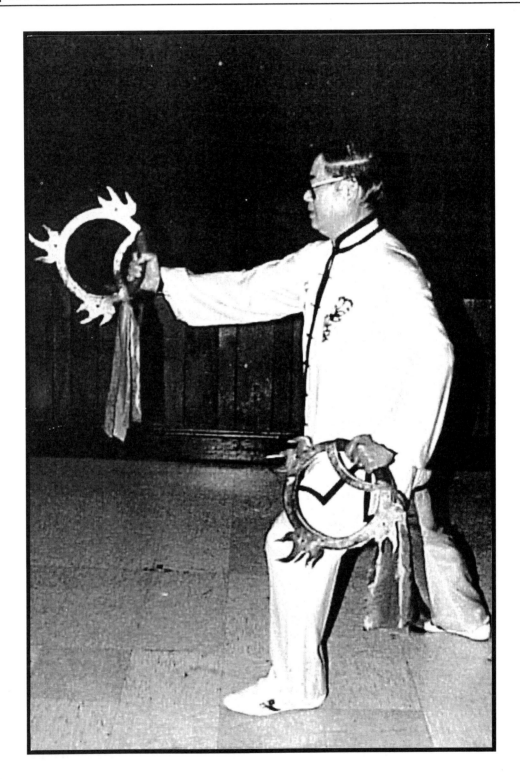

Wind-Fire Wheels in Tai-Chi. As a first form, it is shorter and only requires a moderate amount of strength and grace. The form will, however, help you use the Wheels safely while also building your strength, endurance, and internal power.

As with all the forms in this book, this first form is built on the basic principles, movements, and postures of Yang's Tai-Chi. Although it is simpler than forms covered in later chapters, this form integrates the use of the weapon into such advanced barehanded movements as Embrace Tiger, Flying Diagonal, and Needle at Sea Bottom.

The preamble is now complete and you are ready to examine the pictures that illustrate the form and to digest the text describing each movement's purposes, essentials, and fine points. As you read and practice the movements, you will grow in your ability to tie them together into the harmonious flow that marks advanced practice in Tai-Chi.

5.2 Advanced Form I

1. **Preparatory Posture**
2. **Wind-Fire Commencing**
3. **Left Step Forward Part Wild Horse's Mane**
4. **Turn Right Ward Off, Roll Back, Press and Push**
5. **Left Single Whip**
6. **Right Lifting Hand**
7. **Wind-Fire Turning Wheels**
8. **White Crane Spreads Its Wings And Left Heel Kick**
9. **Left, Right, Left Brush Knee And Step Forward**
10. **Playing The Lute**
11. **Left Slicing And Right Striking**
12. **Wind-Fire Up Blocking And Down Waist Chopping**

13. **Embrace The Tiger And Return To The Mountain**
14. **Fist Under The Elbow**
15. **Reverse Reeling Forearm (3 times)**
16. **Diagonal Flying**
17. **Needle At Sea Bottom**
18. **Fan Through Back**
19. **Right Turn Right Part Wild Horse's Mane**
20. **Left Single Whip**
21. **Wave Hands Like Clouds (3 times)**
22. **Left Single Whip**
23. **High Pat On Horse**
24. **Right Heel Kick And Strike To Ears**
25. **Left Turn Body Left Heel Kick And Strike To Ears**
26. **Brush Knee And Punch Down**
27. **Right Heel Kick And Strike To Ears**
28. **Left Strike The Tiger**
29. **Strike To Ears With Both Fists**
30. **Right Turn Left Part Wild Horse's Mane**
31. **Right Turn Body Fair Lady Shuttles Back And Forth (right 1 time, left 1 time)**
32. **Right Lower Body And Stand On One Leg**
33. **White Snake Spits The Poison**
34. **Wind-Fire High And Low Diagonal Cuts**
35. **Right Step Forward And Left Strike Down**
36. **Left Lower Body And Stand On One Leg**
37. **Wind-Fire Turning Wheels (3 times)**
38. **Step Back And Ride The Tiger**
39. **Right Turn Body Wind-Fire Protecting The Head And Right Heel Kick**
40. **Left Slicing And Right Striking**
41. **Step Forward Left And Right Strikings**
42. **Appears Closed**
43. **Wind-Fire Closing**
44. **Return To Origin**

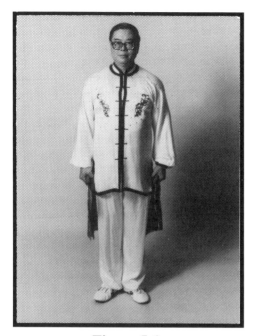

Figure 5-1

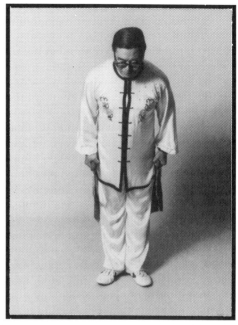

Figure 5-2

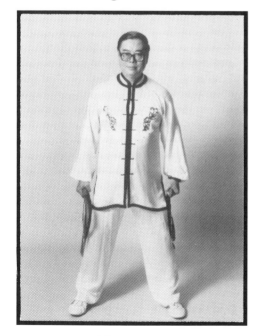

Figure 5-3

1. Preparatory Posture

Movements:

Begin by facing South.

Fig. 5-1: Natural Standing with feet sixty degree outward, back straight, arms relaxed with Wind-Fire Wheels by your side (Facing South, inhale and exhale several times).

Fig. 5-2: Bow to your teachers or spectators politely.

Fig. 5-3: Bend your knees slightly, then step to your left with your left leg.

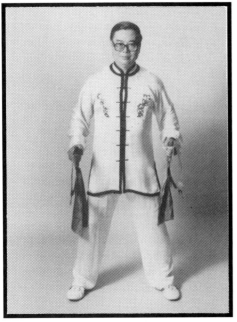
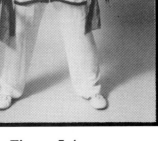
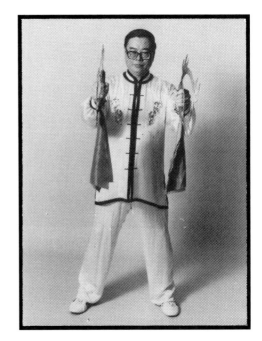

Figure 5-4   Figure 5-5

2. Wind-Fire Commencing

Movements:

Fig. 5-4: Raise your Wind-Fire Wheels in front of you to shoulder height, keeping them parallel to each other.

Fig. 5-5: Rotate the Wind-Fire Wheels outward, down and up three times.

3. Left Step Forward Part Wild Horse's Mane

Movements:

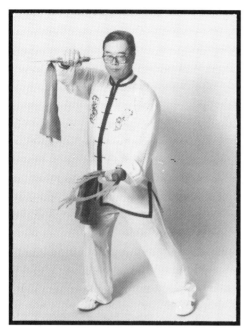

Figure 5-6

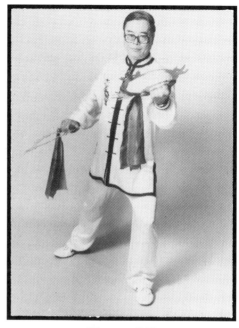

Figure 5-7

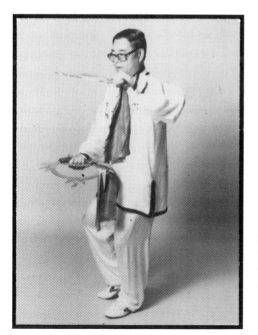

Figure 5-8

Fig. 5-6: Shift your weight to your right foot and bring your left foot next to the right, while turning your body slightly to the right. During the twisting movement, rotate both wheels to face each other. Eyes are looking in the same direction as your right hand.

Fig. 5-7: Step out your left foot into a left Bow Stance, (face South), while slicing your right wheel down next to your hip and extending your left wheel forward to the eye level.

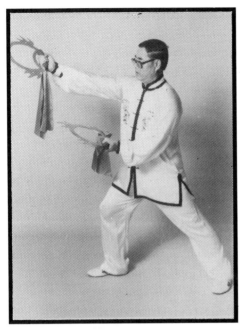 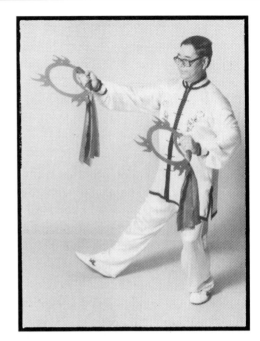

Figure 5-9 Figure 5-10

4. Turn Right Ward Off, Roll Back, Press And Push

Movements:

Fig. 5-8: Turn right and bring both Wind-Fire Wheels to your left facing each other with the right hand downward and the left hand upward. Shift your weight to your left foot and bring the right foot next to the left.

Fig. 5-9: Step forward with your right foot while extending your right wheel forward and upward and draw your left wheel downward and out. Eyes should be focused on your right wheel.

Fig. 5-10: Shift your weight back onto your left leg and roll back right heel while twisting your waist to the left and pulling down with your Wind-Fire Wheels. Keep your eyes focused on the right hand and then focus in the direction of the torso at eye level.

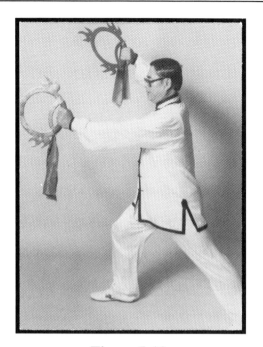

Figure 5-11

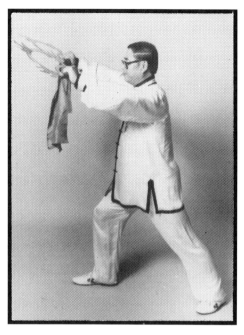

Figure 5-12

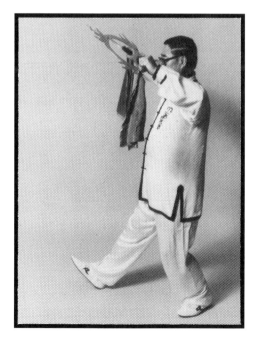

Figure 5-13

Fig. 5-11: Shift your weight forward into a right Bow Stance while right wheel makes an upward blocking and left wheel a forward striking. Eyes focus on the left hand wheel.

Fig. 5-12: Keep the same Bow Stance as shown in Fig. 5-11. Bring the left wheel up to the right wheel level.

Fig. 5-13: Shift your weight back onto your left foot and bring both Wind-Fire Wheels to forehead level (45 degrees above horizontal level). Eyes look straight ahead.

Fig. 5-14: Rotate both wheels down to your waist while shifting your weight onto the right leg. Eyes keep looking ahead.

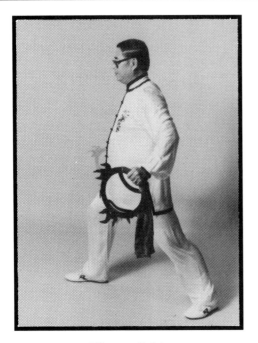

Figure 5-14

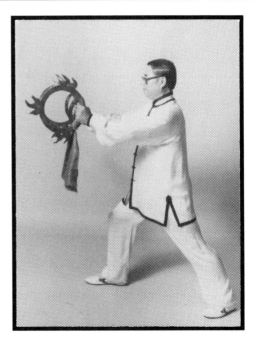

Figure 5-15

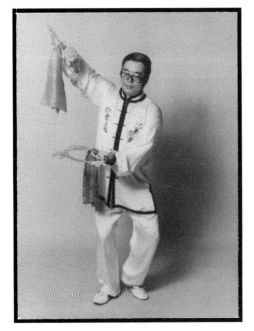

Figure 5-16

Fig. 5-15: Continue shifting your weight onto the right leg and complete Bow Stance. Push forward with both Wind-Fire Wheels and complete the push posture. Eyes continue to look ahead.

5. Left Single Whip

Movements:

Fig. 5-16: Draw the left foot to the right foot and make a "C" Slice with your right-hand wheel while the left-hand wheel rotates from upward to downward and is placed under the right hand wheel. Eyes look to the right hand wheel then move to the left-hand wheel.

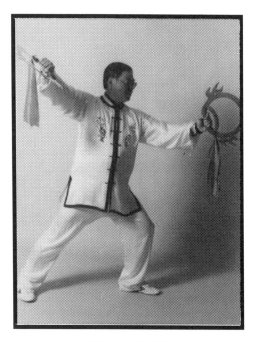

Figure 5-17

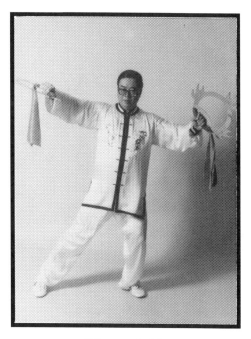

Figure 5-18

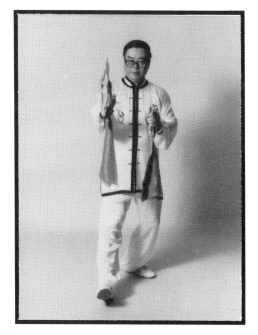

Figure 5-19

Fig. 5-17: Extend your left leg forward and touch down with the heel. Shift your weight to your left foot and complete Bow Stance. Rotate and extend your left wheel forward.

6. Right Lifting Hand

Movements:

Fig. 5-18: Turn your body to your right while rotating at your waist to face South. Both hands are holding Wind-Fire Wheels vertically.

Fig. 5-19: Shift your weight onto your left foot and draw your right foot to

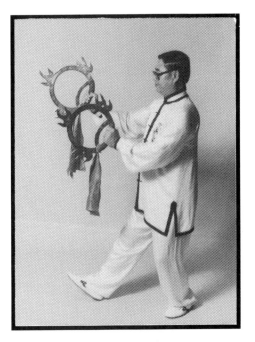

Figure 5-20

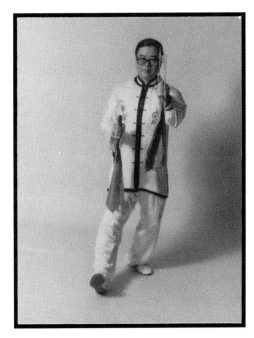

Figure 5-21

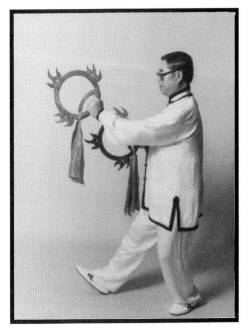

Figure 5-22

your left foot. Step out to the front and touch down with your heel, while drawing the wheels to the center of your chest with your right hand higher than your left hand.

Fig. 5-20: Side view of figure 5-19.

Fig. 5-21: Same stance as Fig. 5-19. Rotate both Wind-Fire Wheels outward once vertically.

Fig. 5-22: Side view of figure 5-21.

Fig. 5-23: After one vertical rotation.

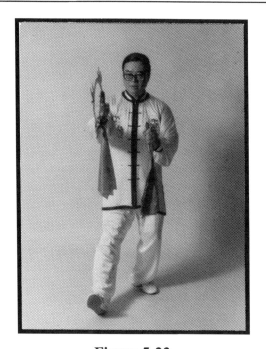

Figure 5-23

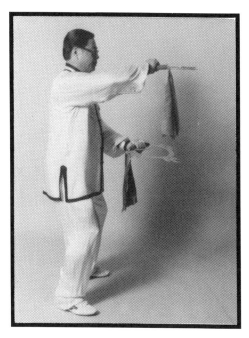

Figure 5-24

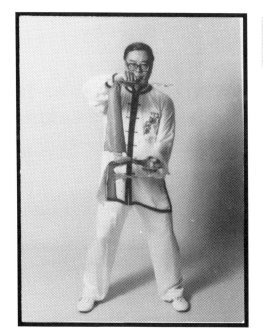

Figure 5-25

7. Wind-Fire Turning Wheels

Movements:

Fig. 5-24: Turn your body to your left while rotating your waist to the left. Both feet are shoulder width apart and slightly bent, while revolving both wheels and slicing your left wheel down and the right wheel up.

Fig. 5-25: Shows front view of Fig. 5-24.

Fig. 5-26: Revolve two wheels once again with the right wheel down and the left wheel up.

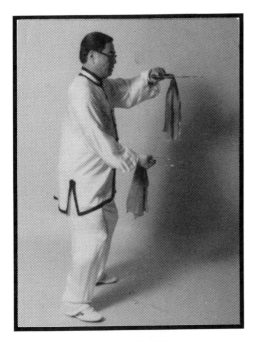

Figure 5-26

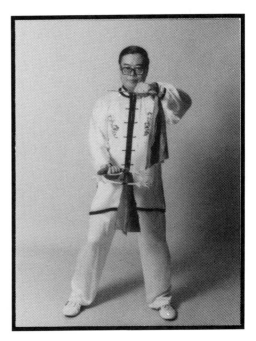

Figure 5-27

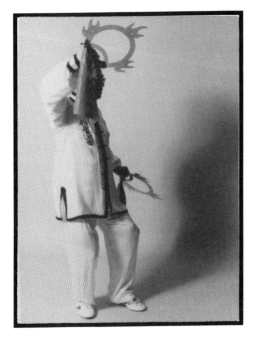

Figure 5-28

Fig. 5-27: Shows front view of Fig. 5-26.

8. White Crane Spreads Its Wings And Left Heel Kick

Movements:

Fig. 5-28: Rotate your waist to the right and step up with your left foot forward as in Cat Stance. Your weight should be in your right leg now. In the meantime, begin raising your right wheel up and slicing your left wheel down.

Fig. 5-29: Lift your left foot up and balance your body.

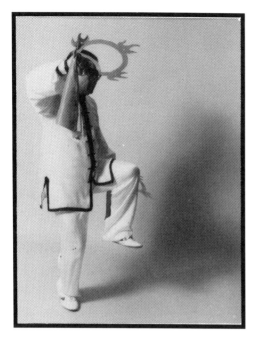
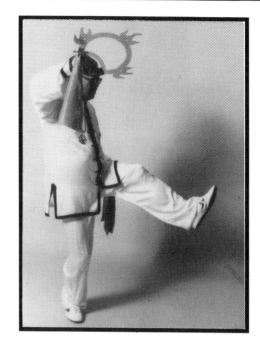

Figure 5-29   **Figure 5-30**

Fig. 5-30: Execute a Heel Kick to the front.

9. Left, Right, Left Brush Knee And Step Forward

Movements:

Fig. 5-31: Bring back your left kicking leg close to your right leg. Turn your body slightly to your left while raising up and slicing your left wheel to the front and bringing down right wheel with blades outward to face height. Turn your body to your right while lowering and slicing your left wheel and slicing your right wheel outward and down, then bring it to ear height vertically, blades pointed to the front.

Step up to left Bow Stance while striking your right wheel forward horizontally, once the blade has passed the head.

Fig. 5-32: Shift your weight to your right foot. Turn your left foot outward and begin turning your body to your left while raising up and slicing your right wheel to the front and bringing down the left wheel with blades outward to face

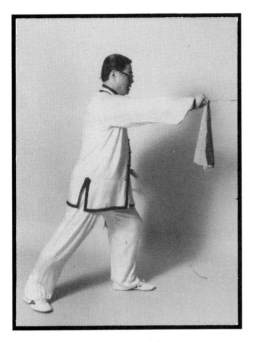

Figure 5-31

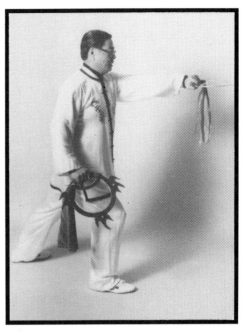

Figure 5-32

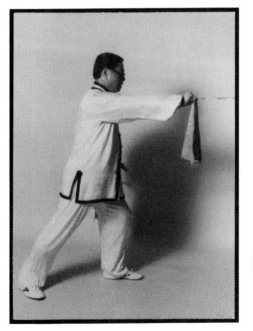

Figure 5-33

height. Turn your body to your left while lowering and slicing your right wheel and slicing your left wheel outward down then bring to left ear height vertically, blades point to the front. Step up your right leg to right Bow Stance while striking up your left wheel forward horizontally.

Fig. 5-33: Repeat the movement described in Figure 5-31.

10. Playing The Lute

Movements:

Fig. 5-34: Shift your weight onto your right foot and bring your right

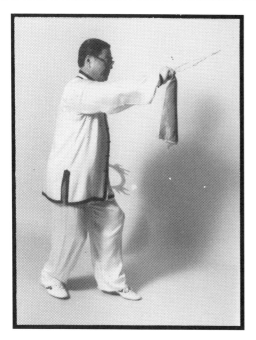

Figure 5-34

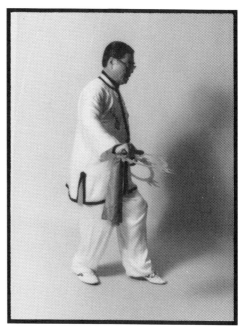

Figure 5-35

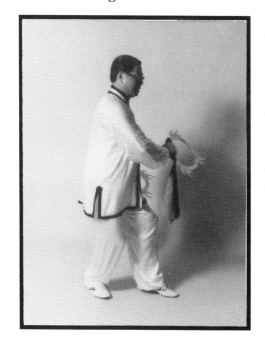

Figure 5-36

wheel to eye level.

Fig. 5-35: Rotate your waist from left to right while lowering your right wheel in a circular motion.

Fig. 5-36: Continue rotating your waist to the left while circling your right wheel up.

Fig. 5-37: Pull your left foot to your right foot and rotate your waist to the right while bringing your right wheel upward and your left wheel downward to face each other.

Fig. 5-38: Step forward with your left foot touching down with your heel while extending your left wheel forward and slicing your right wheel down.

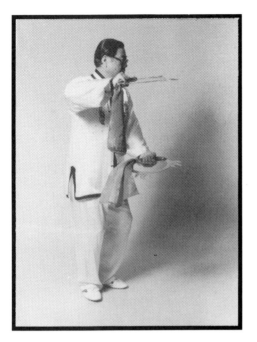

Figure 5-37

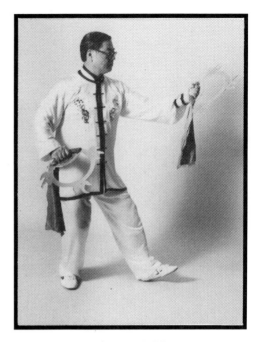

Figure 5-38

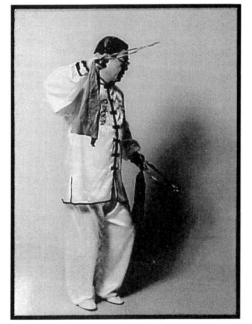

Figure 5-39

11. Left Slicing And Right Striking

Movements:

Fig. 5-39: Bring back your left leg while lowering your left wheel and raising your right wheel to shoulder height.

Fig. 5-40: Slice down your left wheel to your left side waist while striking your right wheel forward vertically.

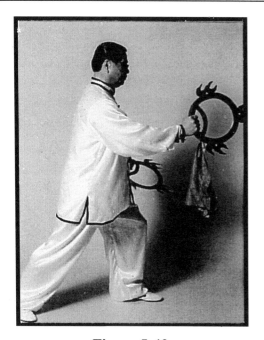

Figure 5-40

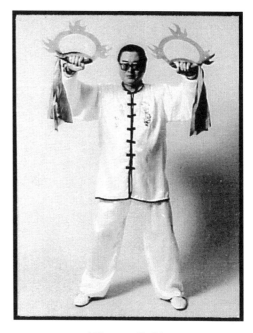

Figure 5-41

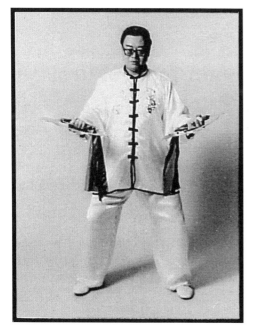

Figure 5-42

12. Wind-Fire Up Blocking And Down Waist Chopping

Movements:

Fig. 5-41: Turn your body to your right while rotating your waist to face south. Raise both wheels arching up blocking about forehead height on either side of the head, palm down.

Fig. 5-42: Bring the wheels in an outward circular motion until the wheels are about the level of the diaphragm, palms up.

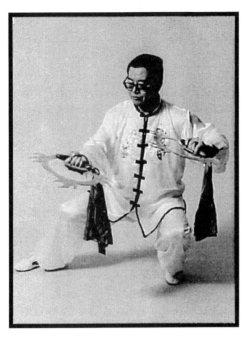

Figure 5-43

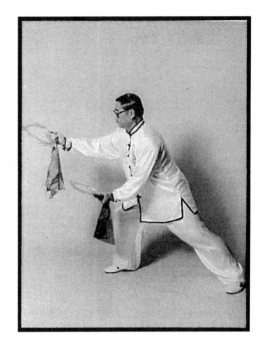

Figure 5-44

13. Embrace The Tiger And Return To The Mountain

Movements:

Fig. 5-43: Drop down your body into a deep Horse Stance and shift your weight onto your left foot. Turn the left wheel so it is palm down, the right wheel is about waist height, the left wheel about diaphragm height.

Fig. 5-44: Shift your weight on your right foot and rise to a normal Bow Stance. Swing the wheels to the right while turning the right wheel to palm out about upper diaphragm height and the left wheel in a forward punching motion of about groin height.

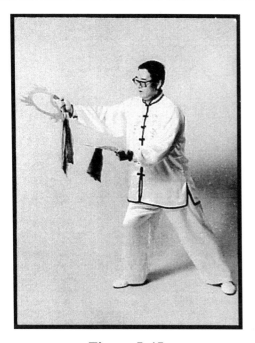

Figure 5-45

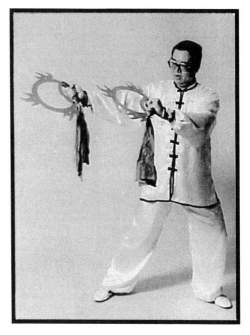

Figure 5-46

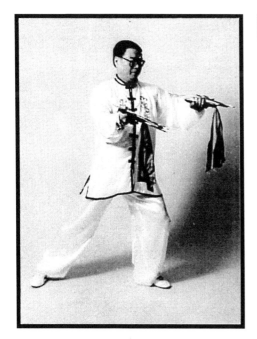

Figure 5-47

14. Fist Under The Elbow

Movements:

Fig. 5-45: Raise the wheels to shoulder height bending the elbows.

Fig. 5-46: Shift your weight on your left foot.

Fig. 5-47: Step into left Bow Stance and rotate your waist to the left while bringing your right wheel upward and your left wheel downward to your left.

Fig. 5-48: Draw your left foot next to your right foot. Swing both wheels in a circular motion downward and bring

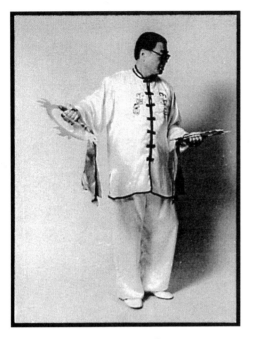

Figure 5-48

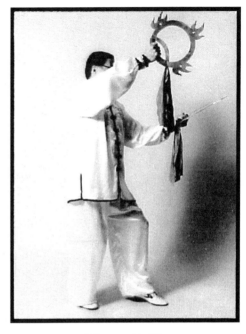

Figure 5-49

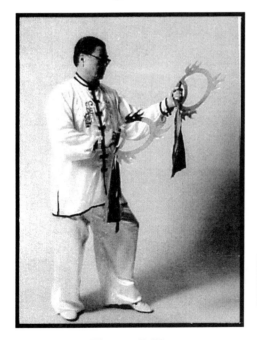

Figure 5-50

your left wheel point out to front at waist height while raising your right wheel to shoulder height.

Fig. 5-49: Step up with your left foot forward as in Cat Stance. Strike the left wheel, the right wheel, palm to center, in a vertical forward cutting motion, to mid abdomen.

Fig. 5-50: Same Cat Stance as in Fig. 5-49. Slice your right wheel down and your left wheel up.

15. Reverse Reeling Forearm (3 times)

Movements:

Fig. 5-51: From Fig. 5-50, slightly

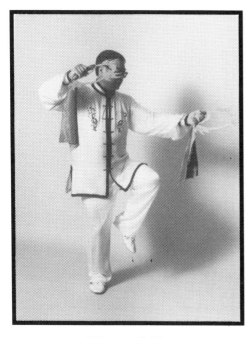
Figure 5-51

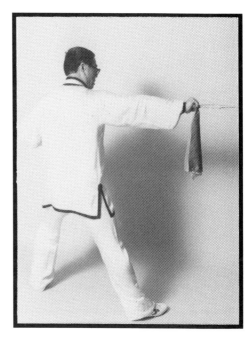
Figure 5-52

lower your left wheel and raise your right wheel from behind to ear height while lifting up your left foot.

Fig. 5-52: Step back with your left foot behind your right foot and pivot on your right foot while pulling your left wheel next to your waist and extending your right wheel forward.

Fig. 5-53: Extend your left wheel out and up while rotating both wheels up.

Fig. 5-54: Bend your left elbow and lift up your right foot.

Fig. 5-55: Step back with your right foot behind your left and pivot on your left foot while pulling your right wheel next to your waist and extending your left wheel forward.

Fig. 5-56: Repeat the movements of Fig. 5-51.

Fig. 5-57: Repeat the movement of Fig. 5-52.

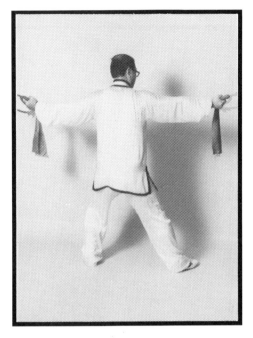

Figure 5-53

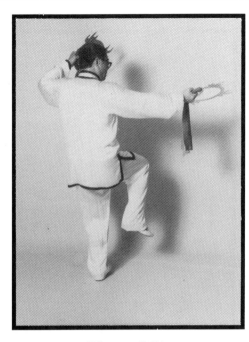

Figure 5-54

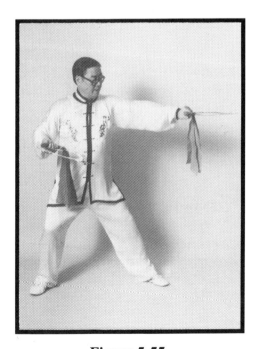

Figure 5-55

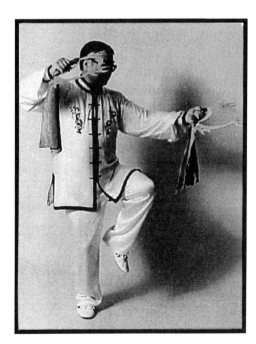

Figure 5-56

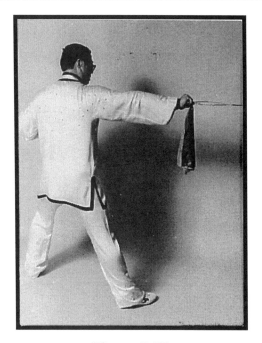

Figure 5-57

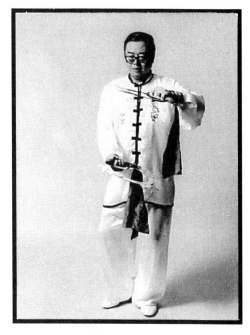

Figure 5-58

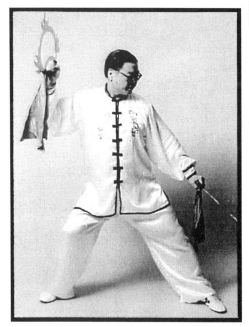

Figure 5-59

16. Diagonal Flying

Movements:

Fig. 5-58: Bring back your right foot next to your left foot. Slowly turn the wheels over in a circular motion bringing the left wheel to the top about shoulder height and the right wheel to the bottom about waist height.

Fig. 5-59: Shift the weight to the left and step out right foot to the right side in a sideways Bow Stance while bringing the right wheel, palm up, in an arc type movement until the right wheel is extended to the right of the body, to about slightly above the head and bringing the left wheel, palm down, in a downward arc pointing towards the floor.

133

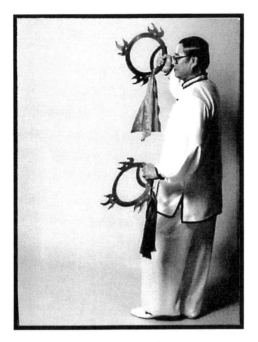

Figure 5-60

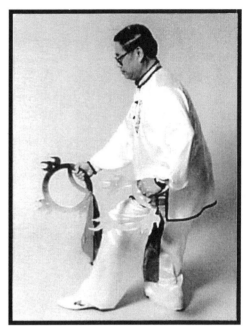

Figure 5-61

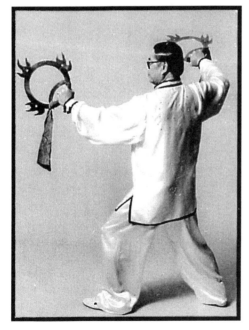

Figure 5-62

17. Needle At Sea Bottom

Movements:

Fig. 5-60: From Fig. 5-59, bring your right foot behind your left and shift all your weight on it, and begin rotating and lowering your left wheel, while lifting your left your left slightly off the floor and circling your right wheel back and up until reaching shoulder height.

Fig. 5-61: Pull your left wheel next to your waist, touch down on your left foot and strike down with your right wheel (Face East)

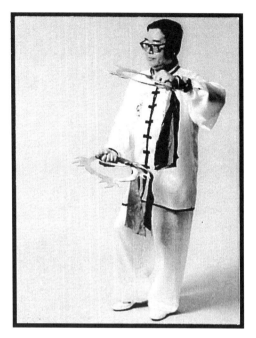

Figure 5-63

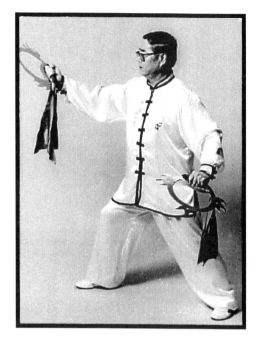

Figure 5-64

18. Fan Through Back

Movements:

Fig. 5-62: From Fig. 5-61, step and slide forward with your left foot into Bow Stance, while raising your right wheel up for blocking and extending your left wheel forward for striking.

19. Right Turn Right Part Wild Horse's Mane

Movements:

Fig. 5-63: Bend down both knees slightly, then shift your weight to your left foot while turning your body to the right. During the twisting moment, rotate both wheels to face each other. Eyes looking in the same direction as your left hand. (Mirror Image)

Fig. 5-64: Step out your right foot into a right Bow Stance, while slicing your left wheel down next to your hip and extending your right wheel forward to the eye level. (Mirror Image)

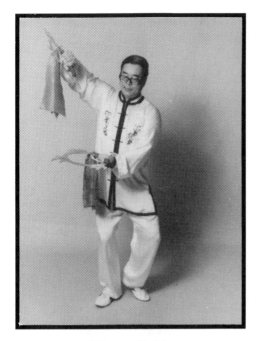

Figure 5-65

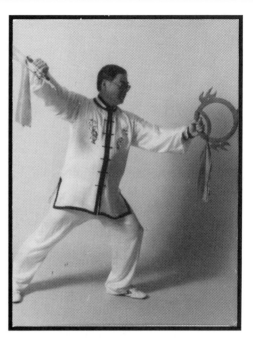

Figure 5-66

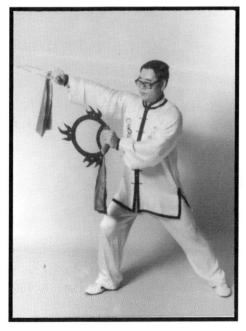

Figure 5-67

20. Left Single Whip

Movements:

Figs. 5-65 and 5-66: Refer to Left Single Whip Posture **5** Figs. 5-16 and 5-17.

21. Wave Hands Like Clouds (3 times)

Movements:

Fig. 5-67: Shift the weight to your right foot while bringing your left wheel to your right and focusing your eyes on your left wheel.

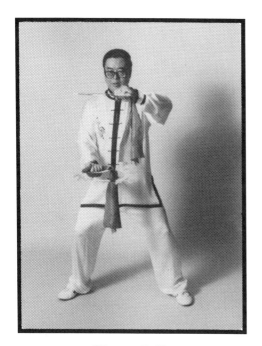

Figure 5-68

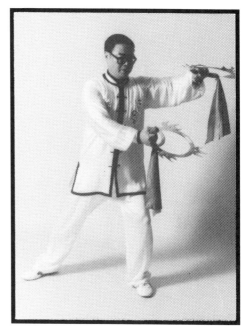

Figure 5-69

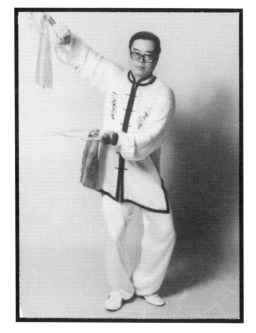

Figure 5-70

Fig. 5-68: Rotate your waist to south and shift your weight onto both legs evenly while lowering your right wheel waist high and raising the left wheel chin high. Both wheels face each other with a slicing motion and the eyes are focused on the left wheel.

Fig. 5-69: Slowly shift your weight to your left foot while continuing slicing both wheels to your left.

22. Left Single Whip

Movements:

Fig. 5-70: Bring the left foot next to your right foot while raising your right

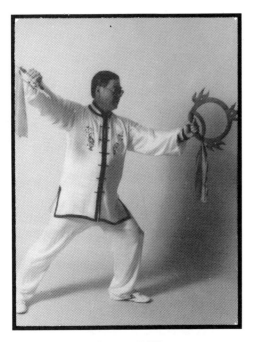

Figure 5-71

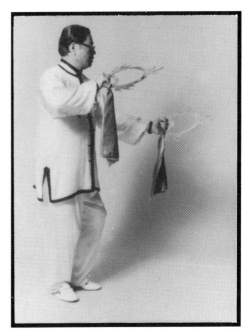

Figure 5-72

wheel to forehead height and lowering your left wheel chest high.

Fig. 5-71: Repeat the motion as described in Fig. 5-17.

23. High Pat On Horse

Movements:

Fig. 5-72: Rotate your waist to the east and step up your right foot next to your left. Deflect with your left wheel face up and bring your right wheel shoulder high and face down.

Fig. 5-73: Step up left foot to Cat Stance while pressing forward to strike with your right wheel. Eyes focus on the right wheel as it passes next to the left upturned wheel.

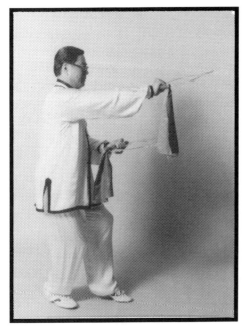

Figure 5-73

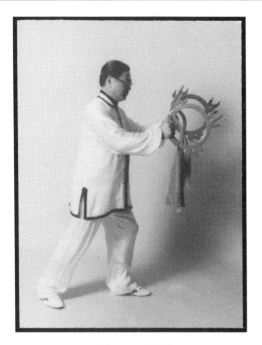

Figure 5-74

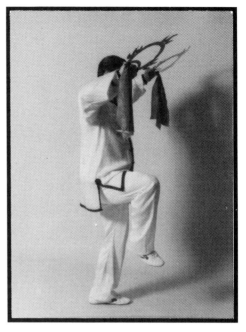

Figure 5-75

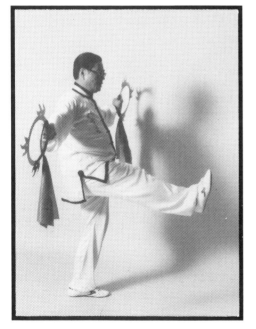

Figure 5-76

24. Right Heel Kick And Strike To Ears

Movements:

Fig. 5-74: Shift your weight to your left foot into Bow Stance while striking with both wheels vertically forward.

Fig. 5-75: Bring your right foot forward to your left, knee high, while rotating both wheels with wheels facing outward at forehead level.

Fig. 5-76: Execute a right Heel Kick to the front while chopping your wheels to both sides of your body. The left knee should bend slightly while doing

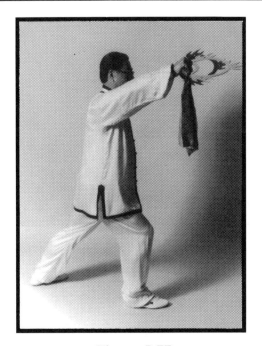

Figure 5-77

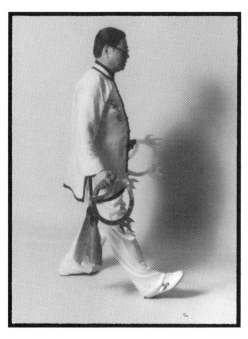

Figure 5-78

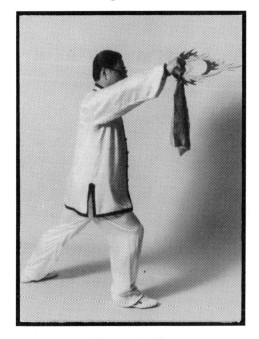

Figure 5-79

this. Eyes looking straight ahead.

Fig. 5-77: Step up with right foot into a Bow Stance, while swinging your wheels upward to face level. Eyes looking between your outstretched wheels.

Fig. 5-78: Shift your weight back onto your left leg and lift the ball of your right foot up, while slicing down your wheels vertically to both sides of your thigh.

Fig. 5-79: Shift your weight onto your right leg into a Bow Stance and swing your whcels upward to ear level.

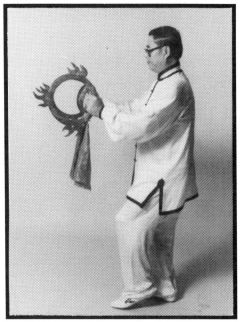

Figure 5-80

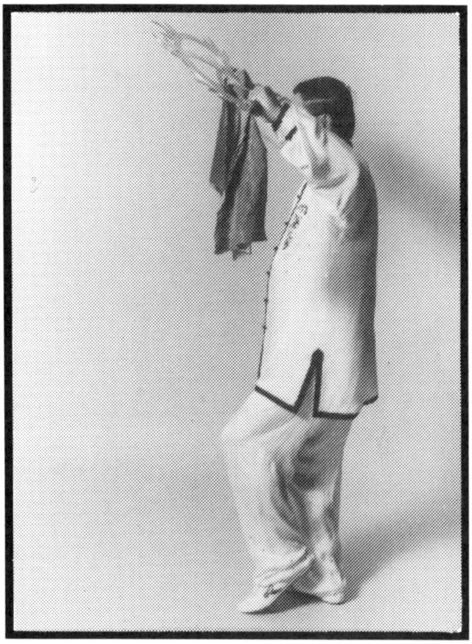

Figure 5-81

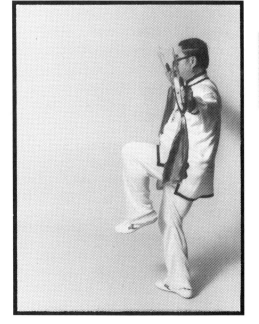

Figure 5-82

25. Left Turn Body Left Heel Kick And Strike To Ears

Movements:

Fig. 5-80: Turn your right foot in and left foot out as you make a 180 degree left turn to face west, while circling both wheels down vertically until they are chest high and chest width apart. Shift your weight on your right foot and bring your left foot next to your right.

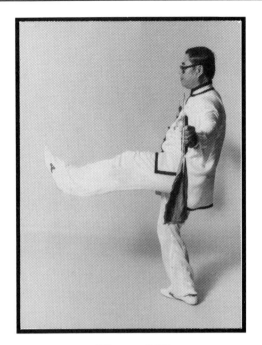

Figure 5-83

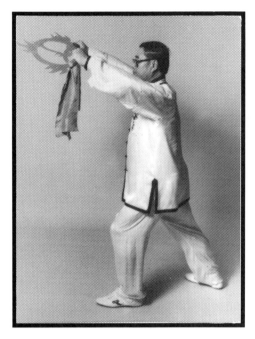

Figure 5-84

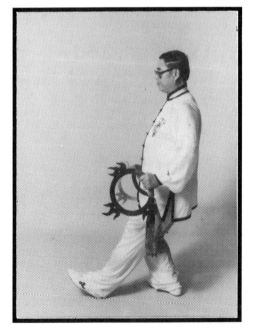

Figure 5-85

Fig. 5-81: Keep same stance and rotate both wheels with wheels facing outward to the forehead level.

Fig. 5-82: Bring your left foot forward to your right knee high.

Fig. 5-83: Execute a left Heel Kick to the front while chopping your wheels to both sides of your body. The right knee should bend slightly while doing this. Eyes looking straight ahead.

Fig. 5-84: Step up with the left foot into a Bow Stance while swinging your wheels upward to face level. Eyes looking between your outstretched wheels.

Fig. 5-85: Shift your weight back on your right leg and lift the ball of your

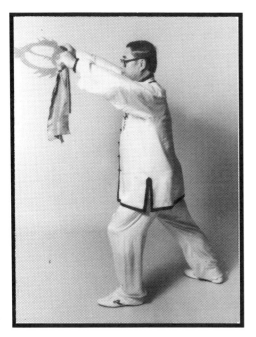

Figure 5-86

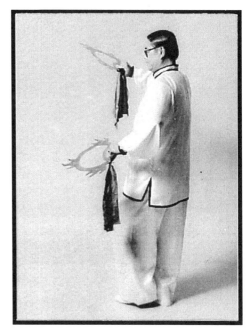

Figure 5-87

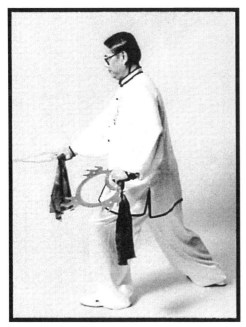

Figure 5-88

left foot up while slicing down your wheels vertically to both sides of your thigh.

Fig. 5-86: Shift your weight onto your right leg to a Bow Stance and swing your wheels upward to ear level.

26. Brush Knee And Punch Down

Movements:

Fig. 5-87: Shift the weight of your body to the right foot and bring the left foot next to your right while lowering your left wheel and raising your right wheel to shoulder height.

143

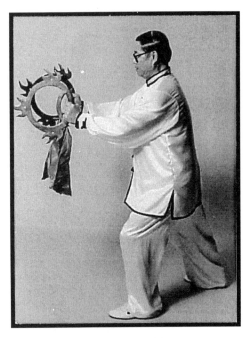
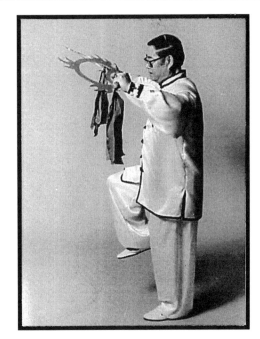

| Figure 5-89 | Figure 5-90 |

Fig. 5-88: Slice down your left wheel to your left side waist while striking your right wheel forward horizontally to the knee level.

27. Right Heel Kick And Stike To Ears

Movements:

Figs. 5-89 to 5-94: Same as posture **24** but in opposite direction. Refer to Figs. 5-74 to 5-79 in this Form.

28. Left Strike The Tiger

Movements:

Fig. 5-95: Step back right foot and stand in left Bow Stance while raising the wheels, parallel to each other, palms facing towards the center, right wheel head height, left wheel shoulder height.

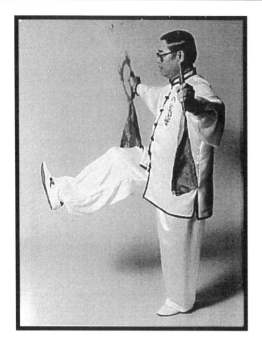

Figure 5-91

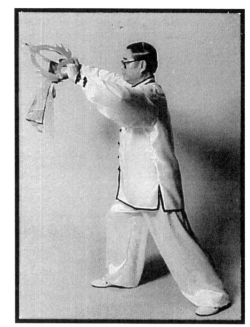

Figure 5-92

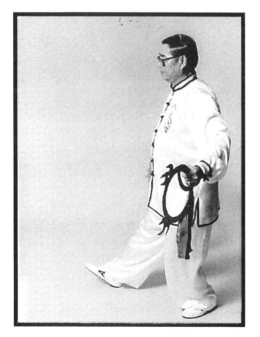

Figure 5-93

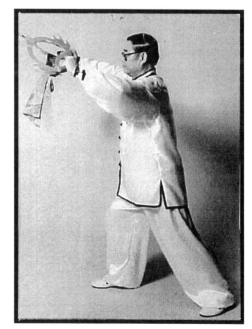

Figure 5-94

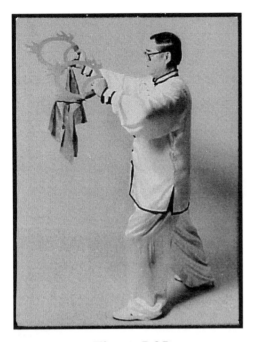

Figure 5-95

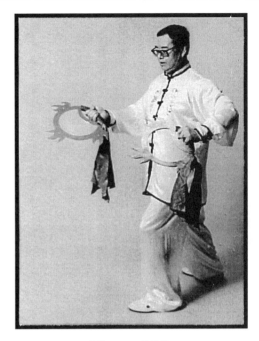

Figure 5-96

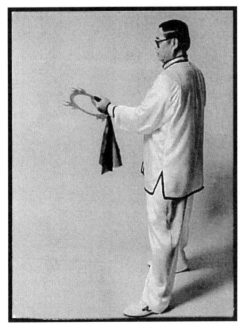

Figure 5-97

Fig. 5-96: Same stance as in Fig. 5-95. Turning with the waist, swing the wheels in a downward arc to the left.

Fig. 5-97: Shift the weight to the right foot into sideways Bow Stance while turning with the waist and swinging the wheels in a downward arc montion to the right.

Fig. 5-98: Turn with the waist to the left into Bow Stance while bringing the left wheel in an upward arc to the height of the head, palm down, and bringing the right wheel in a horizontal arc to the center of the body, palm down.

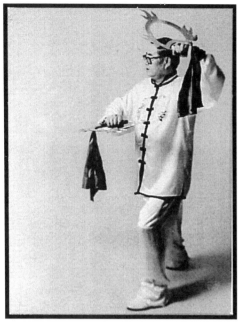

Figure 5-98

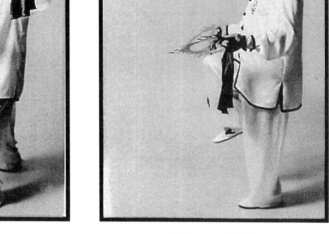
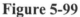

Figure 5-99

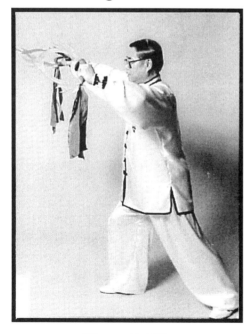

Figure 5-100

29. Strike To Ears with Both Fists

Movements:

Fig. 5-99: Shift the weight to the left foot and lift right to waist height while bringing both wheels downward to waist height both hand palms up.

Fig. 5-100: Step up with your right foot forward in a right Bow Stance while bringing both wheels in an outward arc motion to the head height.

147

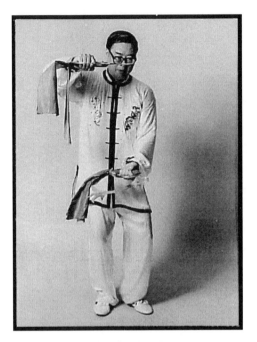

Figure 5-101

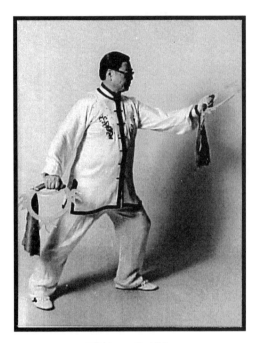

Figure 5-102

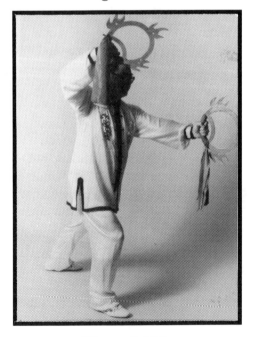

Figure 5-103

30. Right Turn Left Part Wild Horse's Mane

Movements:

Fig. 5-101: Shift your weight to your left foot while turning your body to the left. Shift your weight back to your right foot while bringing your left foot next to your right. (Mirror Image)

Fig. 5-102: Step to the left with your left hell touching down first and shift your weight forward into a left Bow Stance, while extending your left wheel forward to eye level and slicing down with your right wheel next to your hip. (Face East). (Mirror Image)

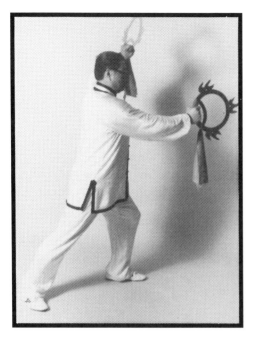

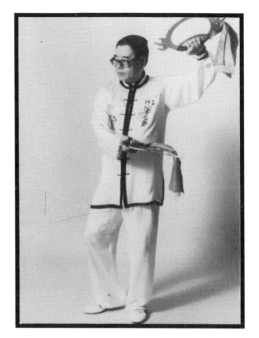

Figure 5-104   **Figure 5-105**

31. Right Turn Body Fair Lady Shuttles Back And Forth (right 1 time, left 1 time)

Movements:

Fig. 5-103: From Fig. 5-102, turn your left foot in and right foot out as you turn 180 degrees to your right. Shift your weight to your left foot and bring your right foot next to your left. Rotate and bring your right wheel to waist height, palm facing up, and lower your left wheel to shoulder height, palm facing down. (Face South East). Step to your front right corner with your right foot while raising your right wheel up for blocking and extending your left wheel forward for striking.

Fig. 5-104: From Fig. 5-103, shift your weight back to your left foot and turn your right foot out slightly. Then shift all your weight to your right foot and bring your left foot next to your right. Bring your left wheel down to waist height, palm facing up, and lower your right wheel to shoulder height, palm facing down (face North East). Step to your front left corner with your left foot while raising

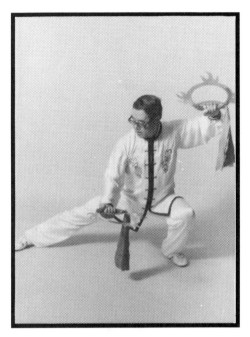

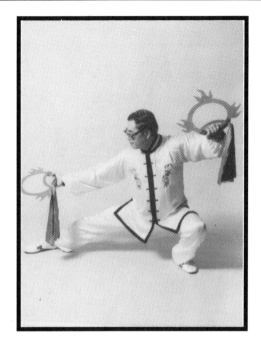

Figure 5-106   **Figure 5-107**

your left wheel up for blocking and extending your right wheel forward for striking.

32. Right Lower Body And Stand On One Leg

Movements:

Fig. 5-105: Put your right foot down in front of you. Slice inward with your left wheel, then lift and extend it to head height while rotating your right wheel to waist height (face South).

Fig. 5-106: Step out with your right foot facing West and bend down your left knee.

Fig. 5-107: Continue lowering your body over your left leg and extend your right wheel along the inside edge of your right leg out to your foot (wheel strike West).

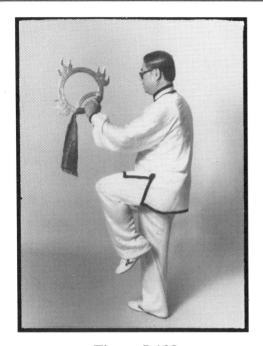

Figure 5-108

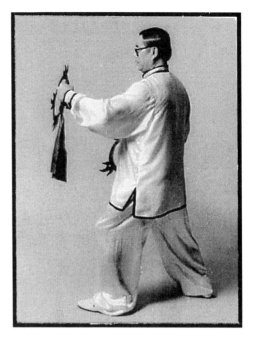

Figure 5-109

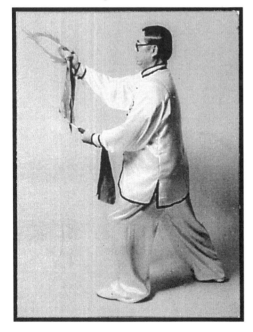

Figure 5-110

Fig. 5-108: Turn your right foot until it points forward. Shift your weight forward into right Bow Stance while lifting your right wheel up and lowering your left leg wheel behind you. Turn your right foot out and stand on it while lifting your leg up. Slice your left wheel down and bring your right wheel up.

33. White Snake Spits The Poison

Movements:

Fig. 5-109: From Fig. 5-108, step up with your left foot forward into left Bow Stance while bringing down your left wheel to mid chest height, parallel to your body.

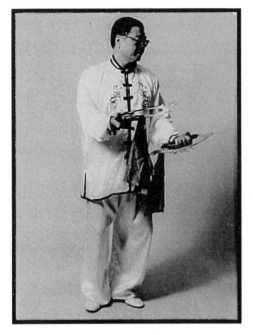

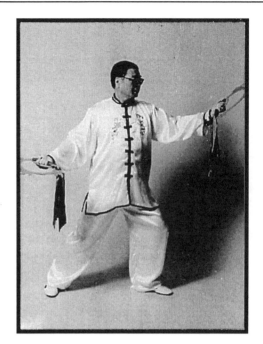

Figure 5-111   Figure 5-112

Fig. 5-110: Same Bow Stance as in Fig. 5-111. Turn the left wheel, palm up, to a 45 degree angle to the floor while raising the right wheel, palm up, in an upward thrusting motion across to top of the left wheel.

34. Wind-Fire High And Low Diagonal Cuts

Movements:

Fig. 5-111: From Fig. 5-110. Shift the weight to the right foot and draw back left foot next to the right foot while bringing both wheels down to about waist height, palms up.

Fig. 5-112: Step forward left foot into left Bow Stance while bringing left wheel high diagonal cut to the throat and right wheel low diagonal cut to the abdomen.

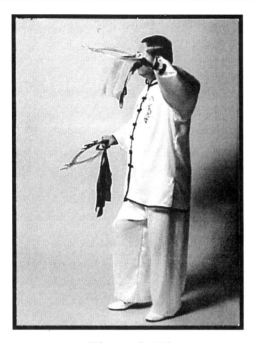

Figure 5-113

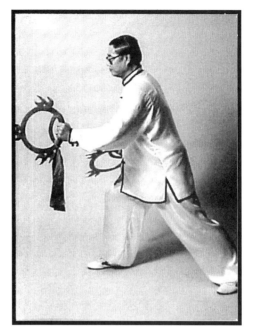

Figure 5-114

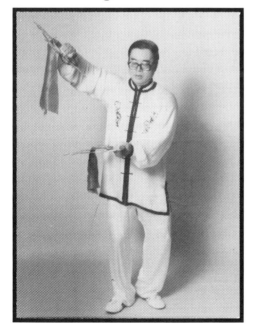

Figure 5-115

35. Right Step Forward And Left Strike Down

Movements:

Fig. 5-113: Shift the weight to your left foot and bring right foot next to your left foot while lowering your right wheel and raising your left wheel to shoulder height.

Fig. 5-114: Slice down your right wheel to your right side waist while striking your left wheel forward vertically to the knee level.

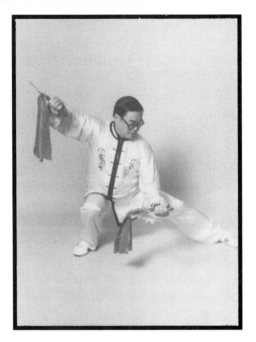

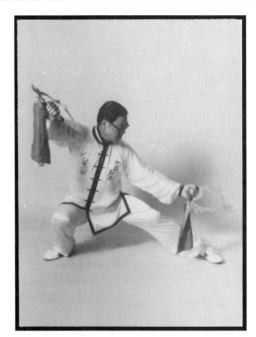

Figure 5-116   **Figure 5-117**

36. Left Lower Body And Stand On One Leg

Movements:

Fig. 5-115: Shift your weight onto your right foot and bring left foot next to right (face North), while rotating right wheel to head height and slicing your left wheel to waist height (mirror image).

Fig. 5-116: Step out with your left foot to the west and bend your right foot, while slicing left wheel down and forward. Eyes looking at your left wheel.

Fig. 5-117: Continue lowering your body weight over your right leg and extend your left wheel along the inside edge of your left leg out to your foot (wheel strike West).

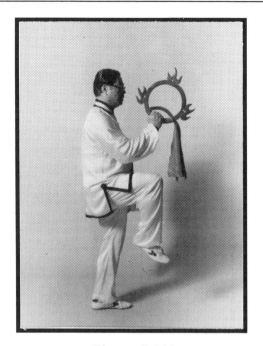

Figure 5-118

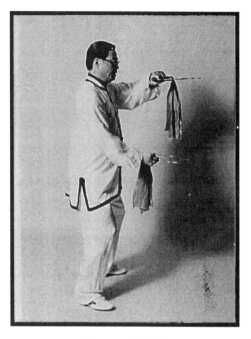

Figure 5-119

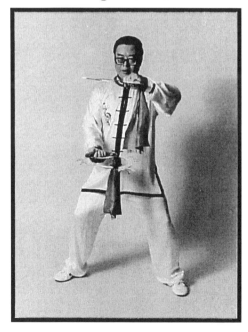

Figure 5-120

Fig. 5-118: Turn your left foot until it points forward. Shift your weight forward into left Bow Stance while lifting your left wheel up and lowering your right wheel behind you. Turn your left foot out and stand on it when lifting your right leg up. Slice your left wheel down and bring your right wheel up.

37. Wind-Fire Turning Wheels (3 times)

Movements:

Figs. 5-119 to 5-122: Same as posture **7**. Refer to Figs. 5-24 to 5-27 in this Form.

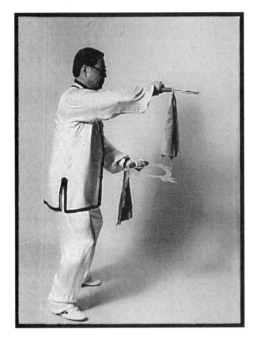

Figure 5-121

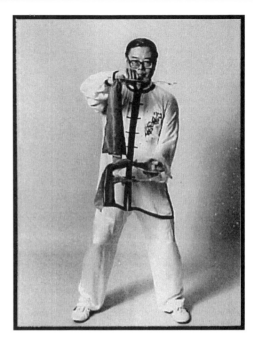

Figure 5-122

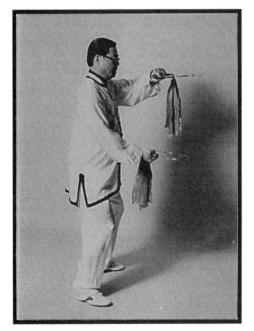

Figure 5-123

38. Step Back And Ride The Tiger

Movements:

Fig. 5-123: Revolve two wheels with the right wheel down and the left wheel up.

Fig. 5-124: Step back the right foot into Cat Stance while bringing the right wheel in an upward arc motion to above the head and bringing the left wheel a downward arc motion to the left side waist of the body.

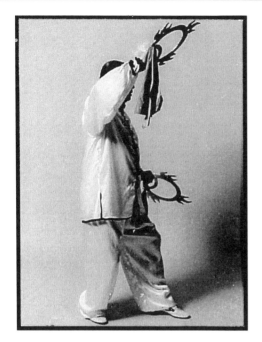

Figure 5-124

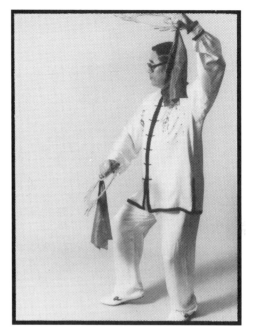

Figure 5-125

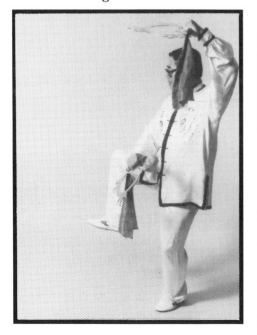

Figure 5-126

39. Right Turn Body Wind-Fire Protecting The Head And Right Heel Kick

Movements:

Fig. 5-125: Shift your weight to your right and make a 180 degree right turn of your body. Shift your weight back to your left foot and bring your right foot to Cat Sance, while raising your left wheel up with blades toward front to protect your head and slicing your right wheel from outward down to your groin area.

Fig. 5-126: Lift your right foot to knee height.

157

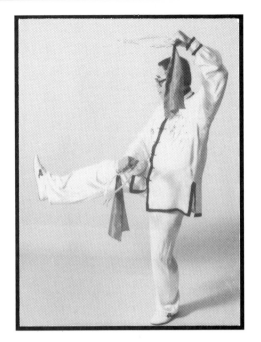

Figure 5-127

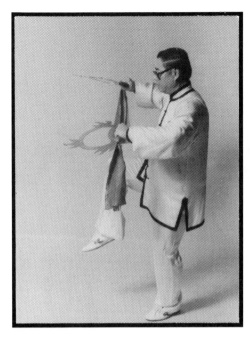

Figure 5-128

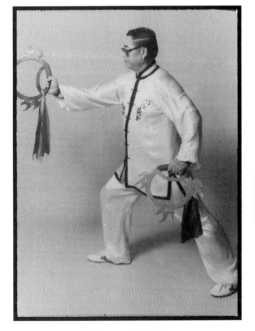

Figure 5-129

Fig. 5-127: Make right heel kick to the front.

40. Left Slicing And Right Striking

Movements:

Figs. 5-128 and 5-129: Same as posture **11**. Refer to Figs. 5-39 and 5-40 in this Form.

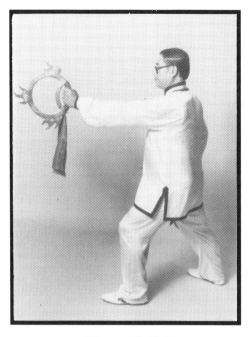

Figure 5-130

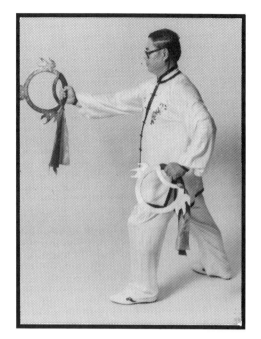

Figure 5-131

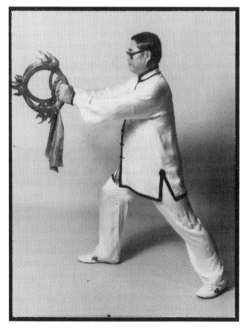

Figure 5-132

41. Step Forward Left And Right Strikings

Movements:

Fig. 5-130: Step left foot forward and make left wheel striking vertically.

Fig. 5-131: Keep same stance and make right wheel striking forward vertically,

42. Appears Closed

Movements:

Fig. 5-132: From Fig. 5-131, step up your right leg and complete Bow Stance while striking left wheel forward vertically.

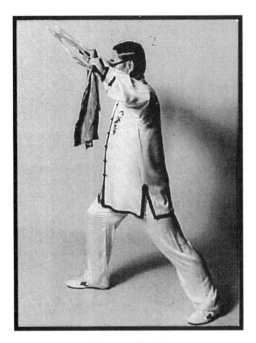

Figure 5-133

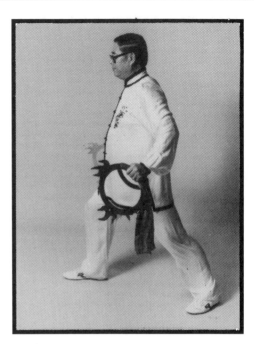

Figure 5-134

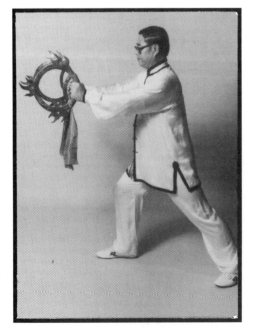

Figure 5-135

Fig. 5-133: Keep the same stance and bring both Wind-Fire Wheels forehead high separately. Eyes Looking staight ahead.

Fig. 5-134: Rotate both wheels down to your waist while keeping the right Bow Stance.

Fig. 5-135: Strike forward with both Wind-Fire Wheels and complete the posture as shown in the picture. Eyes looking ahead, in eye level direction.

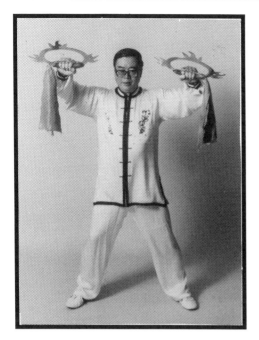

Figure 5-136

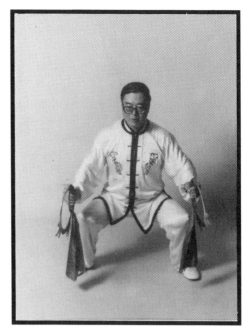

Figure 5-137

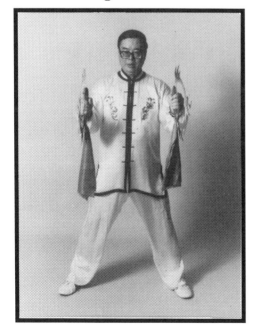

Figure 5-138

43. Wind-Fire Closing

Movements:

Fig. 5-136: From Fig. 5-135, shift your weight to your left foot, lift the ball of your right foot up and begin turning your body 90 degrees to your left while raising both Wind-Fire Wheels outward to forehead height.

Fig. 5-137: Shift your body weight evenly to both feet and begin lowering your body, while bringing down your wheels in a circular motion to knee height.

Fig. 5-138: Stand up gradually, but keep your knees bent slightly while bringing both wheels chest high and shoulder width apart. Then rotate the Wind Fire Wheels outward, down and up three times.

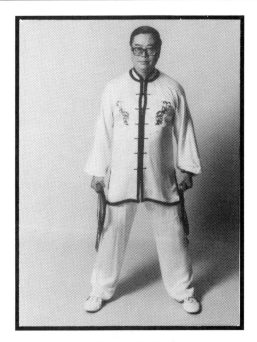

Figure 5-139

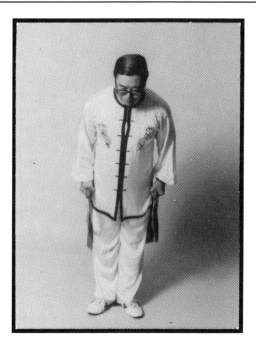

Figure 5-140

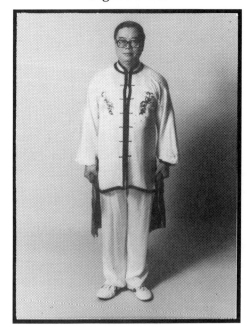

Figure 5-141

44. Return to Origin

Movements:

Fig. 5-139: Bring down both wheels to the sides of your body. Eyes are looking directly ahead.

Fig. 5-140: Bring your left foot next to your right. Bow to your teachers or spectators politely.

Fig. 5-141: Return to your original Preparatory Posture.

CHAPTER 6

ADVANCED FORM II

6.1 Introduction

You now have personal experience with one of the advanced forms for Tai-Chi Wind-Fire Wheels. You have personal experience with the power the wheels impart to the barehanded movements you know so well. Your body feels stronger and more balanced from successfully wielding weights of more than two pounds in each hand. Finally, you have seen how the wheel gives you a new perspective on the role mental intent in Tai-Chi. In short, serious practice with the wheel has built a sound base of strength and awareness of Chi. Now it is time to advance from that base with a longer and more demanding form.

This chapter describes and illustrates a second advanced form for using the wheels in Tai- Chi. As a more advanced form, it is longer than the first and that means it requires greater endurance and physical strength. Therefore, you should tackle this form only after intensively practicing and mastering the first

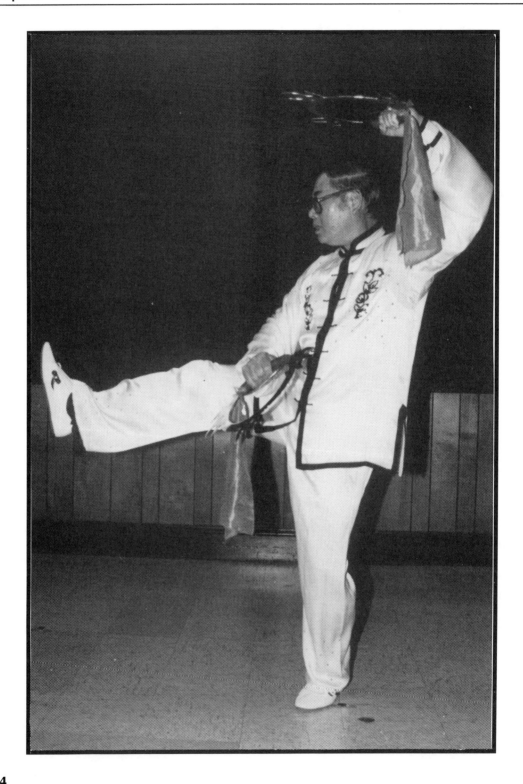

form. Seriously taking these forms in order will produce the internal and physical strength you need for progress to the most advanced form presented in the next chapter.

As before, this second form is built around the principles and techniques of Yang's Tai-Chi. As a more advanced form, it teaches the practitioner the use of the Wind-Fire Wheels in such Tai-Chi movements as A growth in Tai-Chi is also assured in the graceful extension of basics in moves such as Reverse Reeling Forearm, Ride The Tiger, and White Snake Spits The Poison.

The preamble is now complete and you are ready to examine the pictures that describe this second form and to digest the text that describes the purposes, essentials, and fine points of each movement and its place in a total form that will advance your Tai-Chi to new levels of reward and enjoyment.

6.2 Advanced Form II

1. **Preparatory Posture**
2. **Wind-Fire Commencing**
3. **Left Step Forward Part Wild Horse's Mane**
4. **Turn Right Ward Off, Roll Back, Press and Push**
5. **Left Single Whip**
6. **Right Lifting Hand**
7. **Wind-Fire Turning Wheels**
8. **White Crane Spreads Its Wings And Left Heel Kick**
9. **Left, Right, Left Brush Knee And Step Forward**
10. **Playing The Lute**
11. **Left Slicing And Right Striking**
12. **Diagonal Flying**
13. **Fist Under The Elbow**
14. **Reverse Reeling Forearm (4 times)**
15. **Right Turn Body Fair Lady Shuttles Back and Forth** (left 1 time, right 1 time)

16. Left Part Wild Horse's Mane
17. Right Part Wild Horse's Mane
18. Left Single Whip
19. Wave Hands Like Clouds (3 times)
20. Left Single Whip
21. High Pat On Horse
22. Right Heel Kick And Strike To Ears
23. Left Turn Body Left Heel Kick And Strike To Ears
24. Needle At Sea Bottom
25. Fan Through Back
26. White Snake Spits The Poison
27. Wind-Fire High And Low Diagonal Cuts
28. Left Part Wild Horse's Mane
29. Right Heel Kick And Strike To Ears
30. Left Strike The Tiger
31. Right Strike The Tiger
32. Left Part Wild Horse's Mane
33. Right Lower Body And Stand On One Leg
34. Left Step Forward And Right Strike Down
35. Step Forward Ward Off, Roll Back, Press And Push
36. Left Lower Body And Stand On One Leg
37. Wind-Fire Turning Wheels (3 times)
38. Step Back And Ride The Tiger
39. Right Turn Body Wind-Fire Protecting The Head And Right Heel Kick
40. Left Slicing And Right Striking
41. Step Forward Left And Right Strikings
42. Appears Closed
43. Wind-Fire Closing
44. Return To Origin

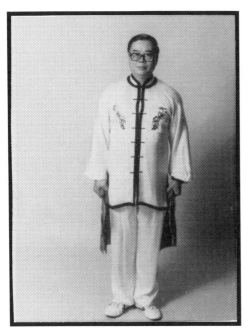

Figure 6-1

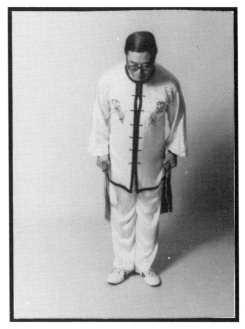

Figure 6-2

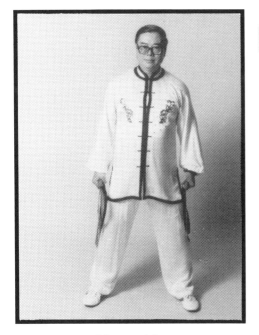

Figure 6-3

1. Preparatory Posture

Movements:

Begin by facing South.

Fig. 6-1: Natural Standing with feet sixty degree outward, back straight, arms relaxed with Wind-Fire Wheels by your side (Facing South, inhale and exhale several times).

Fig. 6-2: Bow to your teachers or spectators politely.

Fig. 6-3: Bend your knees slightly, then step to your left with your left leg.

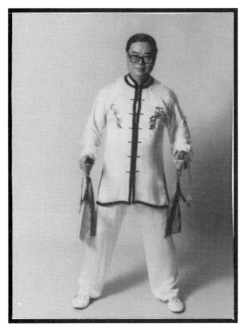

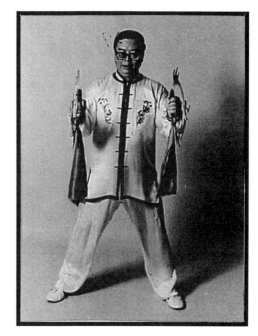

Figure 6-4   Figure 6-5

2. Wind-Fire Commencing

Movements:

Fig. 6-4: Raise your Wind-Fire Wheels in front of you to shoulder height, keeping them parallel to each other.

Fig. 6-5: Rotate the Wind-Fire Wheels outward, down and up three times.

3. Left Step Forward Part Wild Horse's Mane

Movements:

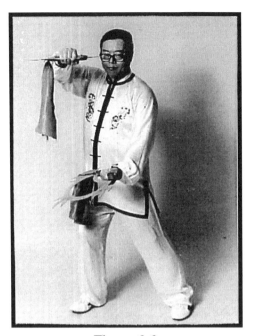

Figure 6-6

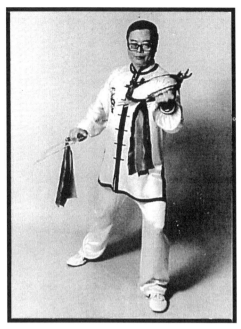

Figure 6-7

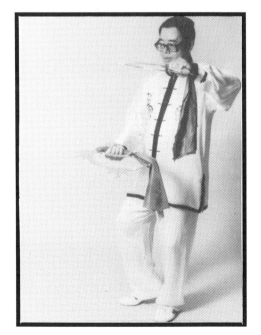

Figure 6-8

Fig. 6-6: Shift your weight to your right foot and bring your left foot next to the right, while turning your body slightly to the right. During the twisting movement, rotate both wheels to face each other. Eyes are looking in the same direction as your right hand.

Fig. 6-7: Step out your left foot into a left Bow Stance, (face South), while slicing your right wheel down next to your hip and extending your left wheel forward to the eye level.

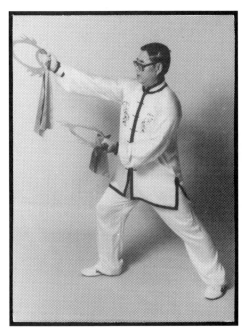

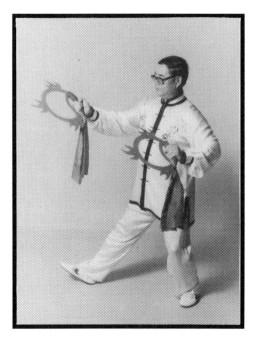

Figure 6-9   Figure 6-10

4.   Turn Right Ward Off, Roll Back, Press And Push

Movements:

Fig. 6-8: Turn right and bring both Wind-Fire Wheels to your left facing each other with the right hand downward and the left hand upward. Shift your weight to your left foot and bring the right foot next to the left.

Fig. 6-9: Step forward with your right foot while extending your right wheel forward and upward and draw your left wheel downward and out. Eyes should be focused on your right wheel.

Fig. 6-10: Shift your weight back onto your left leg and roll back right heel while twisting your waist to the left and pulling down with your Wind-Fire Wheels. Keep your eyes focused on the right hand and then focus in the direction of the torso at eye level.

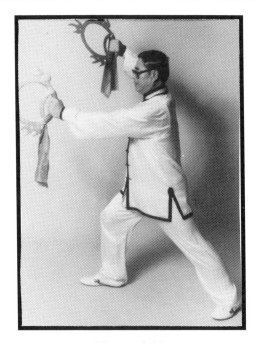

Figure 6-11

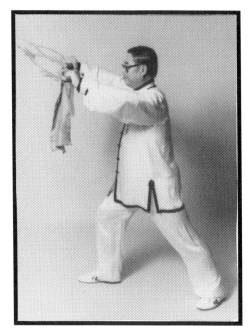

Figure 6-12

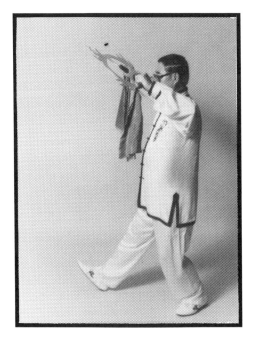

Figure 6-13

Fig. 6-11: Shift your weight forward into a right Bow Stance while right wheel makes an upward blocking and left wheel a forward striking. Eyes focus on the left hand wheel.

Fig. 6-12: Keep the same Bow Stance as shown in Fig. 6-11. Bring the left wheel up to the right wheel level.

Fig. 6-13: Shift your weight back onto your left foot and bring both Wind-Fire Wheels to forehead level (45 degrees above horizontal level). Eyes look straight ahead.

Fig. 6-14: Rotate both wheels down to your waist while shifting your weight onto the right leg. Eyes keep looking ahead.

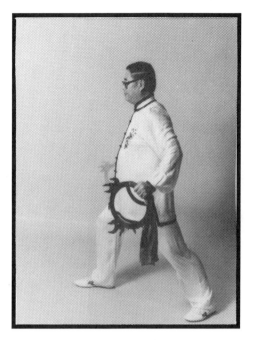

Figure 6-14

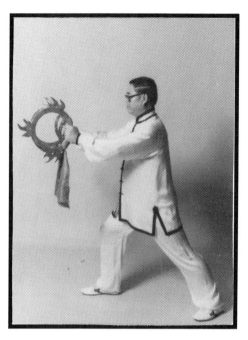

Figure 6-15

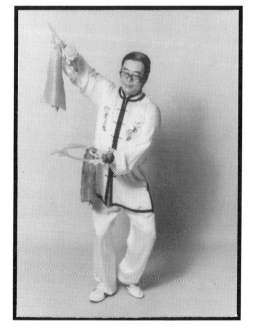

Figure 6-16

Fig. 6-15: Continue shifting your weight onto the right leg and complete Bow Stance. Push forward with both Wind-Fire Wheels and complete the push posture. Eyes focus in the eye level direction.

5. Left Single Whip

Movements:

Fig. 6-16: Draw the left foot to the right foot and make a "C" Slice with your right hand wheel while the left hand wheel rotates from upward to downward and is placed under the right hand wheel. Eyes look to the right hand wheel them move to the left hand wheel.

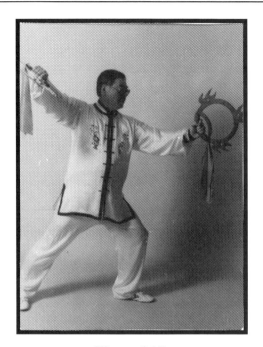

Figure 6-17

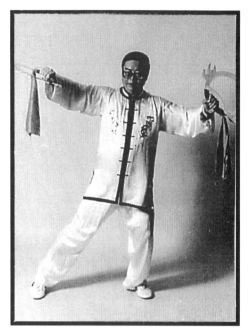

Figure 6-18

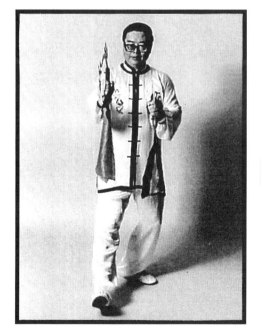

Figure 6-19

Fig. 6-17: Extend your left leg forward and touch down with the heel. Shift your weight to your left foot and complete Bow Stance. Rotate and extend your left wheel forward.

6. Right Lifting Hand

Movements:

Fig. 6-18: Turn your body to your right while rotating at your waist to face South. Both hands are holding Wind-Fire Wheels vertically.

Fig. 6-19: Shift your weight onto your left foot and draw your right foot to touch down with your heel, while

your left foot. Step out to the front and

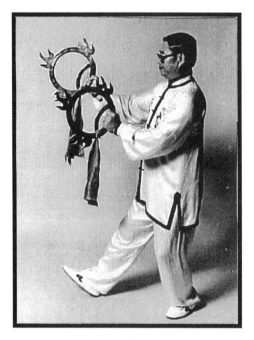

Figure 6-20

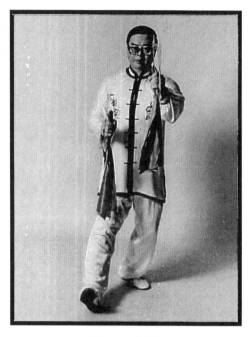

Figure 6-21

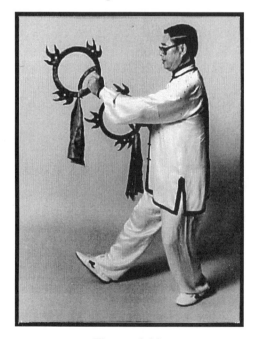

Figure 6-22

drawing the wheels to the center of your chest with your right hand higher than your left hand.

Fig. 6-20: Side view of figure 6-19.

Fig. 6-21: Same stance as Fig. 6-19. Rotate both Wind-Fire Wheels outward once vertically.

Fig. 6-22: Side view of figure 6-21.

Fig. 6-23: After one vertical rotation.

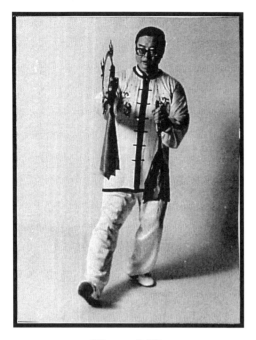

Figure 6-23

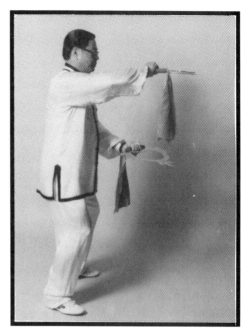

Figure 6-24

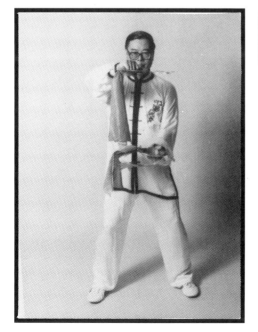

Figure 6-25

7. Wind-Fire Turning Wheels

Movements:

Fig. 6-24: Turn your body to your left while rotating your waist to the left. Both feet are shoulder width apart and slightly bent, while revolving both wheels and slicing your left wheel down and the right wheel up.

Fig. 6-25: Shows front view of Fig. 6-24.

Fig. 6-26: Revolve two wheels once again with the right wheel down and the left wheel up.

175

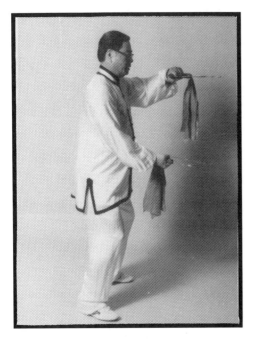

Figure 6-26

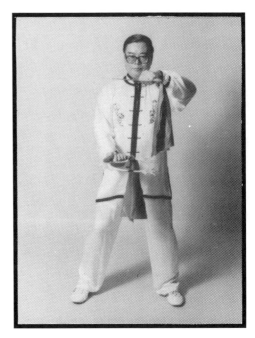

Figure 6-27

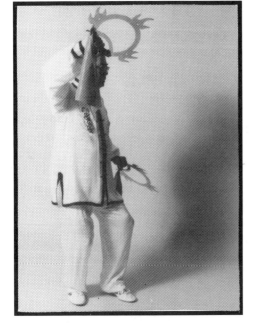

Figure 6-28

Fig. 6-27: Shows front view of Fig. 6-26.

8. White Crane Spreads Its Wings And Left Heel Kick

Movements:

Fig. 6-28: Rotate your waist to the right and step up with your left foot forward as in a Cat Stance. Your weight should be in your right leg now. In the meantime, begin raising your right wheel up and slicing your left wheel down.

Fig. 6-29: Lift your left foot up and balance your body.

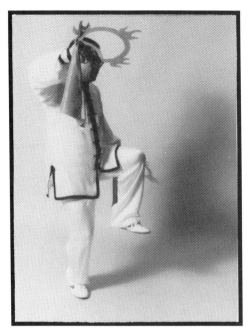
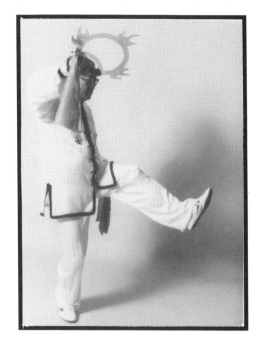

Figure 6-29   Figure 6-30

Fig. 6-30: Execute a Heel Kick to the front.

9. Left, Right, Left Brush Knee And Step Forward

Movements:

Fig. 6-31: Bring back your left kicking leg close to your right leg. Turn your body slightly to your left while raising up and slicing your left wheel to the front and bringing down right wheel with blades outward to face height. Turn your body to your right while lowering and slicing your left wheel and slicing your right wheel outward and down, then bring it to your right ear height vertically, blades pointed to the front.

Step up your left leg to left Bow Stance while striking your right wheel forward horizontally.

Fig. 6-32: Shift your weight to your right foot. Turn your left foot outward and begin turning your body to your left while raising up and slicing your right wheel to the front and bringing down the left wheel with blades outward to face

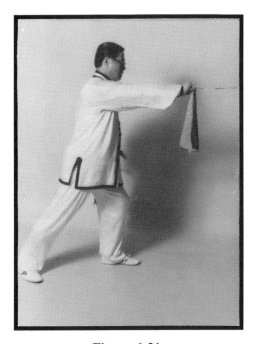

Figure 6-31

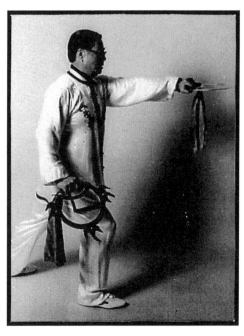

Figure 6-32

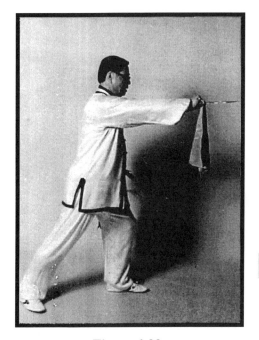

Figure 6-33

height. Turn your body to your left while lowering and slicing your right wheel and slicing your left wheel outward down then bring to left ear height vertically, blades point to the front. Step up your right leg to right Bow Stance while striking up your left wheel forward horizontally.

Fig. 6-33: Repeat the movement described in Figure 6-31.

10. Playing The Lute

Movements:

Fig. 6-34: Shift your weight onto your right foot and bring your right

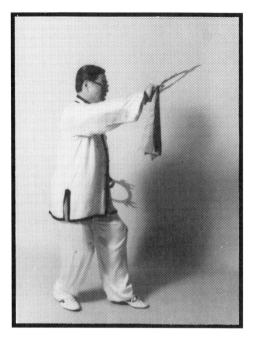

Figure 6-34

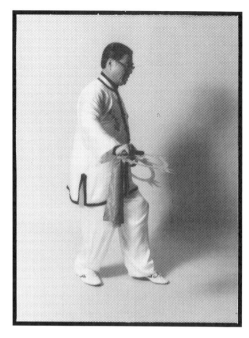

Figure 6-35

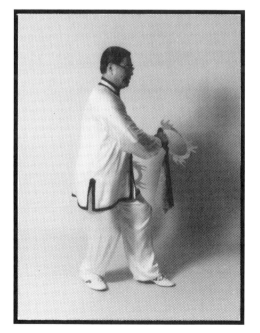

Figure 6-36

wheel to eye level.

Fig. 6-35: Rotate your waist from left to right while lowering your right wheel in a circular motion.

Fig. 6-36: Continue rotating your waist to the left while circling your right wheel up.

Fig. 6-37: Pull your left foot to your right foot and rotate your waist to the right while bringing your right wheel upward and your left wheel downward to face each other.

Fig. 6-38: Step forward with your left foot touching down with your heel while extending your left wheel forward and slicing your right wheel down.

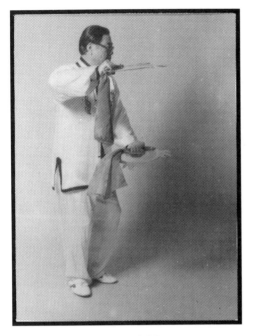

Figure 6-37

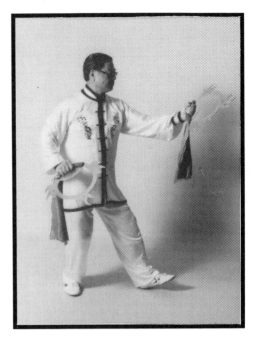

Figure 6-38

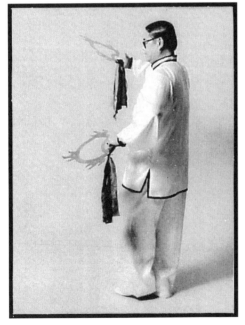

Figure 6-39

11. Left Slicing And Right Striking

Movements:

Fig. 6-39: Bring back your left leg while lowering your left wheel and raising your right wheel to shoulder height.

Fig. 6-40: Slice down your left wheel to your left side waist while striking your right wheel forward vertically.

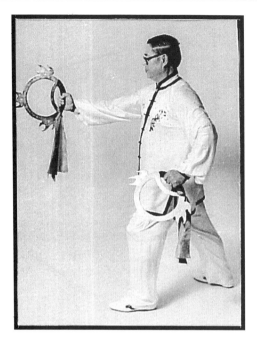

Figure 6-40

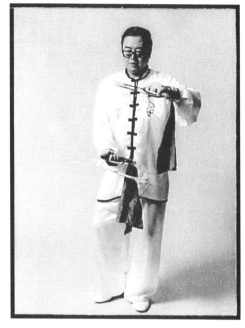

Figure 6-41

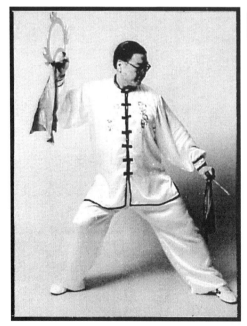

Figure 6-42

12. Diagonal Flying

Movements:

Fig. 6-41: Bring back your right foot next to your left foot. Slowly turn the wheels over in a circular motion bringing the left wheel to the top about shoulder height and the right wheel to the bottom about waist height.

Fig. 6-42: Shift the weight to the left and step out right foot to the right side in a sideways Bow Stance while bringing the right wheel, palm up, in an arc type movement until the right wheel is extended to the right of the body, to about slightly above the head and bringing the left wheel, palm down, in a downward arc pointing towards the floor.

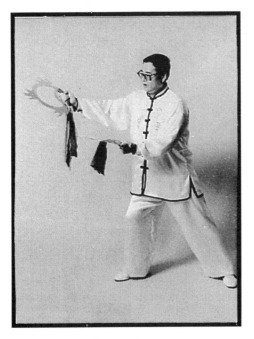

Figure 6-43

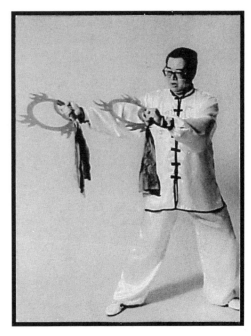

Figure 6-44

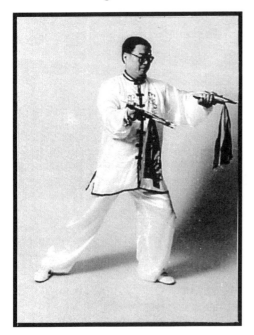

Figure 6-45

13. Fist Under The Elbow

Movements:

Fig. 6-43: Raise the wheels to shoulder height bending the elbows.

Fig. 6-44: Shift your weight on your left foot.

Fig. 6-45: Step into left Bow Stance and rotate your waist to the left while bringing your right wheel upward and your left wheel downward to your left.

Fig. 6-46: Draw your left foot next to your right foot. Swing both wheels in a circular motion downward and bring

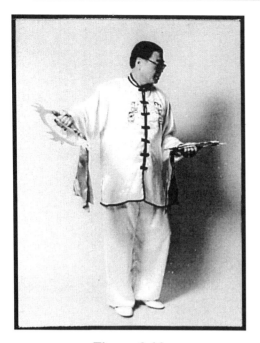

Figure 6-46

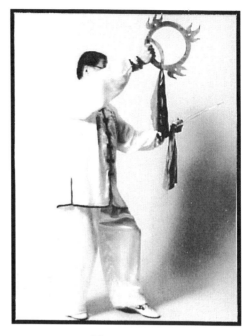

Figure 6-47

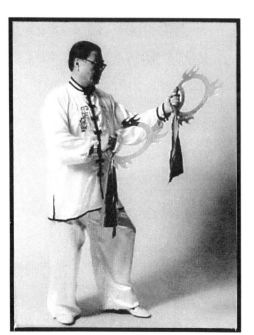

Figure 6-48

your left wheel point out to front at waist height while raising your right wheel to shoulder height.

Fig. 6-47: Step up with your left foot forward as in a Cat Stance. Strike left wheel, the right wheel, palm to center, in a vertical forward cutting motion, to mid abdomen.

Fig. 6-48: Same Cat Stance as in Fig. 6-47. Slice your right wheel down and your left wheel up.

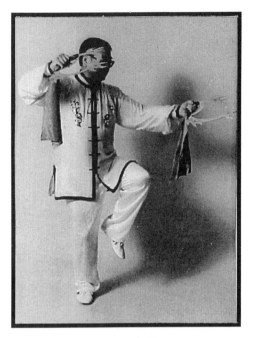

Figure 6-49

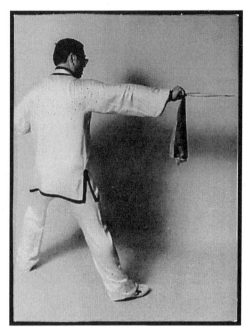

Figure 6-50

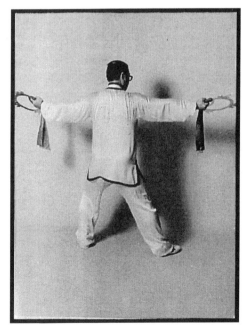

Figure 6-51

14. Reverse Reeling Forearm (4 times)

Movements:

Fig. 6-49: From Fig. 6-48, slightly lower your left wheel and raise your right wheel from behind to ear height while lifting up your left foot.

Fig. 6-50: Step back with your left foot behind your right foot and pivot on your right foot while pulling your left wheel next to your waist and extending your right wheel forward.

Fig. 6-51: Extend your left wheel out and up while rotating both wheels up.

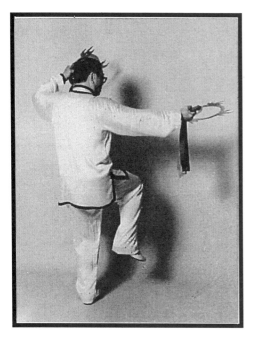
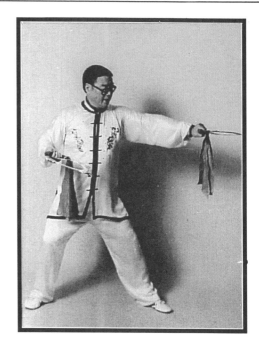

Figure 6-52   **Figure 6-53**

Fig. 6-52: Bend your left elbow and lift up your right foot.

Fig. 6-53: Step back with your right foot behind your left and pivot on your left foot while pulling your right wheel next to your waist and extending your left wheel forward.

15. Right Turn Body Fair Lady Shuttles Back And Forth (left 1 time, right 1 time)

Movements:

Fig. 6-54: From Fig. 6-53, turn your left foot in and right foot out as you turn 180 degrees to your right. Shift your weight back to your left foot and turn your right foot out slightly. Then shift all your weight to your right foot and bring your left foot next to your right. Bring your left wheel down to waist height, palm facing up, and lower your right wheel to shoulder height, palm facing down. (Face South West). Step to your front left corner with your left foot while raising your left wheel up for blocking and extending your right wheel forward for striking.

185

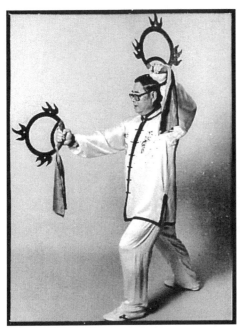

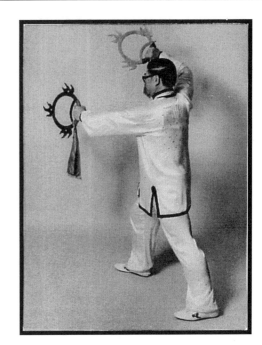

Figure 6-54   **Figure 6-55**

Fig. 6-55: From Fig. 6-54, shift your weight back to your right foot and turn your left foot out slightly. Then shift all your weight to your left foot and bring your right foot next to your left. Bring your right wheel down to waist height, palm facing up, and lower your left wheel to shoulder height, palm facing down (face North East). Step to your front right corner with your right foot while raising your right wheel up for blocking and extending your left wheel forward for striking.

16. Left Part Wild Horse's Mane

Movements:

Fig. 6-56: Shift your weight to your left foot while turning your body to the right. Shift your weight back to your right foot while bringing your left foot next to your right. (Mirror Image)

Fig. 6-57: Step to the left with your left heel touching down first and shift your weight forward into a left Bow Stance, while extending your left wheel forward to eye level and slicing down your right wheel next to your hip. (Face East). (Mirror Image)

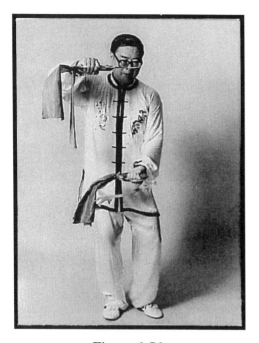

Figure 6-56

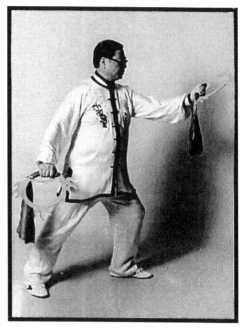

Figure 6-57

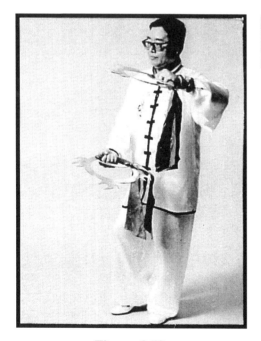

Figure 6-58

17. Right Part Wild Horse's Mane

Movements:

Fig. 6-58: Shift your weight to your right foot while turning your body to the left. Shift your weight back to your left foot while bringing your right foot next to your left.

Fig. 6-59: Step to the right with your right heel touching down first and shift your weight forward into a right Bow Stance, while extending your right wheel forward to eye level and slicing down your left wheel next to your hip. (Face East)

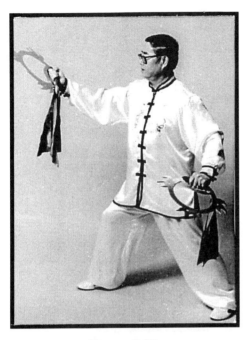

Figure 6-59

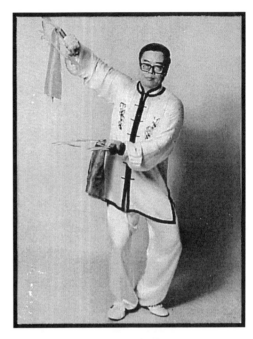

Figure 6-60

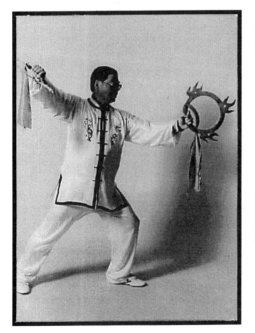

Figure 6-61

18. Left Single Whip

Movements:

Figs. 6-60 and 6-61: Refer to Left Single Whip Posture **5** Figs. 6-17 and 6-18.

19. Wave Hands Like Clouds (3 times)

Movements:

Fig. 6-62: Shift the weight to your right foot while bringing your left wheel to your right and focusing your eyes on your left wheel.

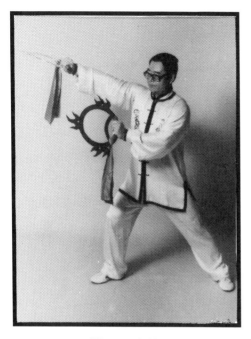

Figure 6-62

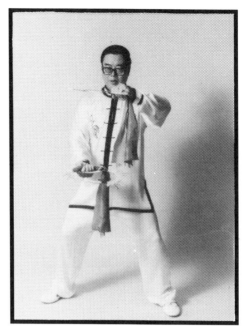

Figure 6-63

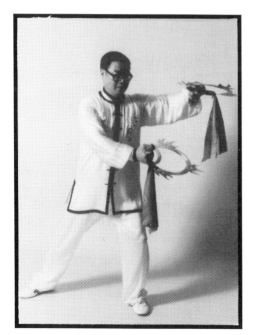

Figure 6-64

Fig. 6-63: Rotate your waist to south and shift your weight onto both legs evenly while lowering your right wheel waist high and raising the left wheel chin high. Both wheels face each other with slicing motion and the eyes are focused on the left wheel.

Fig. 6-64: Slowly shift your weight to your left foot while continuing slicing both wheels to your left.

20. Left Single Whip

Movements:

Fig. 6-65: Bring the left foot next to your right foot while raising your right

189

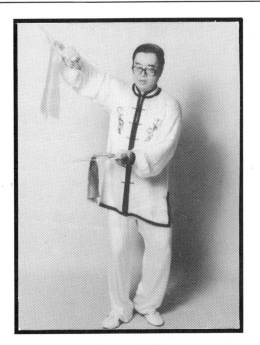

Figure 6-65

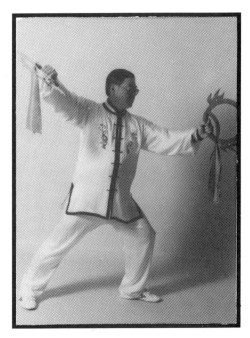

Figure 6-66

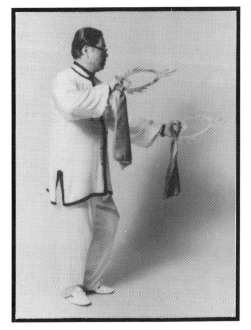

Figure 6-67

wheel to forehead height and lowering your left wheel chest high.

Fig. 6-66: Repeat the motion as described in Fig. 6-18 in the posture **5**.

21. High Pat On Horse

Movements:

Fig. 6-67: Rotate your waist to the east and step up your right foot next to your left. Deflect with your left wheel face up and bring your right wheel shoulder high and face down.

Fig. 6-68: Step up left foot to Cat Stance while pressing forward to strike with your right wheel. Eyes focus on the right wheel as it passes next to the left upturned wheel.

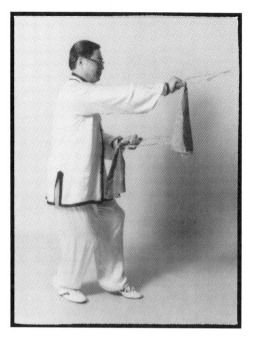

Figure 6-68

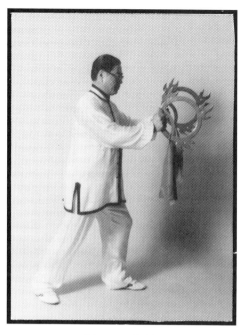

Figure 6-69

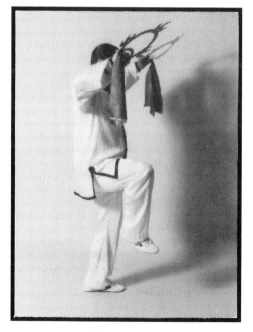

Figure 6-70

22. Right Heel Kick And Strike To Ears

Movements:

Fig. 6-69: Shift your weight to your left foot into Bow Stance while striking with both wheels vertically forward.

Fig. 6-70: Bring your right foot forward to your left, knee high, while rotating both wheels with wheels facing outward at forehead level.

Fig. 6-71: Execute a right Heel Kick to the front while chopping your wheels to both sides of your body. The left knee should bend slightly while doing this. Eyes looking straight ahead.

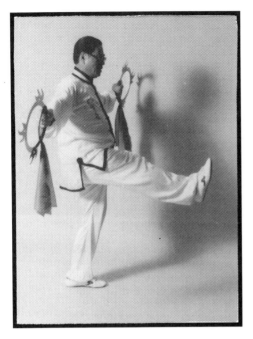

Figure 6-71

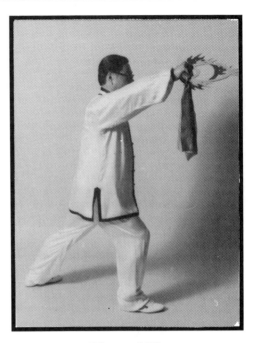

Figure 6-72

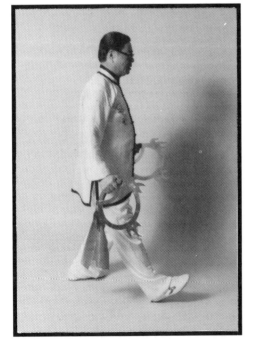

Figure 6-73

Fig. 6-72: Step up with right foot into a Bow Stance, while swinging your wheels upward to face level. Eyes looking between your outstretched wheels.

Fig. 6-73: Shift your weight back onto your left leg and lift the ball of your right foot up, while slicing down your wheels vertically to both sides of your thigh.

Fig. 6-74: Shift your weight onto your right leg into a Bow Stance and swing your wheels upward to ear level.

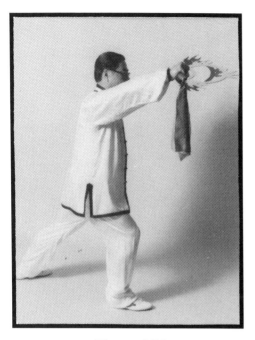

Figure 6-74

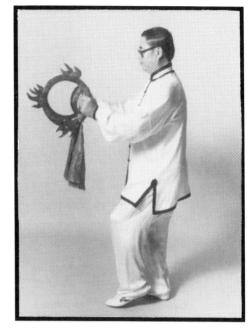

Figure 6-75

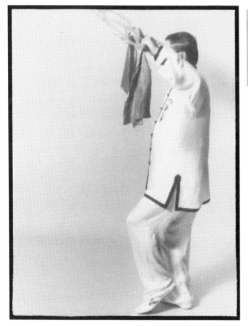

Figure 6-76

23. Left Turn Body Left Heel Kick And Strike To Ears

Movements:

Fig. 6-75: Turn your right foot in and left foot out as you make a 180 degree left turn to face west, while circling both wheels down vertically until they are chest high and chest width apart. Shift your weight on your right foot and bring your left foot next to your right.

Fig. 6-76: Keep same stance and rotate both wheels with wheels facing outward to the forehead level.

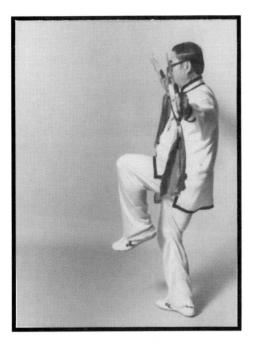

Figure 6-77

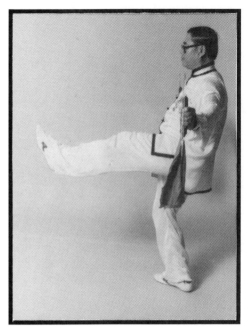

Figure 6-78

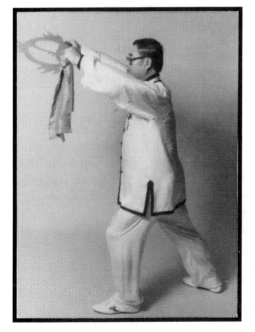

Figure 6-79

Fig. 6-77: Bring your left foot forward to your right, knee high.

Fig. 6-78: Execute a left Heel Kick to the front while chopping your wheels to both sides of your body. The right knee should bend slightly while doing this. Eyes looking straight ahead.

Fig. 6-79: Step up with the left foot into a Bow Stance while swinging your wheels upward to face level. Eyes looking between your outstretched wheels.

Fig. 6-80: Shift your weight back on your right leg and lift the ball of your left foot up while slicing down your wheels vertically to both sides of your thigh.

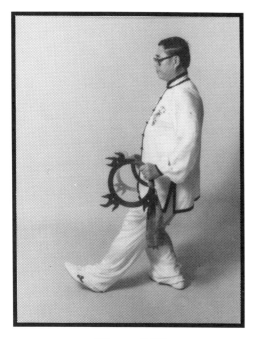

Figure 6-80

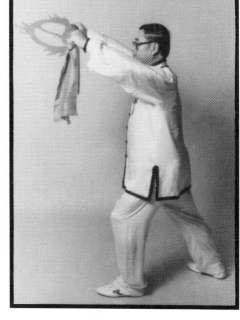

Figure 6-81

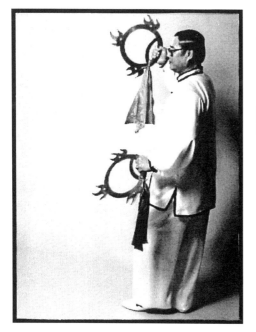

Figure 6-82

Fig. 6-81: Shift your weight onto your right leg to a Bow Stance and swing your wheels upward to ear level.

24. Needle At Sea Bottom

Movements:

Fig. 6-82: From Fig. 6-81, bring your right foot behind your left and shift all your weight on it, and begin rotating and lowering your left wheel, while lifting your left your left slightly off the floor and circling your right wheel back and up until reaching shoulder height.

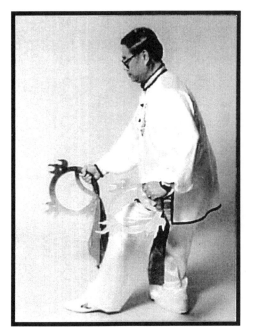
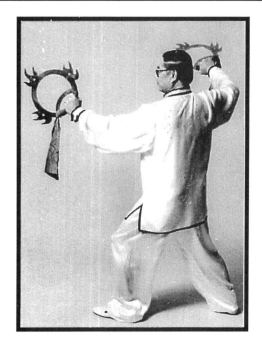

Figure 6-83   Figure 6-84

Fig. 6-83: Pull your left wheel next to your waist, touch down on your left foot and strike down with your right wheel (Face West)

25. Fan Through Back

Movements:

Fig. 6-84: From Fig. 6-83, step and slide forward with your left foot into Bow Stance, while raising your right wheel up for blocking and extending your left wheel forward for striking.

26. White Snake Spits The Poison

Movements:

Fig. 6-85: From Fig. 6-84, step up with your left foot forward into left Bow Stance while bringing down your left wheel to mid chest height, parallel to your body.

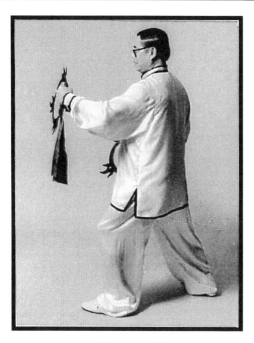

Figure 6-85

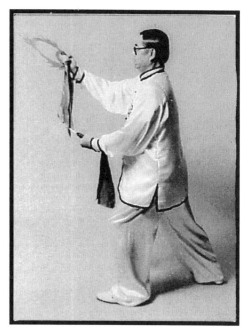

Figure 6-86

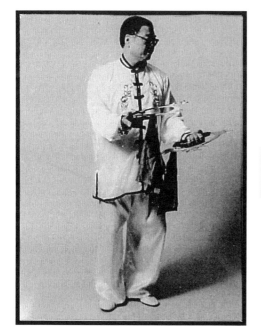

Figure 6-87

Fig. 6-86: Same Bow Stance as in Fig. 6-85. Turn the left wheel, palm up, to a 45 degree angle to the floor while raising the right wheel, palm up, in an upward thrusting motion across to top of the left wheel.

27. Wind-Fire High And Low Diagonal Cuts

Movements:

Fig. 6-87: From Fig. 6-86, shift the weight to the right foot and draw back left foot next to the right foot while bringing both wheels down to about waist height, palms up.

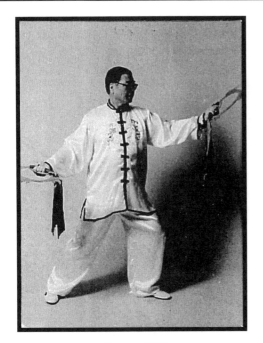

Figure 6-88

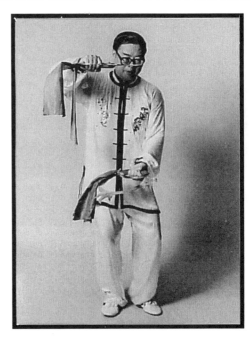

Figure 6-89

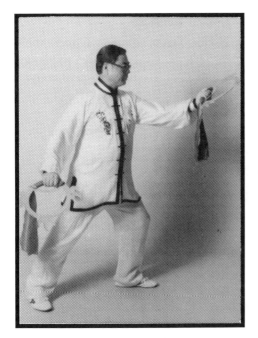

Figure 6-90

Fig. 6-88: Step forward left foot into left Bow Stance while bringing left wheel high diagonal cut to the throat and right wheel low diagonal cut to the abdomen.

28. Left Part Wild Horse's Mane

Movements:

Fig. 6-89: Shift your weight to your left foot while turning your body to the left. Shift your weight back to your right foot while bringing your left foot next to your right. (Mirror Image)

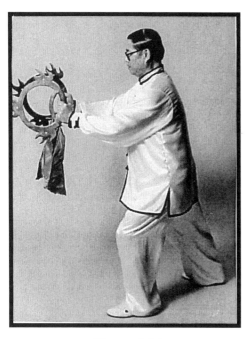 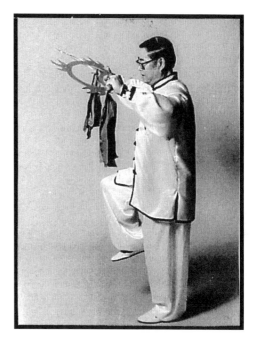

Figure 6-91   **Figure 6-92**

Fig. 6-90: Step to the left with your left heel touching down first and shift your weight forward into a left Bow Stance, while extending your left wheel forward to eye level and slicing down your right wheel next to your hip. (Face East). (Mirror Image)

29. Right Heel Kick And Strike To Ears

Movements:

Fig. 6-91: Shift your weight to your left foot into Bow Stance while striking with both wheels vertically forward.

Fig. 6-92: Bring your right foot forward to your left, knee high, while rotating both wheels with wheels facing outward at forehead level.

Fig. 6-93: Execute a right Heel Kick to the front while chopping your wheels to both sides of your body. The left knee should bend slightly while doing this. Eyes looking straight ahead.

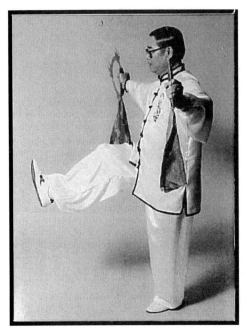

Figure 6-93

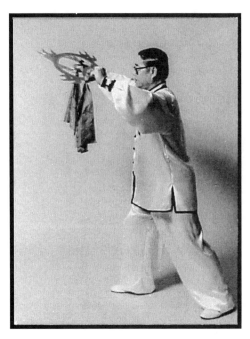

Figure 6-94

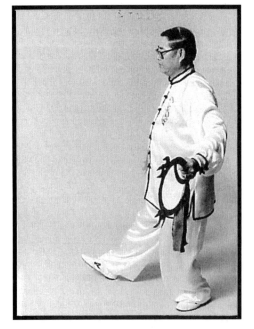

Figure 6-95

Fig. 6-94: Step up with right foot into a Bow Stance, while swinging your wheels upward to face level. Eyes looking between your outstretched wheels.

Fig. 6-95: Shift your weight back onto your left leg and lift the ball of your right foot up, while slicing down your wheels vertically to both sides of your thigh.

Fig. 6-96: Shift your weight onto your right leg into a Bow Stance and swing your wheels upward to ear level.

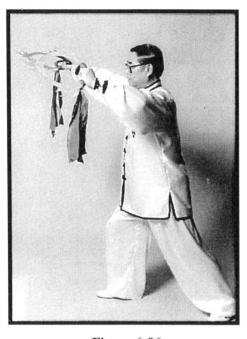

Figure 6-96

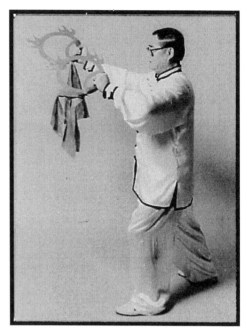

Figure 6-97

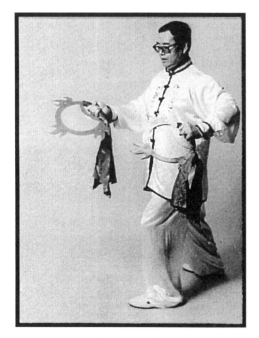

Figure 6-98

30. Left Strike The Tiger

Movements:

Fig. 6-97: Step back right foot and stand in left Bow Stance while raising the wheels, parallel to each other, palms facing towards the center, right wheel head height, left wheel shoulder height.

Fig. 6-98: Same stance as in Fig. 6-97. Turning with the waist, swing the wheels in a downward arc to the left.

Fig. 6-99: Shift the weight to the right foot into sideways Bow Stance while turning with the waist and swinging the wheels in a downward arc motion to the right.

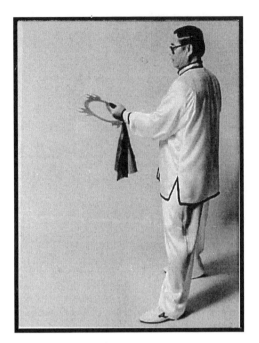

Figure 6-99

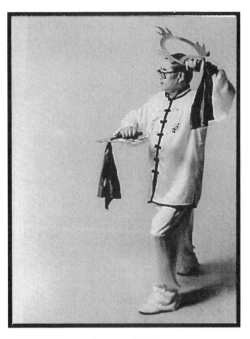

Figure 6-100

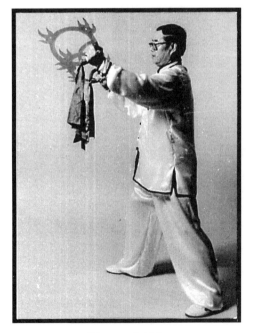

Figure 6-101

Fig. 6-100: Turn with the waist to the left into Bow Stance while bringing the left wheel in an upward arc to the height of the head, palm down, and bringing the right wheel in a horizontal arc to the center of the body, palm down.

31. Right Strike The Tiger

Movements:

Fig. 6-101: Step back left foot and stand in right Bow Stance while raising the wheels, parallel to each other, palms facing towards the center, left wheel head height, right wheel shoulder height.

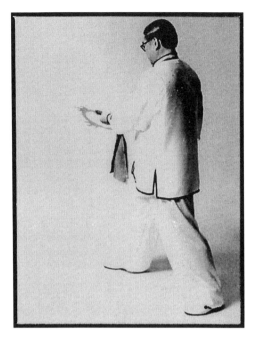

Figure 6-102

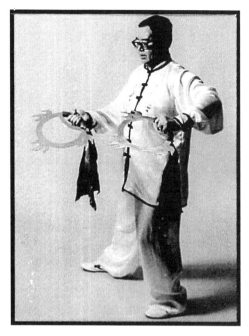

Figure 6-103

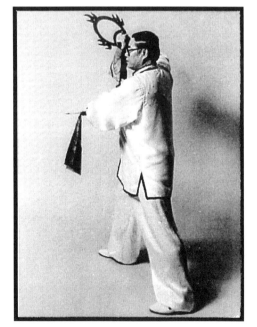

Figure 6-104

Fig. 6-102: Same stance as in Fig. 6-101. Turning with the waist, swing the wheels in a downward arc to the right.

Fig. 6-103: Shift the weight to the left foot into sideways Bow Stance while turning with the waist and swinging the wheels in a downward arc motion to the left.

Fig. 6-104: Turn with the waist to the right into Bow Stance while bringing the right wheel in an upward arc to the height of the head, palm down, and bringing the left wheel in a horizontal arc to the center of the body, palm down.

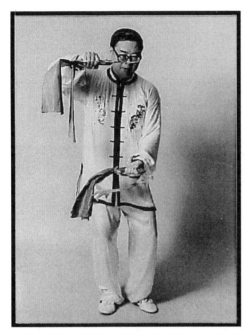
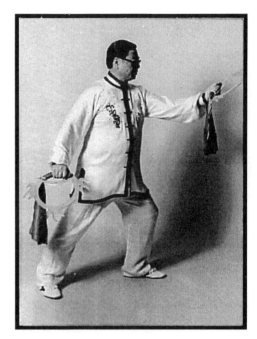

| Figure 6-105 | Figure 6-106 |

32. Left Part Wild Horse's Mane

Movements:

Fig. 6-105: Shift your weight to your left foot while turning your body to the left. Shift your weight back to your right foot while bringing your left foot next to your right.

Fig. 6-106: Step to the left with your left heel touching down first and shift your weight forward into a left Bow Stance, while extending your left wheel forward to eye level and slicing down your right wheel next to your hip. (Face East)

33. Right Lower Body And Stand On One Leg

Movements:

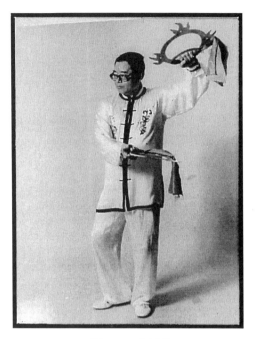

Figure 6-107

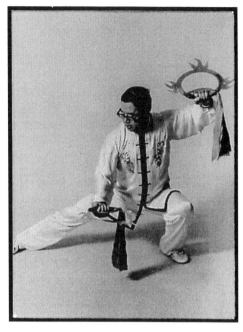

Figure 6-108

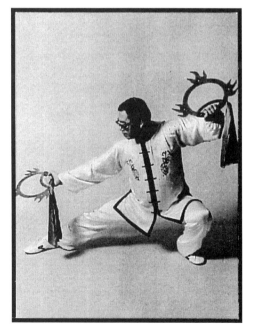

Figure 6-109

Fig. 6-107: Put your right foot down in front of you. Slice inward with your left wheel, then lift and extend it to head height while rotating your right wheel to waist height (face South).

Fig. 6-108: Step out with your right foot facing west and bend down your left knee.

Fig. 6-109: Continue lowering your body over your left leg and extend your right wheel along the inside edge of your right leg out to your foot (wheel strike West).

Fig. 6-110: Turn your right foot until it points forward. Shift your weight

205

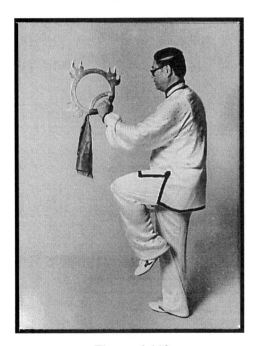

Figure 6-110

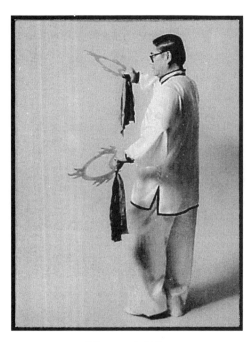

Figure 6-111

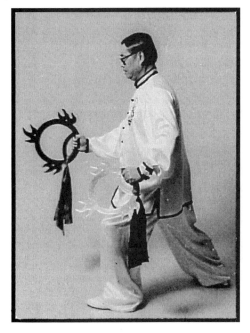

Figure 6-112

forward into right Bow Stance while lifting your right wheel up and lowering your left leg wheel behind you. Turn your right foot out and stand on it while lifting your leg up. Slice your left wheel down and bring your right wheel up.

34. Left Step Forward And Right Strike Down

Movements:

Fig. 6-111: Shift the weight to your left foot and bring right foot next to your left foot while lowering your right

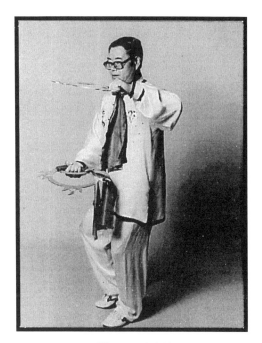

Figure 6-113

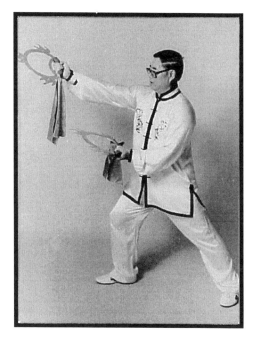

Figure 6-114

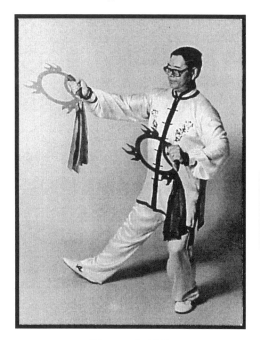

Figure 6-115

wheel and raising your left wheel to shoulder height.

Fig. 6-112: Slice down your right wheel to your right side waist while striking your left wheel forward vertically to the knee level.

35. Step Forward Ward Off, Roll Back, Press And Push

Movements:

Figs. 6-113 to Fig. 6-120: Same as posture **4** in this Form. Refer to Figs. 6-8 to 6-15.

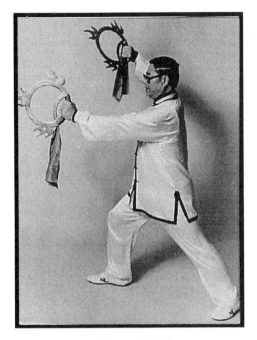

Figure 6-116

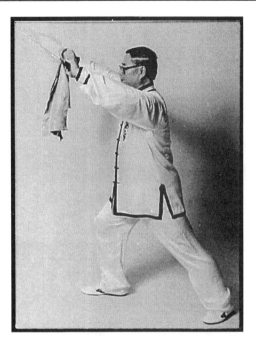

Figure 6-117

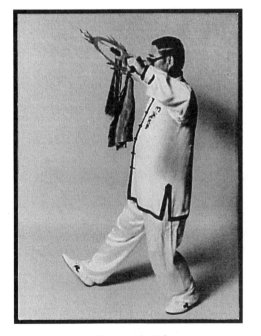

Figure 6-118

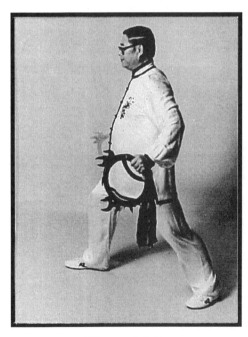

Figure 6-119

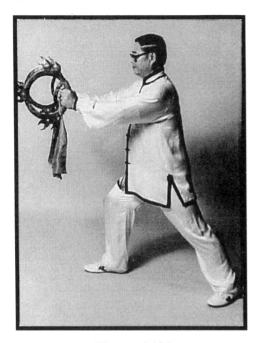

Figure 6-120

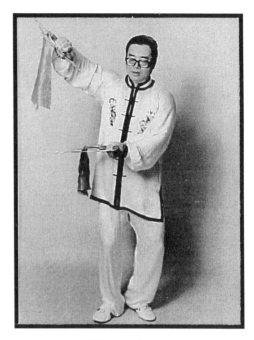

Figure 6-121

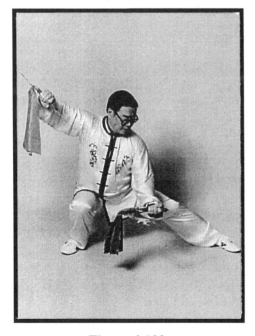

Figure 6-122

36. Left Lower Body And Stand On One Leg

Movements:

Fig. 6-121: Shift your weight onto your right foot and bring left foot next to right (face North), while rotating right wheel to head height and slicing your left wheel to waist height (Mirror Image).

Fig. 6-122: Step out with your left foot to the west and bend your right foot, while slicing left wheel down and forward. Eyes looking at your left wheel.

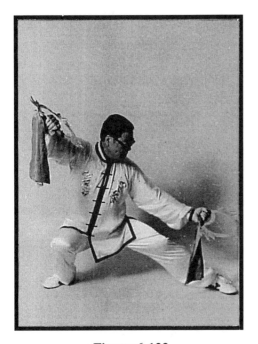

Figure 6-123

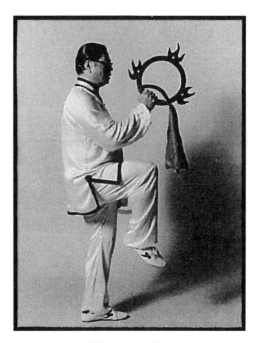

Figure 6-124

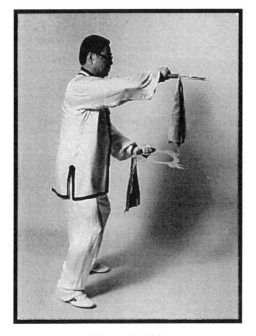

Figure 6-125

Fig. 6-123: Continue lowering your body weight over your right leg and extend your left wheel along the inside edge of your left leg out to your foot (wheel strike West).

Fig. 6-124: Turn your left foot until it points forward. Shift your weight forward into left Bow Stance while lifting your left wheel up and lowering your right wheel behind you. Turn your left foot out and stand on it when lifting your right leg up. Slice your left wheel down and bring your right wheel up.

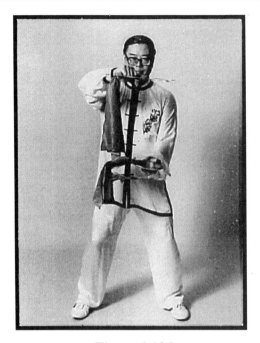

Figure 6-126

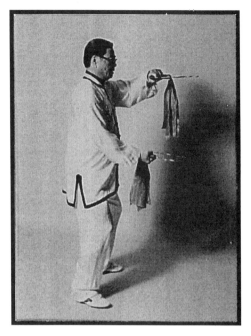

Figure 6-127

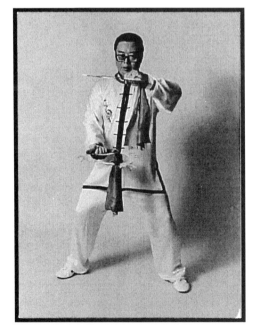

Figure 6-128

37. Wind-Fire Turning Wheels (3 times)

Movements:

Figs. 6-125 to Fig. 6-128: Same as posture **7** in this Form. Refer to Figs. 6-24 to 6-27.

38. Step Back And Ride The Tiger

Movements:

Fig. 6-129: Revolve two wheels with the right wheel down and the left wheel up.

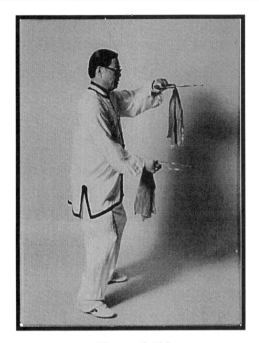

Figure 6-129

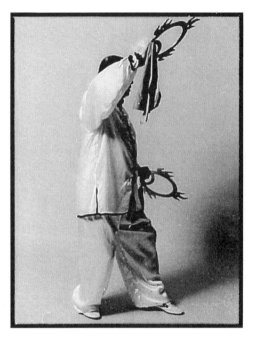

Figure 6-130

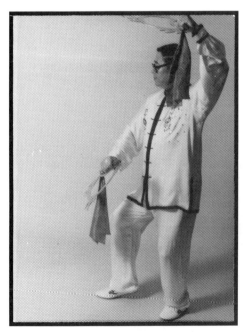

Figure 6-131

Fig. 6-130: Step back the right foot into a Cat Stance while bringing the right wheel in an upward arc motion to above the head and bringing the left wheel a downward arc motion to the left side waist of the body.

39. Right Turn Body Wind-Fire Protecting The Head And Right Heel Kick

Movements:

Fig. 6-131: Shift your weight to your right and make a 180 degree right turn of your body. Shift your weight back to your left foot and bring your right foot to Cat Stance, while raising your left wheel up with blades toward front

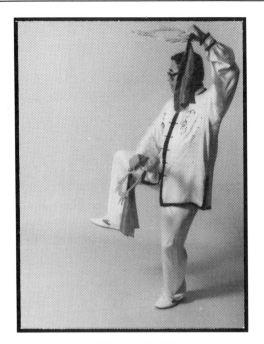

Figure 6-132

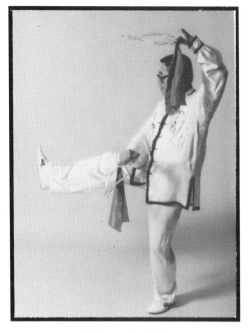

Figure 6-133

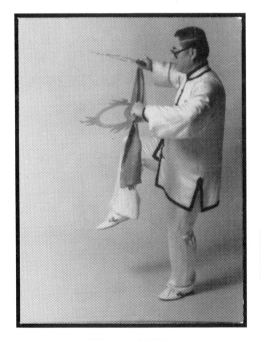

Figure 6-134

to protect your head and slicing your right wheel from outward down to your groin area.

Fig. 6-132: Lift your right foot to knee height.

Fig. 6-133: Make right heel kick to the front.

40. Left Slicing And Right Striking

Movements:

Figs. 6-134 and 6-135: Same as posture **11**. Refer to Figs. 6-39 and 6-40 in this Form.

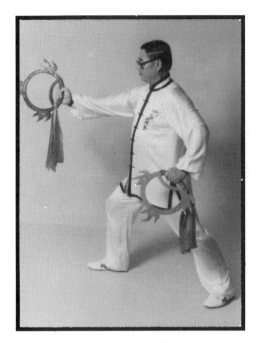

Figure 6-135

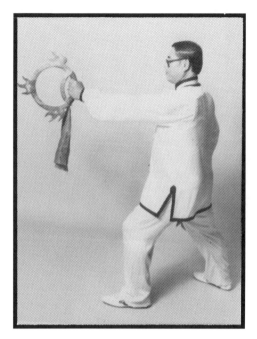

Figure 6-136

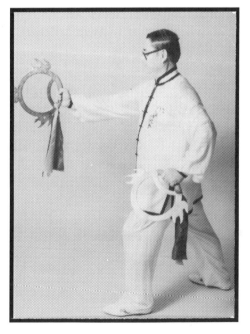

Figure 6-137

41. Step Forward Left And Right Strikings

Movements:

Fig. 6-136: Step left foot forward and make left wheel striking vertically.

Fig. 6-137: Keep same stance and make right wheel striking forward vertically,

42. Appears Closed

Movements:

Fig. 6-138: From Fig. 6-137, step up your right leg and complete Bow

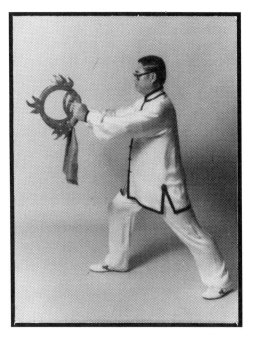

Figure 6-138

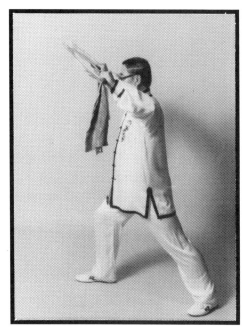

Figure 6-139

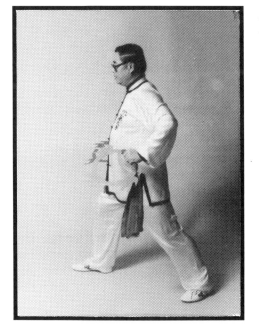

Figure 6-140

Stance while striking left wheel forward vertically.

Fig. 6-139: Keep the same stance and bring both Wind-Fire Wheels forehead high separately. Eyes Looking staight ahead.

Fig. 6-140: Rotate both wheels down to your waist while keeping the right Bow Stance.

Fig. 6-141: Strike forward with both Wind-Fire Wheels and complete the posture as shown in the picture. Eyes looking ahead, in eye level direction.

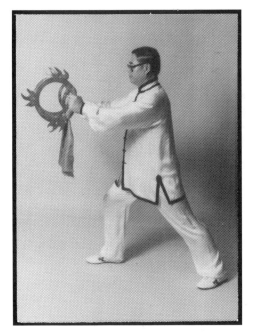

Figure 6-141

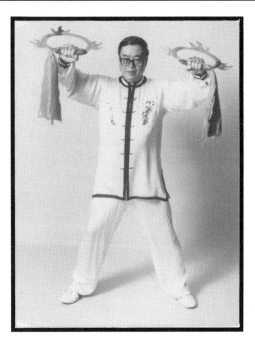

Figure 6-142

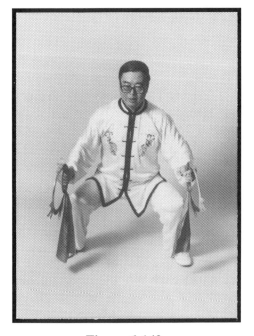

Figure 6-143

43. Wind-Fire Closing

Movements:

Fig. 6-142: From Fig. 6-141, shift your weight to your left foot, lift the ball of your right foot up and begin turning your body 90 degrees to your left while raising both Wind-Fire Wheels outward to forehead height.

Fig. 6-143: Shift your body weight evenly to both feet and begin lowering your body, while bringing down your wheels in a circular motion to knee height.

Fig. 6-144: Stand up gradually, but keep your knees bent slightly while bringing both wheels chest high and

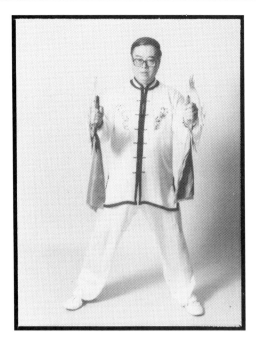

Figure 6-144

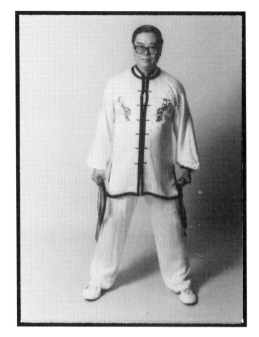

Figure 6-145

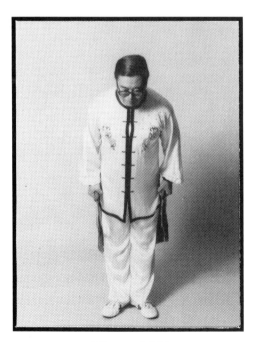
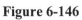

Figure 6-146

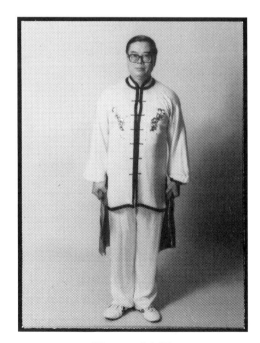

Figure 6-147

shoulder width apart. Then rotate the Wind-Fire Wheels outward, down and up three times.

44. Return to Origin

Movements:

Fig. 6-145: Bring down both wheels to the sides of your body. Eyes are looking directly ahead.

Fig. 6-146: Bring your left foot next to your right and bow to your teachers or spectators politely.

Fig. 6-147: Return to your original Preparatory Posture.

CHAPTER 7

ADVANCED FORM III

7.1 Introduction

As there are many variations on the Yang style, so are there variations of teaching styles. Traditional methods often include the teaching of an entire long form at once. Constant, dedicated repetition of the entire form eventually results in the advancement of skill, endurance and spirit. Our system, however, employs the unique approach of shorter, and then progressively longer variations of the original form.

Eventually, the original form in its entirety is taught and practiced. The Wind-Fire Wheels system is identical in philosophy. The Novice and Intermediate forms actually serve as mental and physical endurance builders for the advanced form. The advanced forms, then, are much more complicated than the others. Time, dedication and endurance are the keys to success. New movements, each

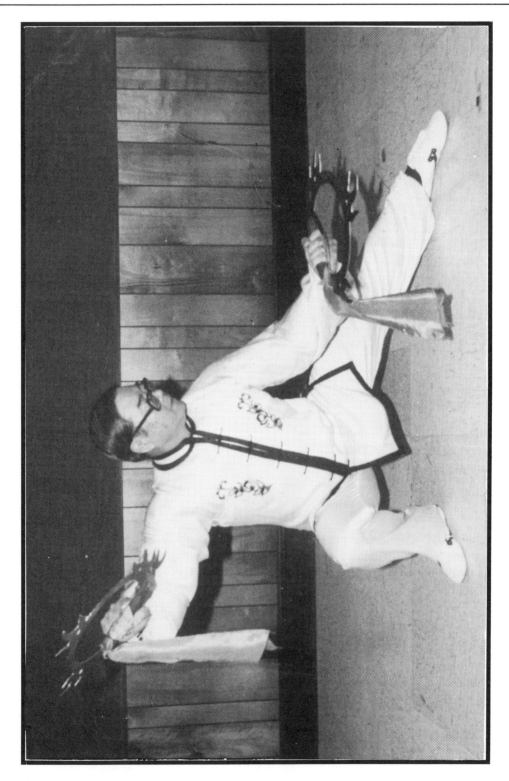

greater in difficulty, are added. More time is required to learn the sequences, thus requiring even more dedication to the system than before. With this complexity, the time needed to complete the form greatly increases. This requires, again more sacrifice from players' busy life schedule, for which they will be amply rewarded. Physical endurance, so important in the shorter forms, is required at a much greater level in the advanced form. The absolute number of movements increases as does the difficulty. Combined, it is understandable that only the more advanced player - that is advanced in barehand techniques as well - is advised to take on these forms. Players must not be discouraged by these requirements. In time, they will acquire the knowledge, skill and endurance to complete the forms. As in all aspects of life, patience and dedication will be rewarded.

7.2 Advanced Form III

1. **Preparatory Posture**
2. **Wind-Fire Commencing**
3. **Left Step Forward Part Wild Horse's Mane**
4. **Turn Right Ward Off, Roll Back, Press And Push**
5. **Left Single Whip**
6. **Wave Hands Like Clouds (3 times)**
7. **Left Single Whip**
8. **Left Lower Body**
9. **Left Golden Rooster Stands By One Leg**
10. **Right Golden Rooster Stands By One Leg**
11. **Reverse Reeling Forearm (3 times)**
12. **Diagonal Flying**
13. **Right Lifting Hand**
14. **Wind-Fire Turning Wheels**
15. **White Crane Spreads Its Wings And Left Heel Kick**
16. **Left Brush Knee And Step Forward**
17. **Needle At Sea Bottom**
18. **Fan Through Back**

19. High Pat On Horse
20. Right Heel Kick And Strike To Ears
21. Left Turn Body Left Heel Kick And Strike To Ears
22. Left Brush Knee And Step Forward
23. Playing The Lute
24. Brush Knee And Punch Down
25. Right Turn Right Part Wild Horse's Mane
26. Left Heel Kick And Strike To Ears
27. Right Strike The Tiger
28. Left Strike The Tiger
29. Right Strike The Tiger
30. Right Lower Body And Stand On One Leg
31. White Snake Spits The Poison
32. Wind-Fire High And Low Diagonal Cuts
33. Left Part Wild Horse's Mane
34. Right Heel Kick And Strike To Ears
35. Left Turn Body Fair Lady Shuttles Back And Forth (forward 1 time, backward 1 time)
36. Left Turn Right Part Wild Horse's Mane
37. Left Turn Body Fist Under The Elbow
38. Step Forward And Strike Down
39. Wind-Fire Turning Wheels (3 times)
40. Step Back And Ride The Tiger
41. Right Turn Body Wind-Fire Protecting The Head And Right Heel Kick
42. Left Slicing And Right Striking
43. Step Forward Left And Right Strikings
44. Appears Closed
45. Wind-Fire Closing
46. Return To Origin

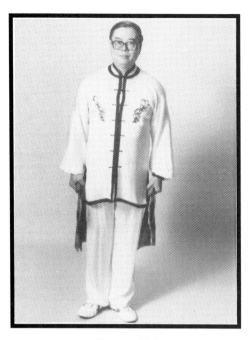

Figure 7-1

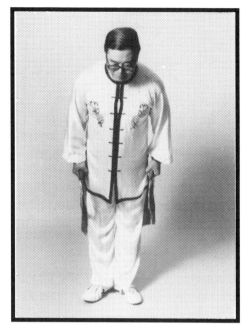

Figure 7-2

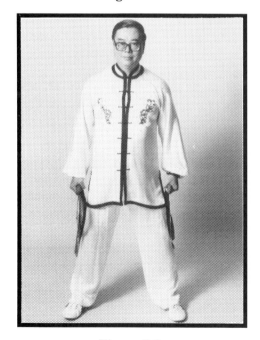

Figure 7-3

1. Preparatory Posture

Movements:

Begin by facing South.

Fig. 7-1: Natural Standing with feet sixty degree outward, back straight, arms relaxed with Wind-Fire Wheels by your side (Facing South, inhale and exhale several times).

Fig. 7-2: Bow to your teachers or spectators politely.

Fig. 7-3: Bend your knees slightly, then step to your left with your left leg.

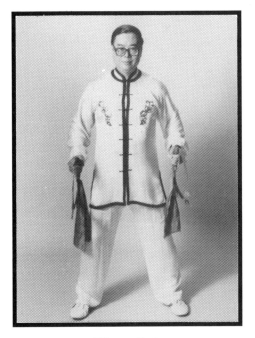
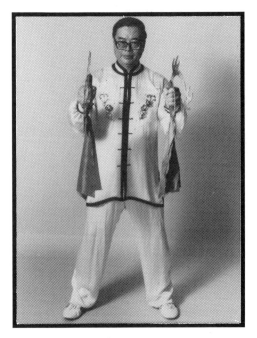

Figure 7-4   Figure 7-5

2. Wind-Fire Commencing

Movements:

Fig. 7-4: Raise your Wind-Fire Wheels in front of you to shoulder height, keeping them parallel to each other.

Fig. 7-5: Rotate the Wind-Fire Wheels outward, down and up three times.

3. Left Step Forward Part Wild Horse's Mane

Movements:

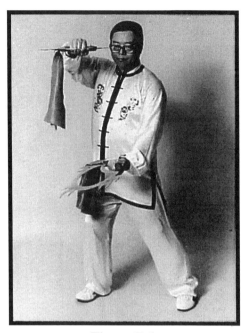

Figure 7-6

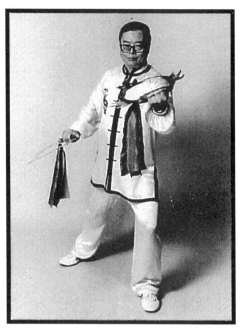

Figure 7-7

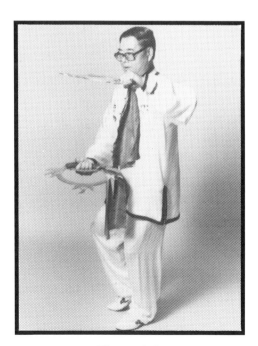

Figure 7-8

Fig. 7-6: Shift your weight to your right foot and bring your left foot next to the right, while turning your body slightly to the right. During the twisting movement, rotate both wheels to face each other. Eyes looking in the same direction as your right hand.

Fig. 7-7: Step out your left foot into left Bow Stance, (face South), while slicing your right wheel down next to your hip and extending your left wheel forward to the eye level.

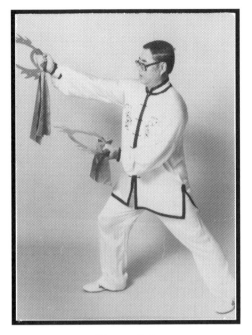 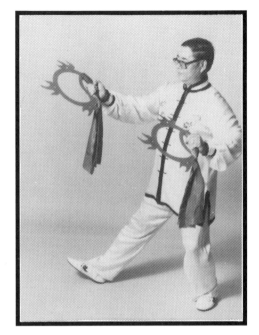

Figure 7-9   Figure 7-10

4. Turn Right Ward Off, Roll Back, Press And Push

Movements:

Fig. 7-8: Turn right and bring both Wind-Fire Wheels to your left facing each other with right hand downward and left hand upward. Shift your weight to your front foot and bring back your right foot next to your left.

Fig. 7-9: Step forward with your right foot while extending your right wheel forward and upward and draw your left wheel downward and out. Eyes should be focused on your right wheel.

Fig. 7-10: Shift your weight back onto your left leg and right heel while twisting your waist to the left and pulling down with your Wind-Fire Wheels. Keep your eyes focused on the right hand and then focus in the direction of the torso at eye level.

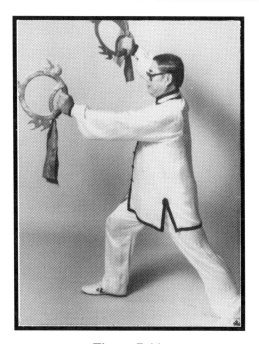

Figure 7-11

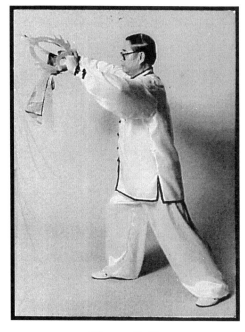

Figure 7-12

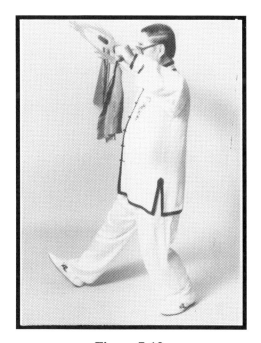

Figure 7-13

Fig. 7-11: Shift your weight forward into a right Bow Stance while right wheel makes an upward blocking and left wheel a forward striking. Eyes focus on the left hand wheel.

Fig. 7-12: Keep the same Bow Stance as shown in Fig. 7-11. Bring the left wheel up to the right wheel level.

Fig. 7-13: Shift your weight back onto your left foot and bring both wind-fire wheels to forehead level (45 degrees above horizontal level). Eyes look straight ahead.

Fig. 7-14: Rotate both wheels down to your waist while shifting your weight onto the right leg. Eyes keep looking ahead.

227

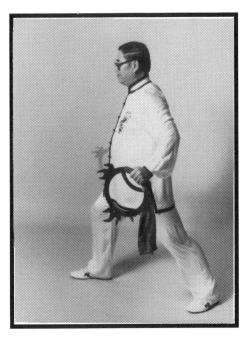

Figure 7-14

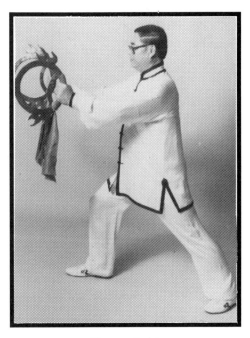

Figure 7-15

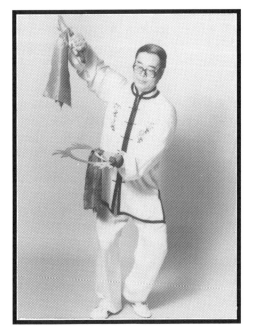

Figure 7-16

Fig. 7-15: Continue shifting your weight onto the right leg and complete Bow Stance. Push forward with both wind-fire wheels and complete the push posture. Eyes continue to look ahead.

5. Left Single Whip

Movements:

Fig. 7-16: Draw the left foot to the right foot and make a "C" Slice with your right-hand wheel while the left-hand wheel rotates from upward to downward and is placed under the right hand wheel. Eyes look to the right hand wheel then move to the left-hand wheel.

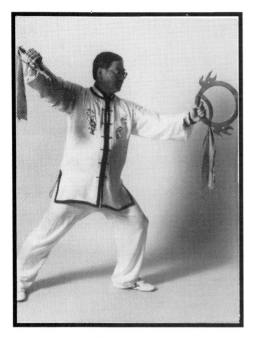
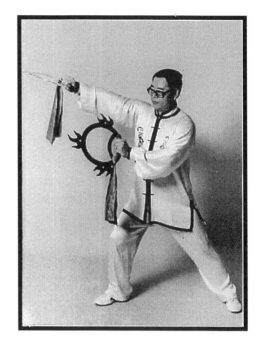

Figure 7-17   Figure 7-18

Fig. 7-17: Extend your left leg touching down with the heel and shift your weight to your left foot and complete Bow Stance. Rotate and extend your left wheel forward.

6. Wave Hands Like Clouds (3 times)

Movements:

Fig. 7-18: Shift the weight to your right foot while bringing your left wheel to your right and focusing your eyes on your left wheel.

Fig. 7-19: Rotate your waist to south and shift your weight onto both legs evenly while lowering your right wheel waist high and raising the left wheel chin high. Both wheels face each other with slicing motion and the eyes are focused on the left wheel.

Fig. 7-20: Slowly shift your weight to your left foot while continuing slicing both wheels to your left.

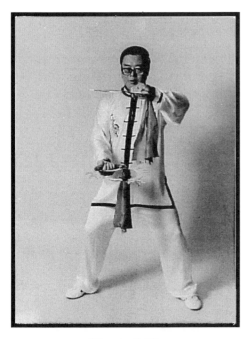

Figure 7-19

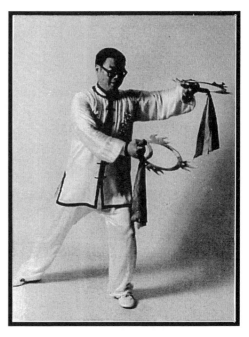

Figure 7-20

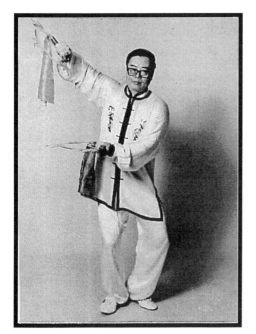

Figure 7-21

7. Left Single Whip

Movements:

Fig. 7-21: Bring the right foot next to your left foot while raising your right wheel to forehead height and lowering your left wheel chest high.

Fig. 7-22: Repeat the motion as described in Fig. 7-17 in this form.

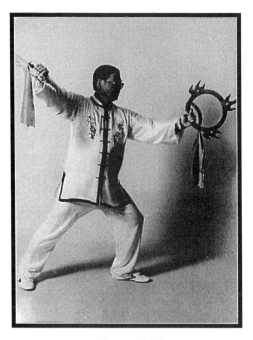

Figure 7-22

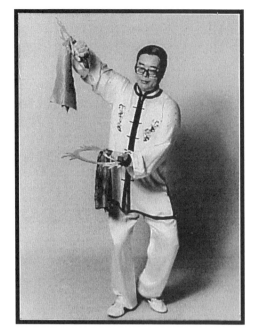

Figure 7-23

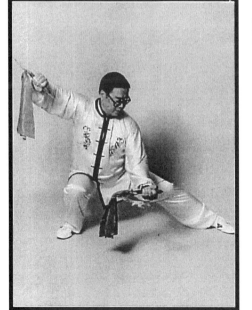

Figure 7-24

8. Left Lower Body

Movements:

Fig. 7-23: Shift your weight onto your right foot and bring left foot next to right (face South), while rotating right wheel to head height and slicing your left wheel to waist height (Mirror Image).

Fig. 7-24: Step out with your left foot to the West and bend your right foot, while slicing left wheel down and forward. Eyes looking at your left wheel.

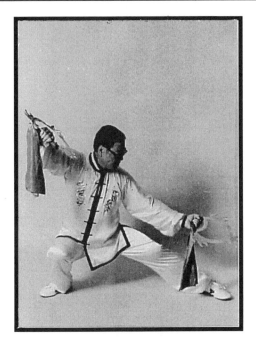

Figure 7-25

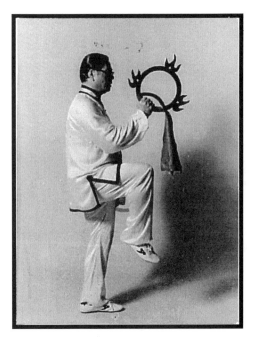

Figure 7-26

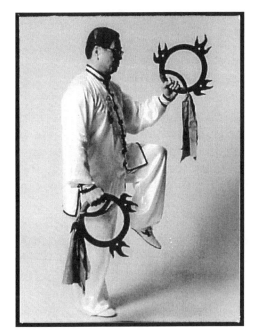

Figure 7-27

Fig. 7-25: Continue lowering your body weight over your right leg and extend your left wheel along the inside edge of your left leg out to your foot (wheel strike East).

9. Left Golden Rooster Stands By One Leg

Movements:

Fig. 7-26: Turn your left foot until it points forward. Shift your weight forward into left Bow Stance while lifting your left wheel up and lowering your right wheel behind you. Turn your left foot out and stand on it when lifting your right leg up. Slice your left wheel down and bring your right wheel up.

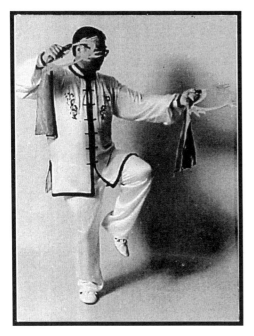 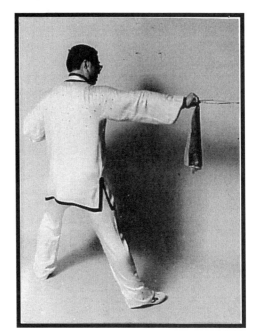

Figure 7-28   Figure 7-29

10. Right Golden Rooster Stands By One Leg

Movements:

Fig. 7-27: Step back your right foot and stand on it when lifting your left leg up. Slice your right wheel down and bring your left wheel up.

11. Reverse Reeling Forearm (3 times)

Movements:

Fig. 7-28: From Fig. 7-27, slightly lower your left wheel and raise your right wheel from behind to ear height while lifting up your left foot.

Fig. 7-29: Step back with your left foot behind your right foot and pivot on your right foot while pulling your left wheel next to your waist and extending your right wheel forward.

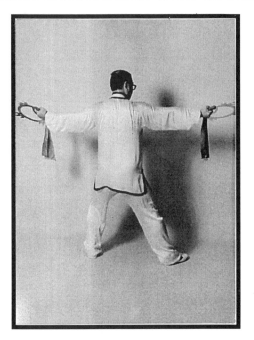

Figure 7-30

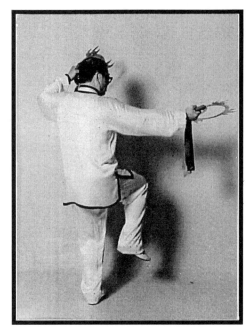

Figure 7-31

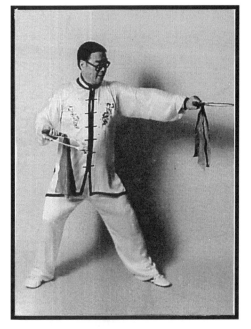

Figure 7-32

Fig. 7-30: Extend your left wheel out and up while rotating both wheels up.

Fig. 7-31: Bend your left elbow and lift up your right foot.

Fig. 7-32: Step back with your right foot behind your left and pivot on your left foot while pulling your right wheel next to your waist and extending your left wheel forward.

Fig. 7-33: Same as Fig. 7-28. Repeat the movement one time.

Fig. 7-34: Same as Fig. 7-29. Repeat the movement one time.

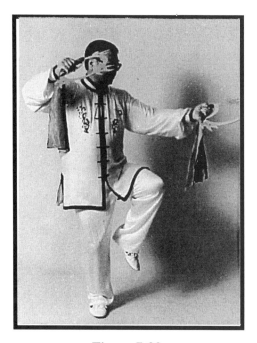

Figure 7-33

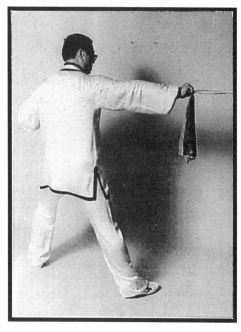

Figure 7-34

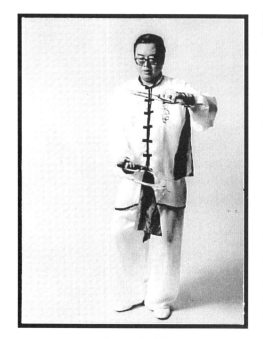

Figure 7-35

12. Diagonal Flying

Movements:

Fig. 7-35: Bring back your right foot next to your left foot. Slowly turn the wheels over in a circular motion bringing the left wheel to the top about shoulder height and the right wheel to the bottom about waist height.

Fig. 7-36: Shift the weight to the left and step out right foot to the right side in a sideways Bow Stance while bringing the right wheel, palm up, in an arc type movement until the right wheel is extended to the right of the body, to about slightly above the head and bringing the left wheel, palm down, in a downward arc pointing towards the floor.

235

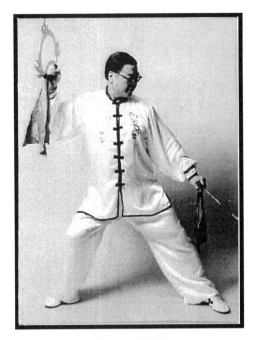

Figure 7-36

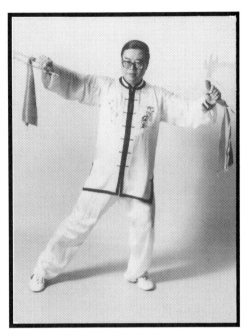

Figure 7-37

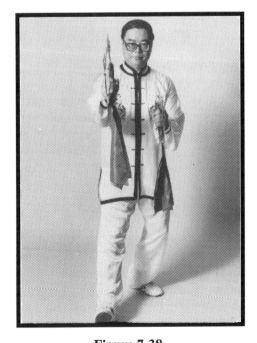

Figure 7-38

13. Right Lifting Hand

Movements:

Fig. 7-37: Turn your body to your right, while rotating your waist to face south. Both hands are holding Wind-Fire Wheels vertically.

Fig. 7-38: Shift your weight on your left foot and draw your right foot to your left foot. Step out to the front touching down with your heel. While drawing wheels to the center in front of your chest with your right hand higher than your left hand.

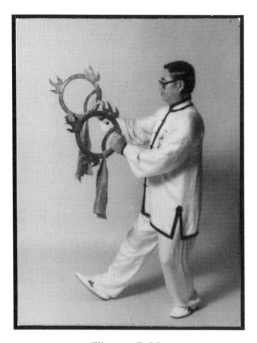

Figure 7-39

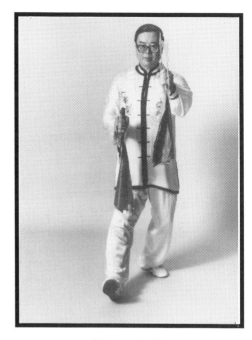

Figure 7-40

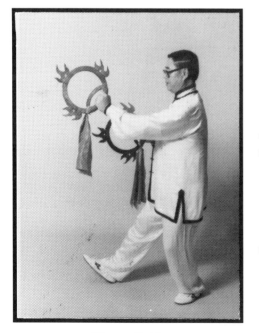

Figure 7-41

Fig. 7-39: Side view of figure 7-38.

Fig. 7-40: Same stance as Fig. 7-41. Rotate both Wind-Fire Wheels outward one time vertically.

Fig. 7-41: Side view of figure 7-40.

Fig. 7-42: Shows completion of one time vertical rotation.

237

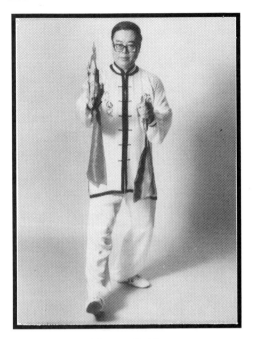

Figure 7-42

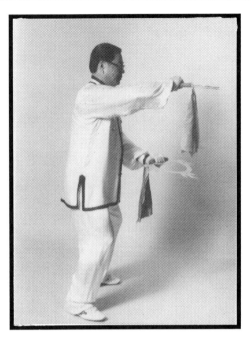

Figure 7-43

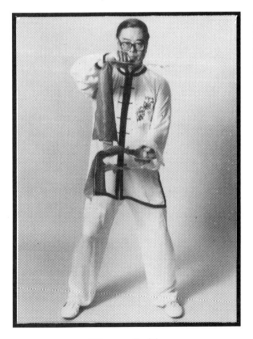

Figure 7-44

14. Wind-Fire Turning Wheels

Movements:

Fig. 7-43: Turn your body to your left while rotating your waist to the left. Both feet are shoulder width apart and slightly bent, while revolving both wheels and slicing your left wheel down and the right wheel up.

Fig. 7-44: Shows front view of Fig. 7-43.

Fig. 7-45: Revolve two wheels once again with the right wheel down and the left wheel up.

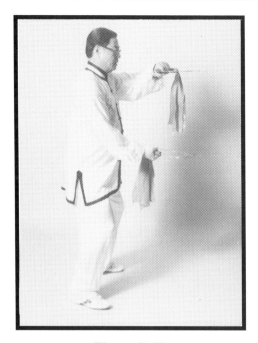

Figure 7-45

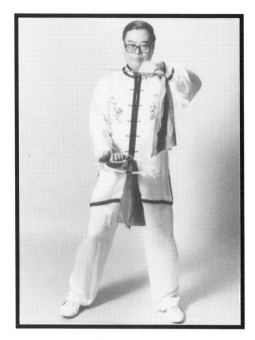

Figure 7-46

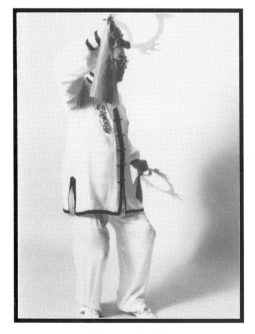

Figure 7-47

Fig. 7-46: Shows front view of Fig. 7-45.

15. White Crane Spreads Its Wings And Left Heel Kick

Movements:

Fig. 7-47: Rotate your waist to the right and step up with your left foot forward as in a Cat Stance. Your weight should be in your right leg now. In the meantime, begin raising your right wheel up and slicing your left wheel down.

Fig. 7-48: Lift your left foot up and balance your body.

239

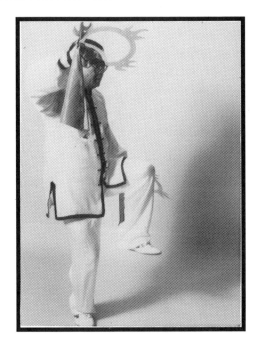

Figure 7-48

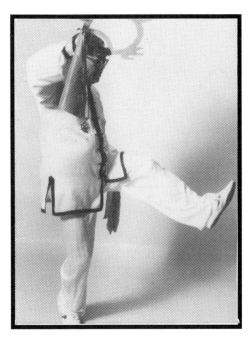

Figure 7-49

Fig. 7-49: Execute a Heel Kick to the front.

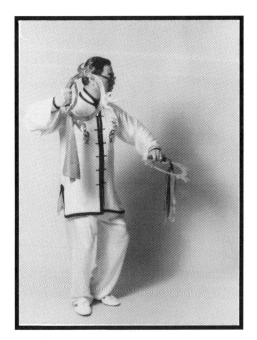

Figure 7-50

16. Left Brush Knee And Step Forward

Movements:

Fig. 7-50: Bring back your left kicking leg close to your right leg. Turn your body slightly to your left while raising up and slicing your left wheel to the front and bringing down right wheel with blades outward to face height. Turn your body to your right while lowering and slicing your left wheel and slicing your right wheel outward and down, then bring it to your right ear height vertically, blades pointed to the front.

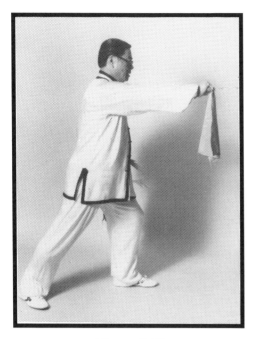

Figure 7-51

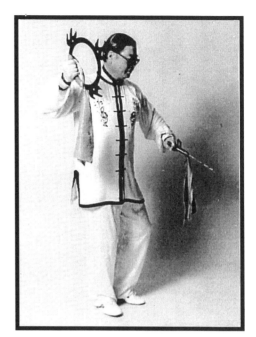

Figure 7-52

Fig. 7-51: Step up your left leg to left Bow Stance while striking your right wheel forward horizontally.

17. Needle At Sea Bottom

Movements:

Fig. 7-52: From Fig. 7-51, Bring your right foot behind your left and shift all your weight on it, and begin rotating and lowering your left wheel, while lifting your left foot slightly off the floor and circling your right wheel back and up until reaching shoulder height.

Fig. 7-53: Pull your left wheel next to your waist, touch down on your left foot and strike down with your right wheel (Face East)

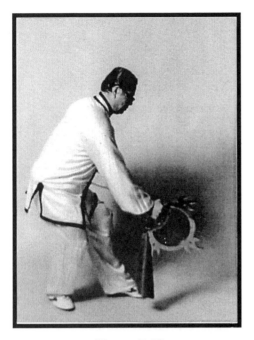

Figure 7-53

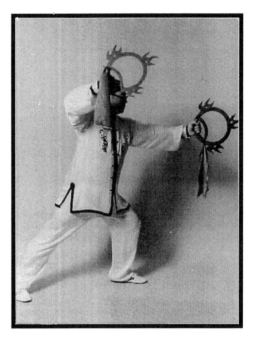

Figure 7-54

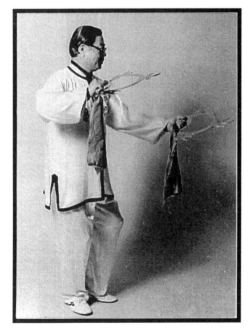

Figure 7-55

18. Fan Through Back

Movements:

Fig. 7-54: From Fig. 7-53, step and slide forward with your left foot into Bow Stance, while raising your right wheel up for blocking and extending your left wheel forward for striking.

19. High Pat On Horse

Movements:

Fig. 7-55: Rotate your waist to the east and step up your right foot next to your left. Deflect with your left wheel face up and bring your right wheel shoulder high and face down.

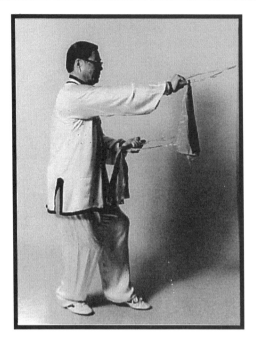

Figure 7-56

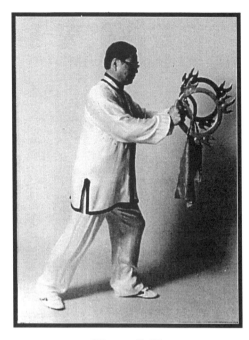

Figure 7-57

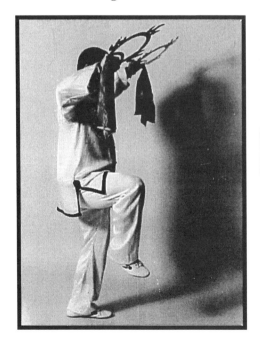

Figure 7-58

Fig. 7-56: Step up left foot to Cat Stance while pressing forward to strike with your right wheel. Eyes focus on the right wheel as it passes next to the left upturned wheel.

20. Right Heel Kick And Strike To Ears

Movements:

Fig. 7-57: Shift your weight to your left foot into Bow Stance while striking with both wheels vertically forward.

Fig. 7-58: Bring your right foot forward to your left, knee high, while rotating both wheels with wheels facing outward at forehead level.

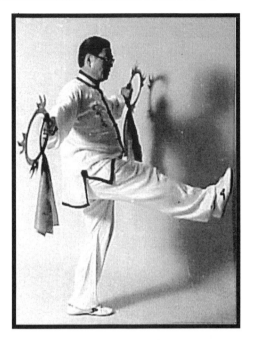

Figure 7-59

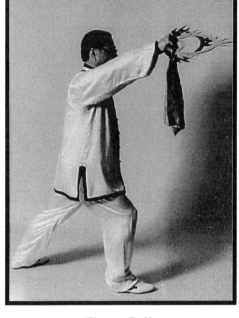

Figure 7-60

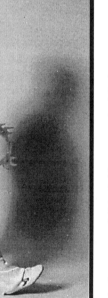

Figure 7-61

Fig. 7-59: Execute a right Heel Kick to the front while chopping your wheels to both sides of your body. The left knee should bend slightly while doing this. Eyes looking straight ahead.

Fig. 7-60: Step up with right foot into a Bow Stance, while swinging your wheels upward to face level. Eyes looking between your outstretched wheels.

Fig. 7-61: Shift your weight back onto your left leg and lift the ball of your right foot up, while slicing down your wheels vertically to both sides of your thigh.

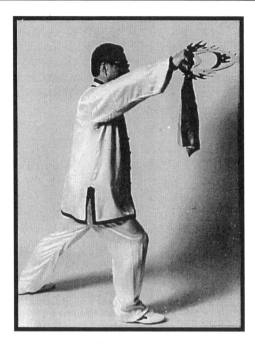

Figure 7-62

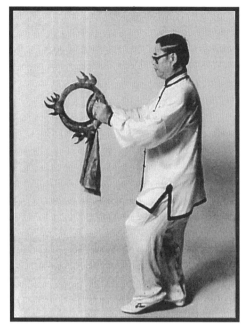

Figure 7-63

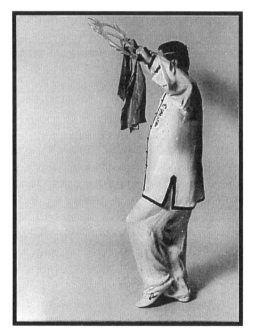

Figure 7-64

Fig. 7-62: Shift your weight onto your right leg into a Bow Stance and swing your wheels upward to ear level.

21. Left Turn Body Left Heel Kick And Strike To Ears

Movements:

Fig. 7-63: Turn your right foot in and left foot out as you make a 180 degree left turn to face West, while circling both wheels down vertically until they are chest high and chest width apart. Shift your weight on your right foot and bring your left foot next to your right.

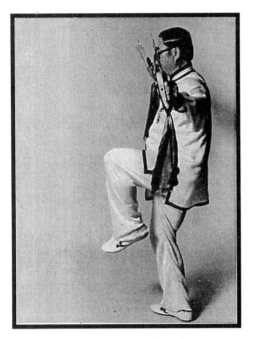

Figure 7-65

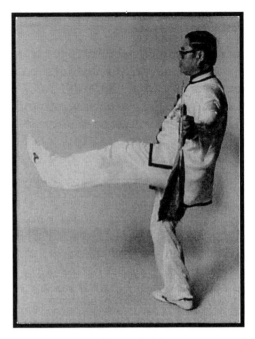

Figure 7-66

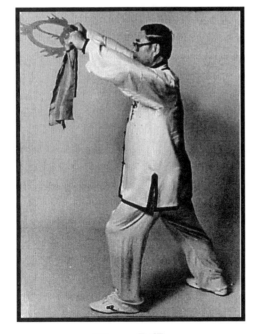

Figure 7-67

Fig. 7-64: Keep same stance and rotate both wheels with wheels facing outward to the forehead level.

Fig. 7-65: Bring your left foot forward to your right, knee high.

Fig. 7-66: Execute a left Heel Kick to the front while chopping your wheels to both sides of your body. The right knee should bend slightly while doing this. Eyes looking straight ahead.

Fig. 7-67: Step up with the left foot into a Bow Stance while swinging your wheels upward to face level. Eyes looking between your outstretched wheels.

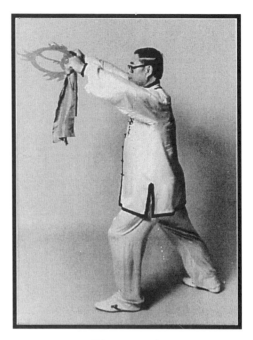

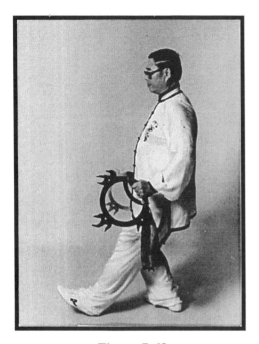

Figure 7-68

Figure 7-69

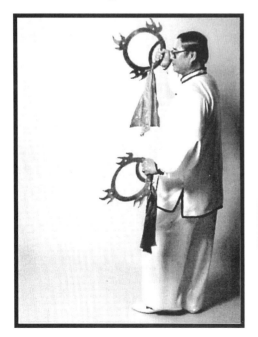

Figure 7-70

Fig. 7-68: Shift your weight back on your right leg and lift the ball of your left foot up while slicing down your wheels vertically to both sides of your thigh.

Fig. 7-69: Shift your weight onto your right leg to a Bow Stance and swing your wheels upward to ear level.

22. Left Brush Knee And Step Forward

Movements:

Fig. 7-70: Bring back your left leg close to your right leg. Turn your body slightly to your left while raising up and slicing your left wheel to the front and

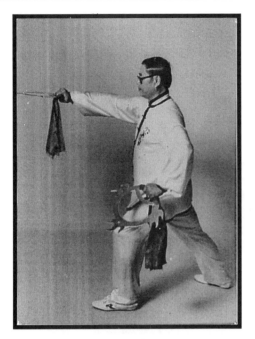 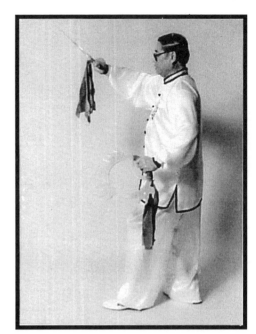

Figure 7-71	Figure 7-72

bringing down right wheel with blades outward to face height. Turn your body to your right while lowering and slicing your left wheel and slicing your right wheel outward and down, then bring it to your right ear height vertically, blades pointed to the front.

Fig. 7-71: Step up your left leg to left Bow Stance while striking your right wheel forward horizontally.

23. Playing The Lute

Movements:

Fig. 7-72: Shift your weight onto your right foot and bring your right wheel to eye level.

Fig. 7-73: Rotate your waist from left to right while lowering your right wheel in a circular motion.

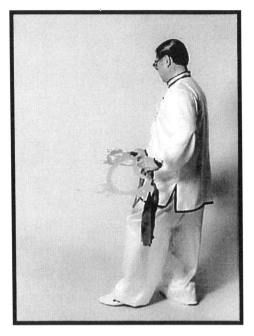
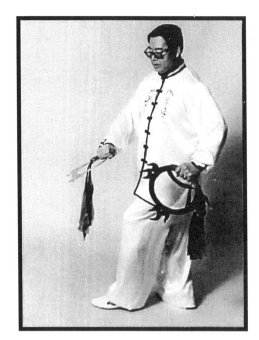

Figure 7-73   **Figure 7-74**

Fig. 7-74: Continue rotating your waist to the left while circling your right wheel up.

Fig. 7-75: Pull your left foot to your right foot and rotate your waist to the right while bringing your right wheel upward and your left wheel downward to face each other.

Fig. 7-76: Step forward with your left foot touching down with your heel while extending your left wheel forward and slicing your right wheel down.

24. Brush Knee And Punch Down

Movements:

Fig. 7-77: Shift the weight of your body to the right foot and bring left foot next to your right while lowering your left wheel and raising your right wheel to shoulder height.

Fig. 7-78: Slice down your left wheel to your left side waist while striking your right wheel forward horizontally to the knee level.

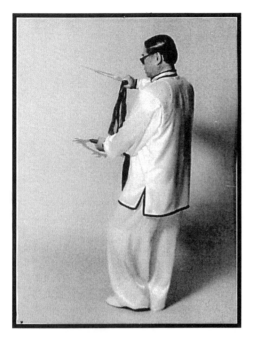

Figure 7-75

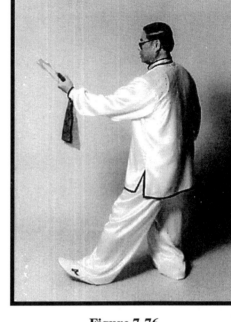

Figure 7-76

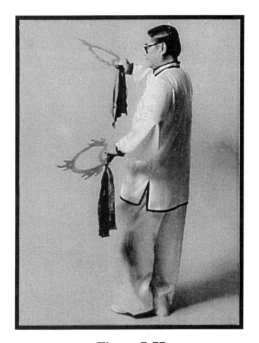

Figure 7-77

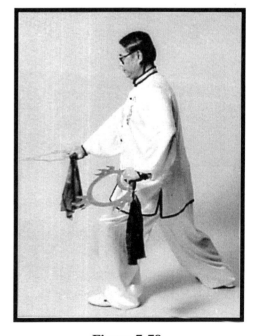

Figure 7-78

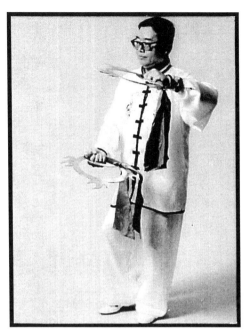 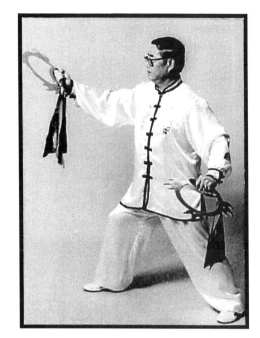

Figure 7-79   Figure 7-80

25. Right Turn Right Part Wild Horse's Mane

Movements:

Fig. 7-79: Bend down both knees slightly, then shift your weight to your left foot while turning your body to the left. During the twisting moment, rotate both wheels to face each other. Eyes looking in the same direction as your left hand.

Fig. 7-80: Step out your right foot into a right Bow Stance, while slicing your left wheel down next to your hip and extending your right wheel forward to the eye level.

26. Left Heel Kick And Strike To Ears

Movements:

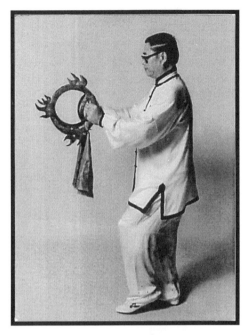

Figure 7-81

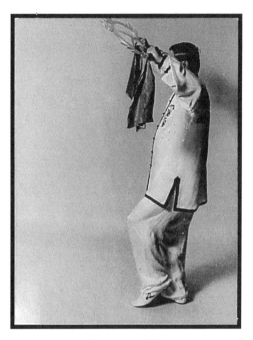

Figure 7-82

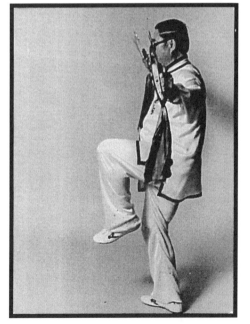

Figure 7-83

Fig. 7-81: Same as Fig. 7-63, repeat the Movement one time.

Fig. 7-82: Same as Fig. 7-64, repeat the Movement one time.

Fig. 7-83: Same as Fig. 7-65, repeat the Movement one time.

Fig. 7-84: Same as Fig. 7-66, repeat the Movement one time.

Fig. 7-85: Same as Fig. 7-67, repeat the Movement one time.

Fig. 7-86: Same as Fig. 7-68, repeat the Movement one time.

Fig. 7-87: Same as Fig. 7-69, repeat the Movement one time.

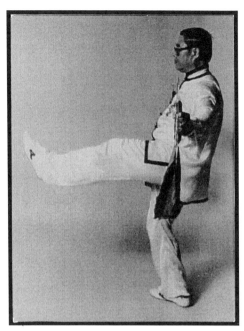

Figure 7-84

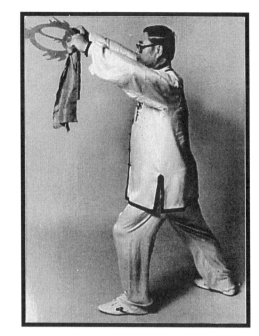

Figure 7-85

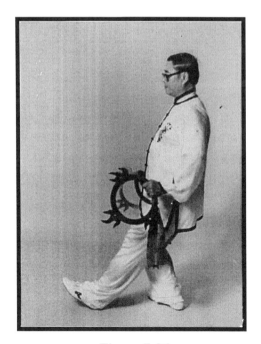

Figure 7-86

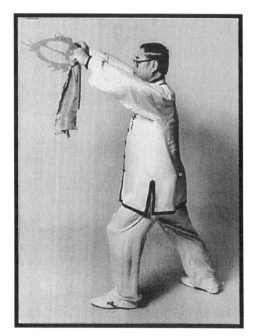

Figure 7-87

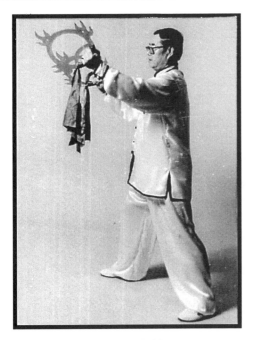

Figure 7-88

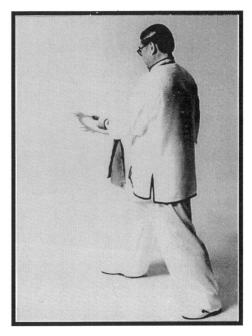

Figure 7-89

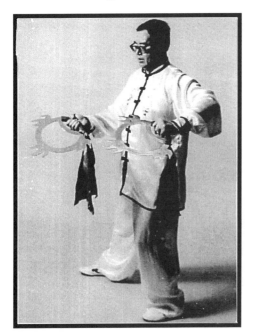

Figure 7-90

27. Right Strike The Tiger

Movements:

Fig. 7-88: Step back left foot and stand in right Bow Stance while raising the wheels, parallel to each other, palms facing towards the center, left wheel head height, right wheel shoulder height.

Fig. 7-89: Same stance as in Fig. 7-88. Turning with the waist, swing the wheels in a downward arc to the right.

Fig. 7-90: Shift the weight to the left foot into sideways Bow Stance while turning with the waist and swinging the wheels in a downward arc montion to the left.

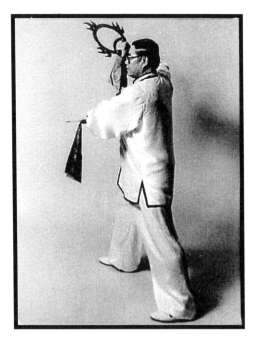

Figure 7-91

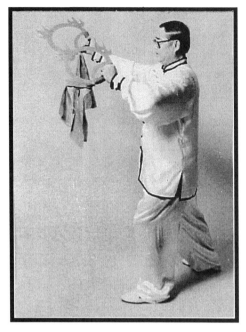

Figure 7-92

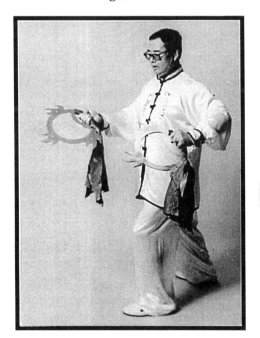

Figure 7-93

Fig. 7-91: Turn with the waist to the right into Bow Stance while bringing the right wheel in an upward arc to the height of the head, palm down, and bringing the left wheel in a horizontal arc to the center of the body, palm down.

28. Left Strike The Tiger

Movements:

Fig. 7-92: Step back right foot and stand in left Bow Stance while raising the wheels, parallel to each other, palms facing towards the center, right wheel head height, left wheel shoulder height.

255

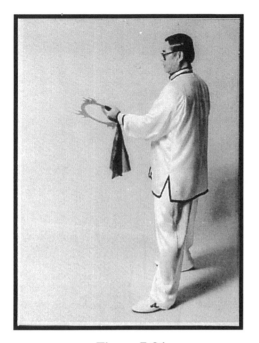

Figure 7-94

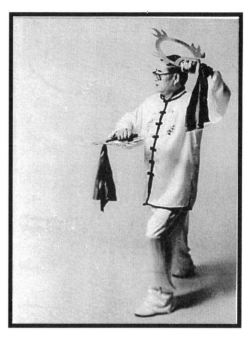

Figure 7-95

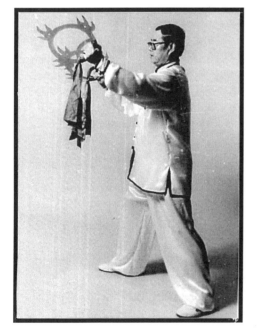

Figure 7-96

Fig. 7-93: Same stance as in Fig. 7-92. Turning with the waist, swing the wheels in a downward arc to the left.

Fig. 7-94: Shift the weight to the right foot into sideways Bow Stance while turning with the waist and swinging the wheels in a downward arc montion to the right.

Fig. 7-95: Turn with the waist to the left into Bow Stance while bringing the left wheel in an upward arc to the height of the head, palm down, and bringing the right wheel in a horizontal arc to the center of the body, palm down.

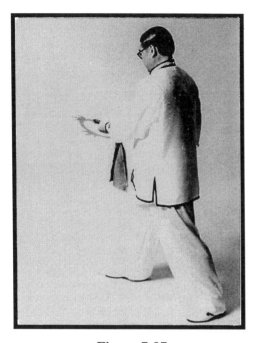

Figure 7-97

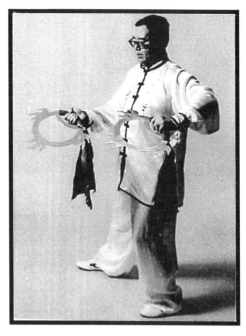

Figure 7-98

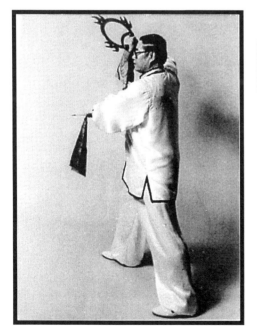

Figure 7-99

29. Right Strike The Tiger

Movements:

Fig. 7-96: Same as Fig. 7-88, repeat the movement one time.

Fig. 7-97: Same as Fig. 7-89, repeat the movement one time.

Fig. 7-98: Same Fig. 7-90, repeat the movement one time.

Fig, 7-99: Same as Fig. 7-91, repeat the movement one time.

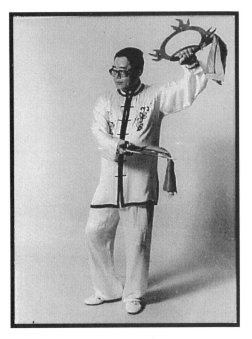

Figure 7-100

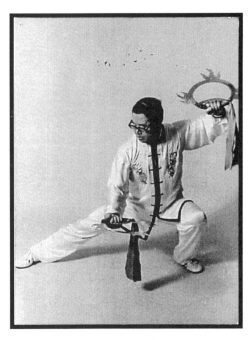

Figure 7-101

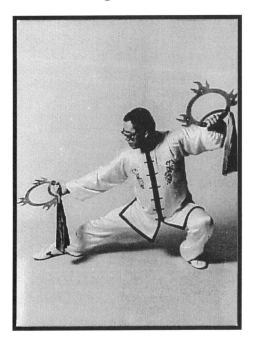

Figure 7-102

30. Right Lower Body And Stand On One Leg

Movements:

Fig. 7-100: Put your right foot down in front of you. Slice inward with your left wheel, then lift and extend it to head height while rotating your right wheel to waist height (face South).

Fig. 7-101: Step out with your right foot facing West and bend down your left knee.

Fig. 7-102: Continue lowering your body over your left leg and extend your right wheel along the inside edge of your right leg out to your foot (wheel strike West).

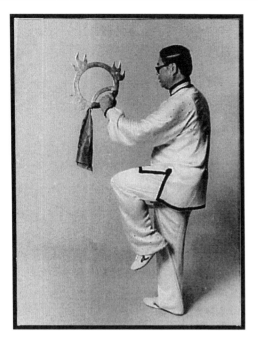

Figure 7-103

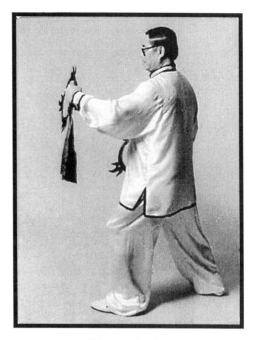

Figure 7-104

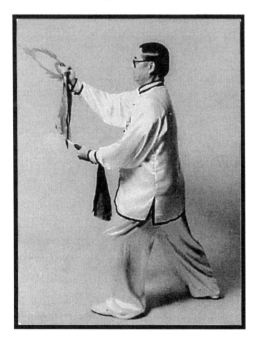

Figure 7-105

Fig. 7-103: Turn your right foot until it points forward. Shift your weight forward into right Bow Stance while lifting your right wheel up and lowering your left leg wheel behind you. Turn your right foot out and stand on it while lifting your leg up. Slice your left wheel down and bring your right wheel up.

31. White Snake Spits The Poison

Movements:

Fig. 7-104: From Fig. 7-103, step up with your left foot forward into left Bow Stance while bringing down your left wheel to mid chest height, parallel to your body.

259

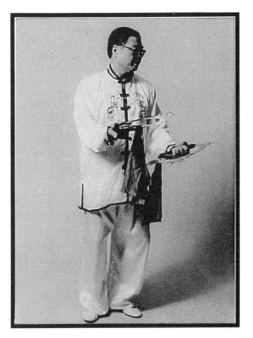
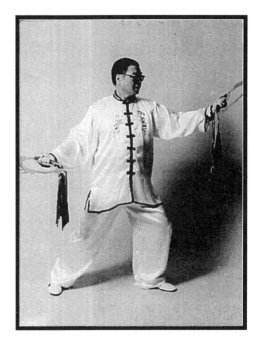

Figure 7-106   **Figure 7-107**

Fig. 7-105: Same Bow Stance as in Fig. 7-104. Turn the left wheel, palm up, to a 45 degree angle to the floor while raising the right wheel, palm up, in an upward thrusting motion across to top of the left wheel.

32. Wind-Fire High And Low Diagonal Cuts

Movements:

Fig. 7-106: From Fig. 7-105, shift the weight to the right foot and draw back left foot next to the right foot while bringing both wheels down to about waist height, palms up.

Fig. 7-107: Step forward left foot into left Bow Stance while bringing left wheel high diagonal cut to the throat and right wheel low diagonal cut to the abdomen.

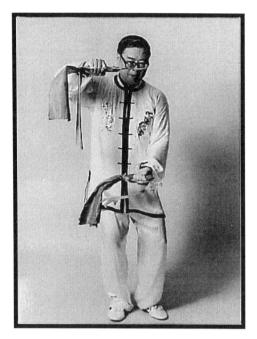

Figure 7-108

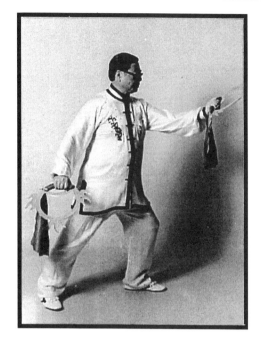

Figure 7-109

33. Left Part Wild Horse's Mane

Movements:

Fig. 7-108: Shift your weight to your left foot while turning your body to the left. Shift your weight back to your right foot while bringing your left foot next to your right.

Fig. 7-109: Step to the left with your left heel touching down first and shift your weight forward into left Bow Stance, while extending your left wheel forward to eye level and slicing down your right wheel next to your hip. (Face East)

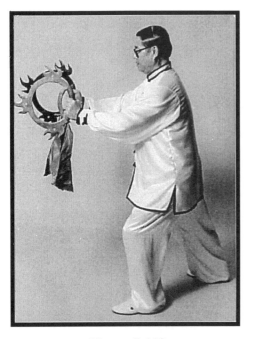

Figure 7-110

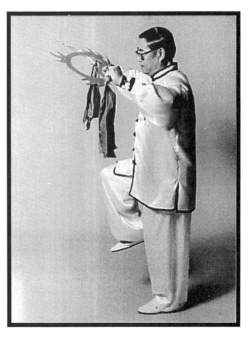

Figure 7-111

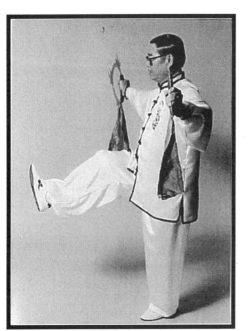

Figure 7-112

34. Right Heel Kick And Strike To Ears

Movements:

Fig. 7-110: Shift your weight to your left foot into Bow Stance while striking with both wheels vertically forward.

Fig. 7-111: Bring your right foot forward to your left, knee high, while rotating both wheels with wheels facing outward at forehead level.

Fig. 7-112: Execute a right Heel Kick to the front while chopping your wheels to both sides of your body. The left knee should bend slightly while doing this. Eyes looking straight ahead.

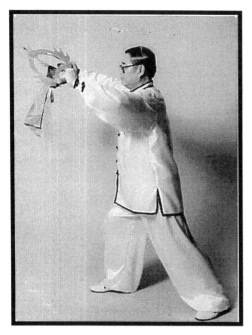

Figure 7-113

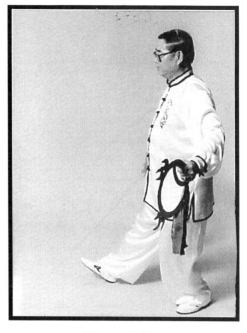

Figure 7-114

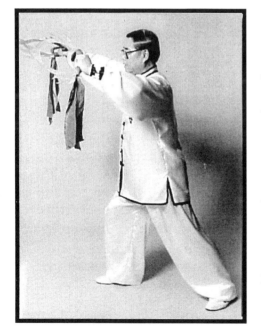

Figure 7-115

Fig. 7-113: Step up with right foot into a Bow Stance, while swinging your wheels upward to face level. Eyes looking between your outstretched wheels.

Fig. 7-114: Shift your weight back onto your left leg and lift the ball of your right foot up, while slicing down your wheels vertically to both sides of your thigh.

Fig. 7-115: Shift your weight onto your right leg into a Bow Stance and swing your wheels upward to ear level.

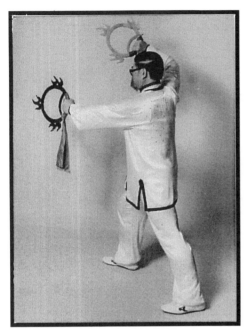 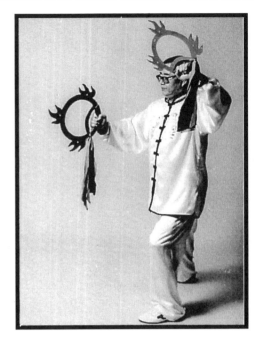

Figure 7-116   Figure 7-117

35. Left Turn Body Fair Lady Shuttles Back And Forth (forward 1 time, backward 1 time)

Movements:

Fig. 7-116: From Fig. 7-115, step down to your front left corner with your left foot. Bring your right wheel to waist height, palm facing up, and lower your left wheel to shoulder height, palm facing down. Shift your weight onto your left foot and bring your right foot next to your left (face north west). Step to your front right corner with your right foot while raising your right wheel up for blocking and extending your left wheel forward for striking.

Fig. 7-117: From Fig. 7-116, shift your weight back to your left foot and turn your right foot out slightly. Then shift all your weight to your right foot and bring your left foot next to your right. Bring your left wheel down to waist height, palm facing up, and lower your right wheel to shoulder height, palm facing down. (Face South West). Step to your front left corner with your left foot while raising your left wheel up for blocking and extending your right wheel forward for striking.

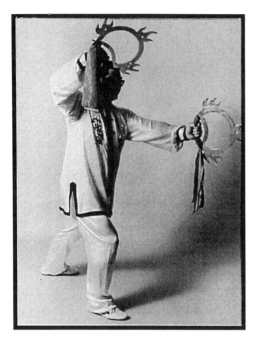

Figure 7-118

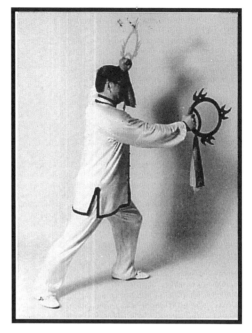

Figure 7-119

Fig. 7-118: From Fig. 7-117, turn your left foot in and right foot out as you turn 180 degrees to your right. Shift your weight to your left foot and bring your right foot next to your left. Rotate and bring your right wheel to waist height, palm facing up, and lower your left wheel to shoulder height, palm facing down. (Face South East). Step to your front right corner with your right foot while raising your right wheel up for blocking and extending your left wheel forward for striking.

Fig. 7-119: From Fig. 7-118, shift your weight back to your left foot and turn your right foot out slightly. Then shift all your weight to your right foot and bring your left foot next to your right. Bring your left wheel down to waist height, palm facing up, and lower your right wheel to shoulder height, palm facing down (face North East). Step to your front left corner with your left foot while raising your left wheel up for blocking and extending your right wheel forward for striking.

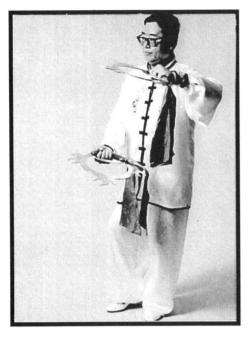

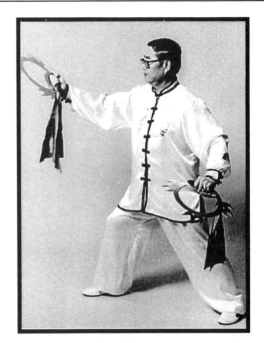

Figure 7-120   **Figure 7-121**

36. Left Turn Right Part Wild Horse's Mane

Movements:

Fig. 7-120: Bend down both knees slightly, then shift your weight to your left foot while turning your body to the left. During the twisting moment, rotate both wheels to face each other. Eyes looking in the same direction as your left hand.

Fig. 7-121: Step out your right foot into a right Bow Stance, while slicing your left wheel down next to your hip and extending your right wheel forward to the eye level.

37. Left Turn Body Fist Under The Elbow

Movements:

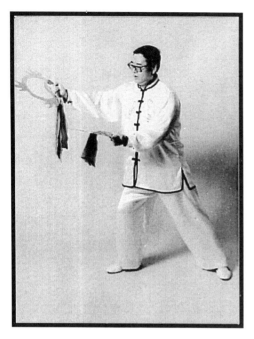

Figure 7-122

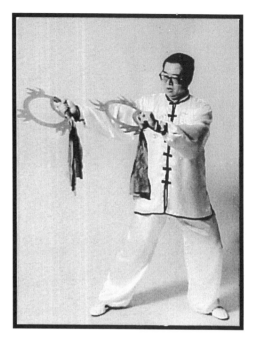

Figure 7-123

Fig. 7-122: Raise the wheels to shoulder height bending the elbows.

Fig. 7-123: Shift your weight on your left foot.

Fig. 7-124: Step into left Bow Stance and rotate your waist to the left while bringing your right wheel upward and your left wheel downward to your left.

Fig. 7-125: Draw your left foot next to your right foot. Swing both wheels in a circular motion downward and bring your left wheel point out to front at waist height while raising your right wheel to shoulder height.

Fig. 7-126: Step up with your left foot forward as in a Cat Stance. Strike left wheel, the right wheel, palm to center, in a vertical forward cutting motion, to mid abdomen.

Fig. 7-127: Same Cat Stance as in Fig. 7-126. Slice your right wheel down and your left wheel up.

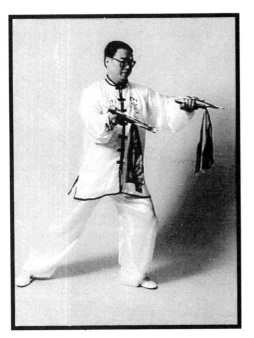

Figure 7-124

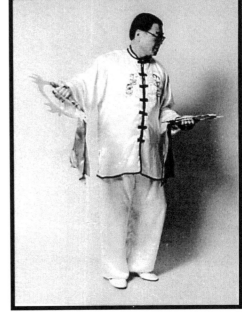

Figure 7-125

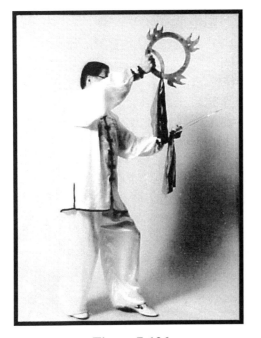

Figure 7-126

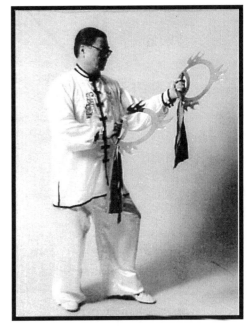

Figure 7-127

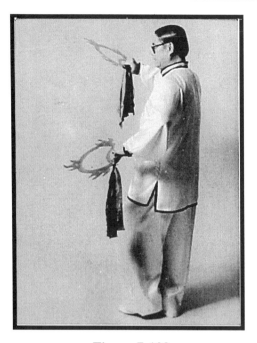

Figure 7-128

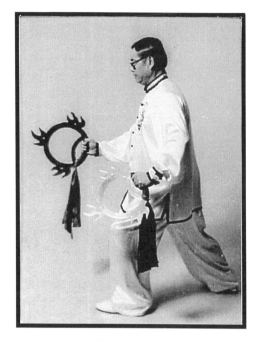

Figure 7-129

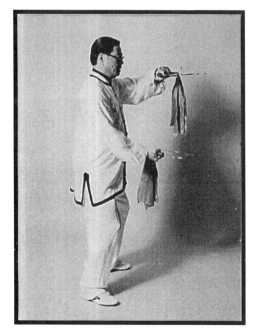

Figure 7-130

38. Step Forward And Strike Down

Movements:

Fig. 7-128: Shift the weight to your left foot and bring right foot next to your left foot while lowering your right wheel and raising your left wheel to shoulder height.

Fig. 7-129: Slice down your right wheel to your right side waist while striking your left wheel forward vertically to the knee level.

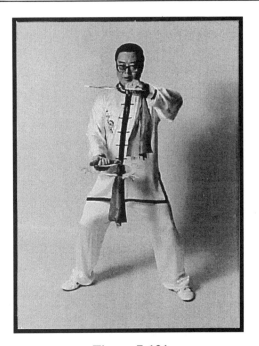

Figure 7-131

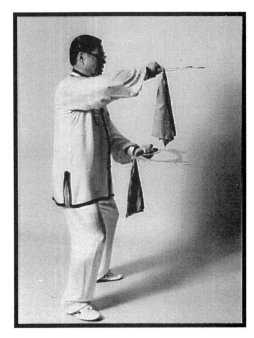

Figure 7-132

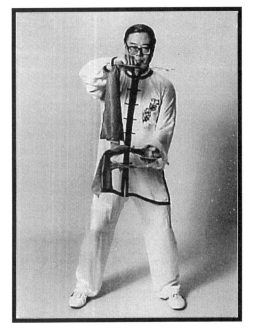

Figure 7-133

39. Wind-Fire Turning Wheels (3 times)

Movements:

Figs. 7-130 to 7-133 same as posture **14** in this Form. Refer to Figs. 7-43 to 7-45.

40. Step Back And Ride The Tiger

Movements:

Fig. 7-134: Revolve two wheels with the right wheel down and the left wheel up.

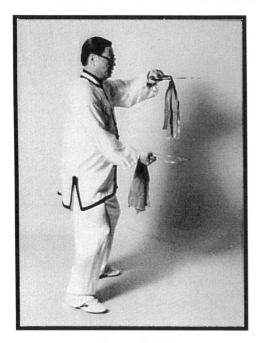

Figure 7-134

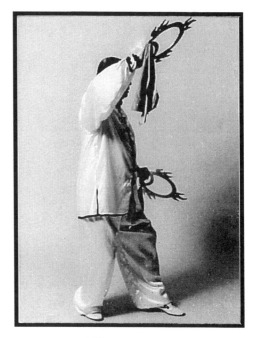

Figure 7-135

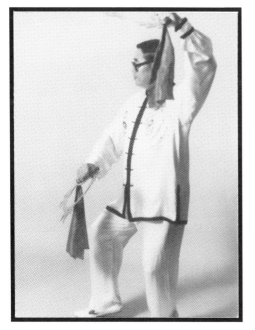

Figure 7-136

Fig. 7-135: Step back the right foot into a Cat Stance while bringing the right wheel in an upward arc motion to above the head and bringing the left wheel a downward arc motion to the left side waist of the body.

41. Right Turn Body Wind-Fire Protecting The Head And Right Heel Kick

Movements:

Fig. 7-136: Shift your weight to your right and make a 180 degree right turn of your body. Shift your weight back to your left foot and bring your right foot to Cat Stance, while raising your left wheel up with blades toward front

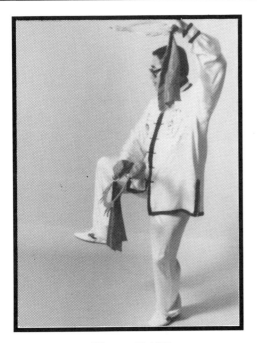

Figure 7-137

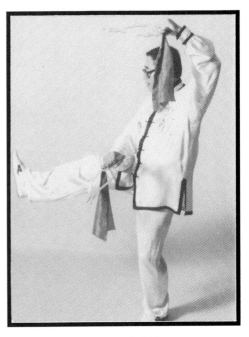

Figure 7-138

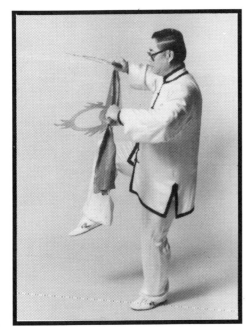

Figure 7-139

to protect your head and slicing your right wheel from outward down to your groin area.

Fig. 7-137: Lift your right foot to knee height.

Fig. 7-138: Make right heel kick to the front.

42. Left Slicing And Right Striking

Movements:

Fig. 7-139: Bring back your left leg while lowering your left wheel and raising your right wheel to shoulder height.

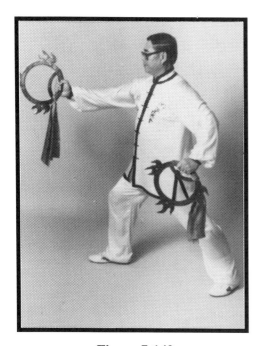

Figure 7-140

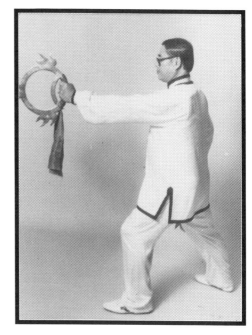

Figure 7-141

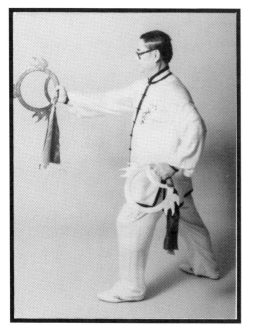

Figure 7-142

Fig. 7-140: Slice down your left wheel to your left side waist while striking your right wheel forward vertically.

43. Step Forward Left And Right Strikings

Movements:

Fig. 7-141: Step left foot forward and make left wheel striking vertically.

Fig. 7-142: Keep same stance and make right wheel striking forward vertically.

273

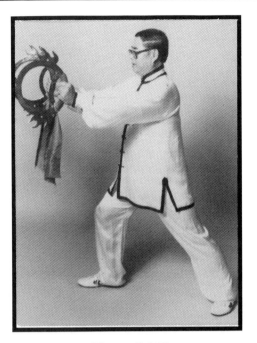

Figure 7-143

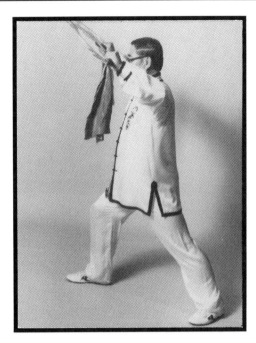

Figure 7-144

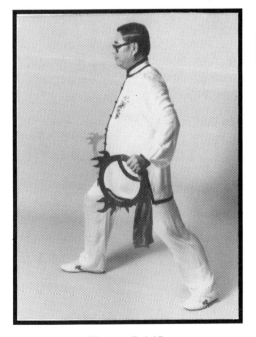

Figure 7-145

44. Appears Closed

Movements:

Fig. 7-143: From Fig. 7-142, step up your right leg and complete Bow Stance while striking left wheel forward vertically.

Fig. 7-144: Keep the same stance and bring both Wind-Fire Wheels forehead high separately. Eyes Looking straight ahead.

Fig. 7-145: Rotate both wheels down to your waist while keeping the right Bow Stance.

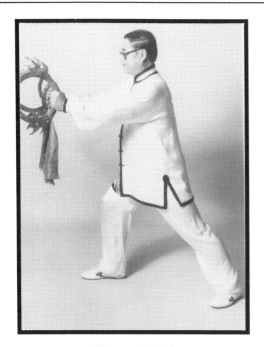

Figure 7-146

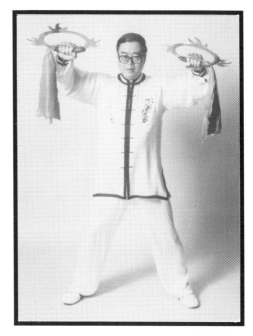

Figure 7-147

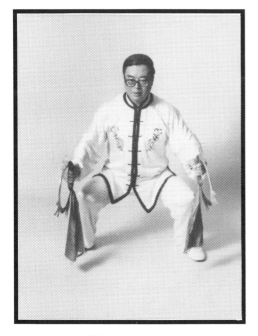

Figure 7-148

Fig. 7-146: Strike forward with both Wind-Fire wheels and complete the posture as shown in the picture. Eyes looking ahead, in eye level direction.

45. Wing-Fire Closing

Movements:

Fig. 7-147: From Fig. 7-146, shift your weight to your left foot, lift the ball of your right foot up and begin turning your body 90 degrees to your left while raising both wind fire wheels outward to forehead height.

Fig. 7-148: Shift your body weight evenly to both feet and begin lowering your body, while bringing down your wheels in a circular motion to knee height.

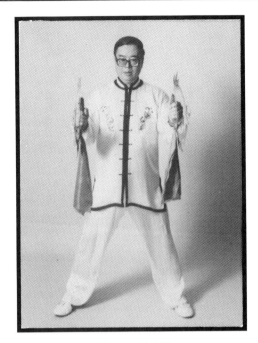

Figure 7-149

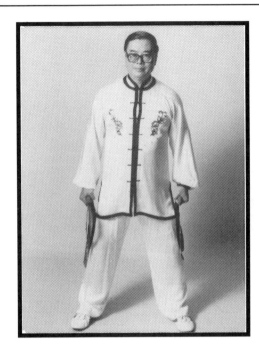

Figure 7-150

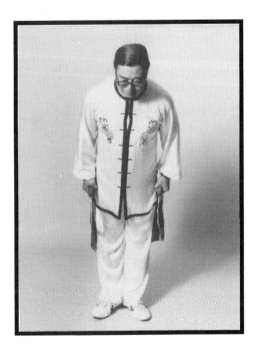

Figure 7-151

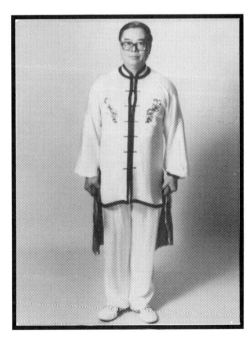

Figure 7-152

Fig. 7-149: Stand up gradually, but keep your knees bent slightly while bringing both wheels chest high and shoulder width apart. Then rotate the Wind Fire Wheels outward, down and up three times.

46. Return to Origin

Movements:

Fig. 7-150: Bring down both wheels to the sides of your body. Eyes are looking directly ahead.

Fig. 7-151: Bring your left foot next to your right and bow to your teachers or spectators politely.

Fig. 7-152: Return to your original Preparatory Posture.

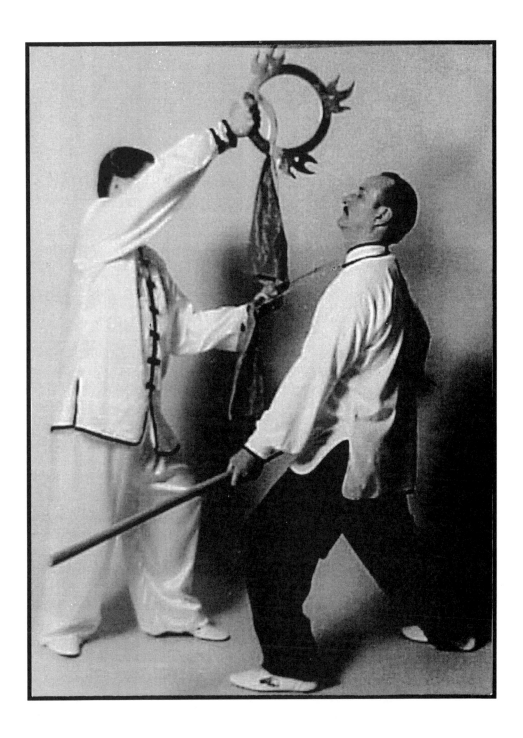

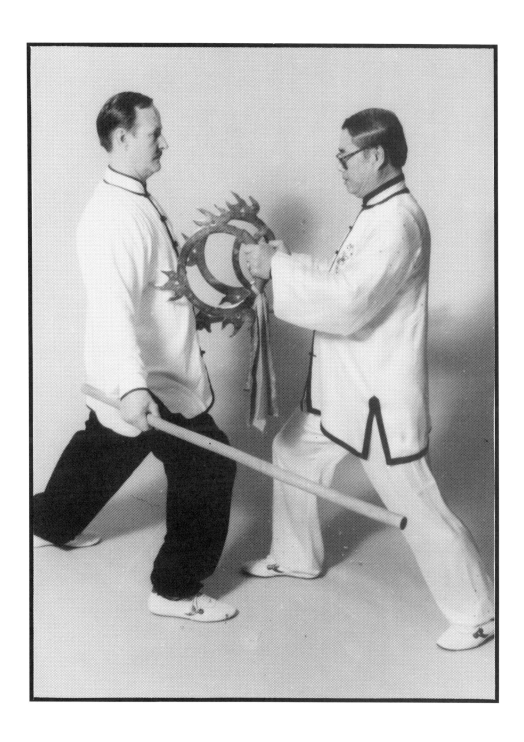

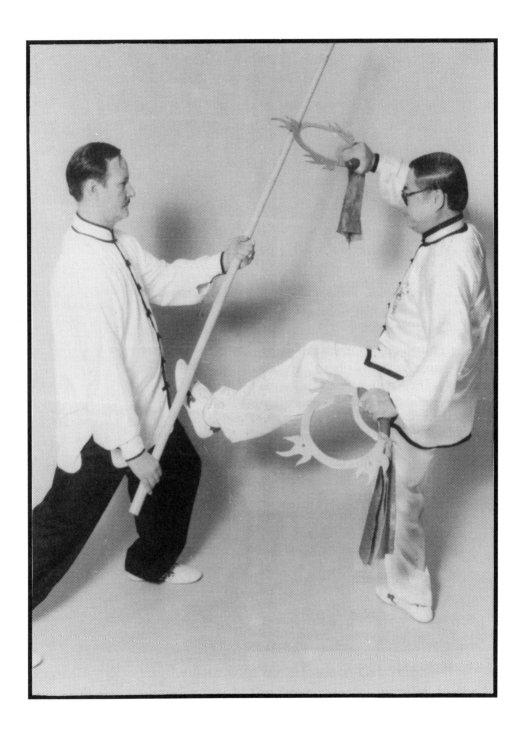

CHAPTER 8

SELF-DEFENSE APPLICATIONS

8.1 Introduction

The self-defense applications presented here are intended to provide examples of how the Wind-Fire Wheels could be used in different martial techniques. The effective execution of these combined techniques depends upon the depth of understanding and degree of skill developed in the previous chapters.

In this chapter, applications of Wind-Fire Wheels are demonstrated. These applications represent a wide range of techniques that can be used in a variety of typical weapon fighting situations. It is advisable that the reader practice a technique repeatedly and at full speed. The reaction should be automatic

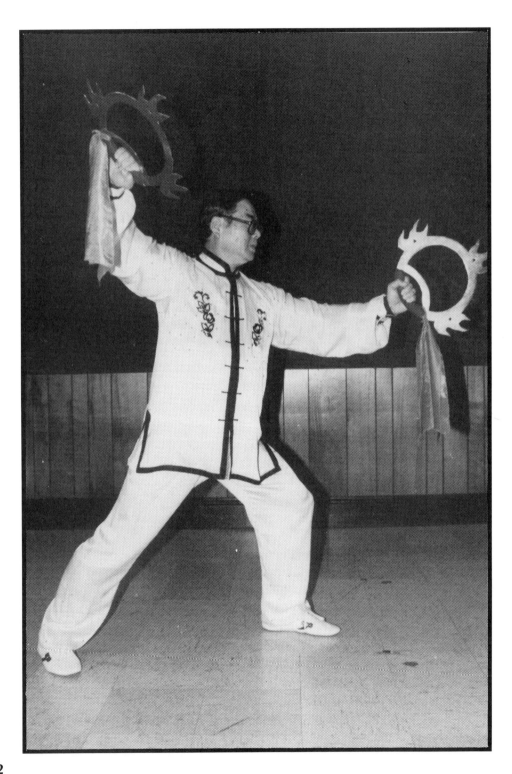

because, in a real fighting situation, there is no time to think of the mechanics of a technique.

The key to mastery of the Wind-Fire Wheels is constant practice, but always with correct posture, proper stances and good breathing. Persons trained in Tai-Chi Chuan should use their Tai-Chi basics as a foundation for the Wind-Fire techniques. Though this has always been true with the performance of the barehand forms, this is more emphatic when using weapons. With more practice, the players could expand on these applications by creating combinations in addition to those developed in this chapter.

8.2 Self-Defense Applications

1. Application Of "Wind-Fire Commencing" And "Ward Off"
2. Application Of "Wind-Fire Commencing" And "Roll Back And Press"
3. Application Of "Push"
4. Application Of "Single Whip"
5. Application Of "Single Whip-Alternative Method"
6. Application Of "Lifting Hand"
7. Application Of "Wind-Fire Commencing And Wind-Fire Turning Wheels"
8. Application Of "Wind-Fire Turning Wheels - Alternative Method"
9. Application Of "White Crane Spreads Its Wings And Heel Kick"
10. Application Of "Brush Knee And Step Forward"
11. Application Of "Brush Knee And Step Forward - Alternative

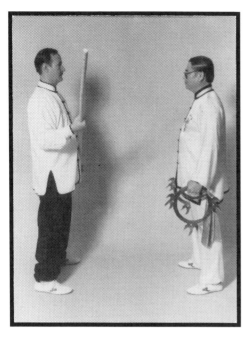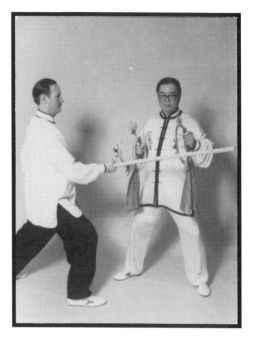

| Figure 8-1 | Figure 8-2 |

1. Application Of "Wind-Fire Commencing" And "Ward Off"

** The attacker (wearing black pants) will be denoted as B in the following photographs and text. The defender (wearing white) will be denoted as W.

Fig. 8-1: (B) and (W) are facing each other.

Fig. 8-2: (B) tries a straight thrust strike with the cudgel to (W's) midsection of the body. (W) quickly steps to the right side into a Horse Stance and parries with a block using a "Wind Fire Commencing" technique.

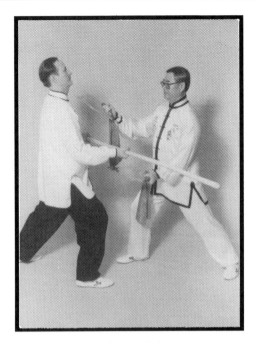

Figure 8-3

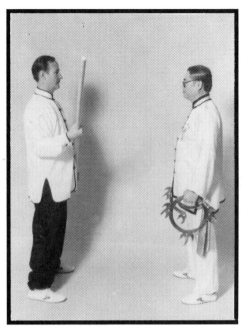

Figure 8-4

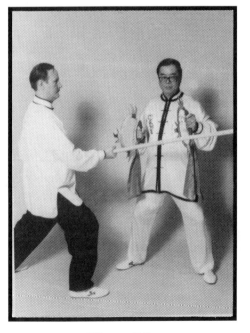

Figure 8-5

Fig. 8-3: (W) presses the cudgel outward and down and strikes to (B's) throat and abdomen by using the "Ward Off" technique while shifting stance into a right Bow Stance.

2. Application Of "Wind-Fire Commencing" And "Roll Back And Press"

Fig. 8-4: Refer to Fig. 8-1.

Fig. 8-5: Refer to Fig. 8-2.

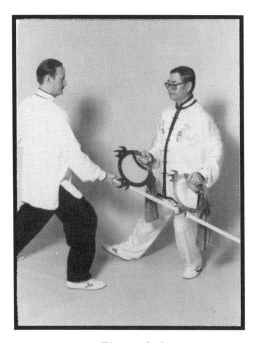

Figure 8-6

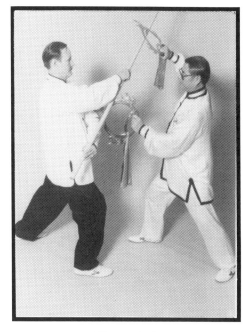

Figure 8-7

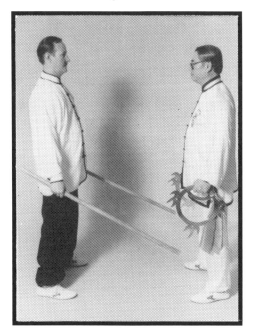

Figure 8-8

Fig. 8-6: (W) presses down the cudgel by using "Roll Back " technique.

Fig. 8-7: (B) moves the cudgel up and tries a reverse strike to (W's) right temple (W) quickly executes a "Press" technique while shifting stance into a right Bow Stance.

3. Application Of "Push"

Fig. 8-8: Refer to Fig. 8-1.

Fig. 8-9: (B) tries a double sticks strike to both sides of (W's) temple.

(W) quickly shifts back the weight to the left leg and tips the right heel

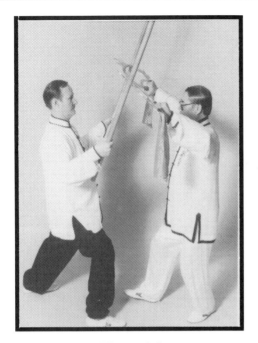

Figure 8-9

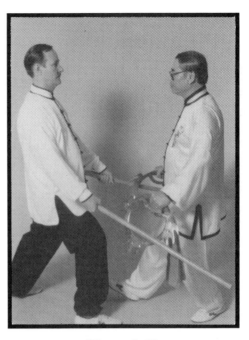

Figure 8-10

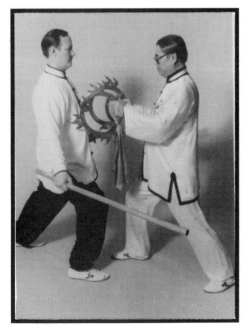

Figure 8-11

while blocking (B's) sticks upward with both wheels.

Fig. 8-10: (W) brings down the sticks with Wind-Fire Wheels and pushes them away.

Fig. 8-11: (W) immediately executes a "Push" technique and strikes to (B's) chest.

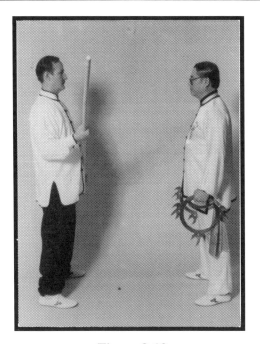

Figure 8-12

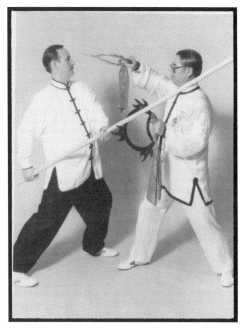

Figure 8-13

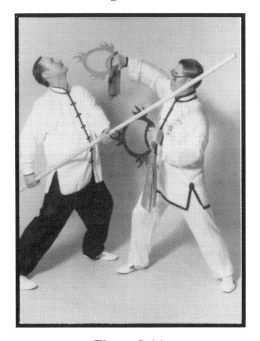

Figure 8-14

4. Application Of "Single Whip"

Fig. 8-12: Refer to Fig. 8-1.

Fig. 8-13: (B) tries a straight thrust strike with the cudgel to (W's) eyes or face. (W) quickly steps to the right side into a right Bow Stance and deflects the cudgel using the left wheel while striking to (B's) eyes with the right wheel.

Fig. 8-14: By making use of the "Single Whip", (W) cuts (B's) throat with the right wheel.

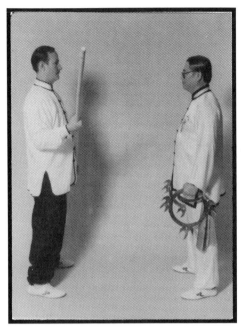 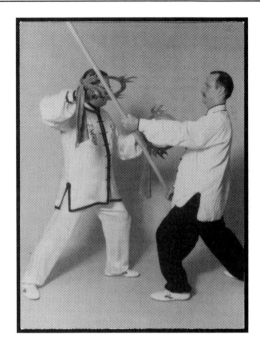

Figure 8-15   **Figure 8-16**

5. Application Of "Single Whip-Alternative Method"

Fig. 8-15: Refer to Fig. 8-1.

Fig. 8-16: (B) attempts a high strike with the cudgel to (W's) head. (W) quickly intercepts the strike and controls the cudgel with the right wheel while striking to (B's) chest with the left wheel completing the " Single Whip" technique (picture shown on the other side).

6. Application Of "Lifting Hand"

Fig. 8-17: Refer to Fig. 8-1.

Fig. 8-18: (B) tries an upward thrust strike with the cudgel aiming for (W's) eyes or face while making a low knee stance. (W) quickly steps to the right

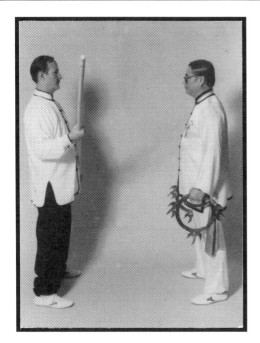

Figure 8-17

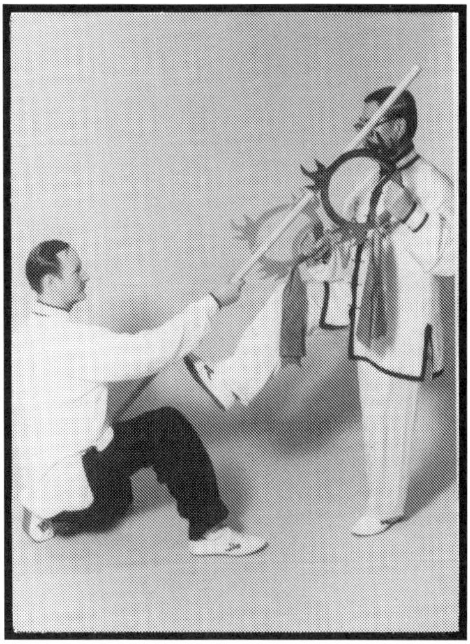

Figure 8-18

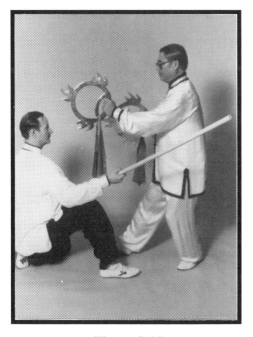

Figure 8-19

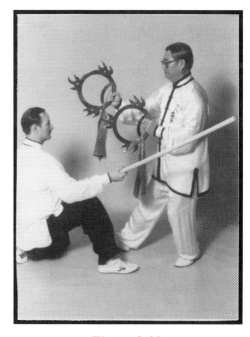

Figure 8-20

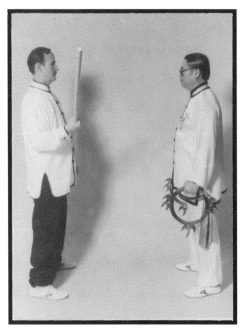 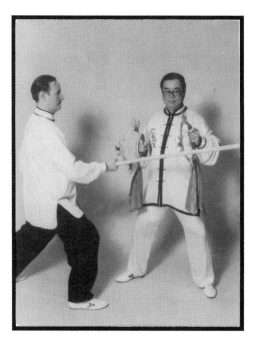

Figure 8-21   **Figure 8-22**

side and blocks the cudgel in between the two wheels while simultaneously making a snap right toe kick to (B).

Fig. 8-19: (W) brings down the left wheel while pushing away the cudgel to the left side with the right wheel. Immediately (W) brings the left wheel up and cuts to (B's) face.

Fig. 8-20: (W) rotates both Wind-Fire Wheels outward one time vertically to strike (B's) face.

7.   Application Of "Wind-Fire Commencing" And "Wind-Fire Turning Wheels"

Fig. 8-21: Refer to Fig. 8-1.

Fig. 8-22: Refer to Fig. 8-2.

Fig. 8-23: (W) then turns right wheel up to block the cudgel and pushes it away while turning left wheel down to slice (B).

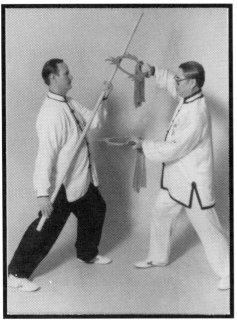

Figure 8-23

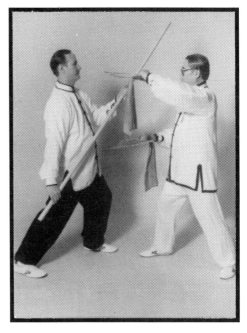

Figure 8-24

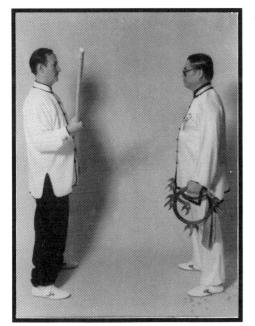

Figure 8-25

Fig. 8-24: (W) revolves two wheels once again with right wheel down and left wheel up to complete "Wind-Fire Turning Wheels".

8. Application Of "Wind-Fire Turning Wheels - Alternative Method"

Fig. 8-25: Refer to Fig. 8-1.

Fig. 8-26: (B) assumes a low knee stance with an upward thrust strike of the cudgel to (W's) eyes or face. (W) quickly makes a Horse Stance and intercepts the strike with a "Turning Wheels" technique of the right wheel blocking and the left wheel striking.

293

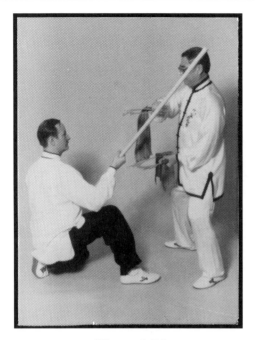

Figure 8-26

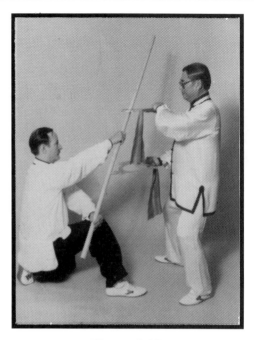

Figure 8-27

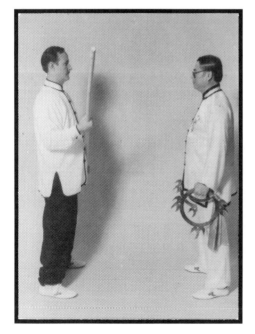

Figure 8-28

Fig. 8-27: (W) immediately revolves two wheels once again to block the reverse cudgel strike and strike to (B's) hand.

9. Application Of "White Crane Spreads Its Wings And Heel Kick"

Fig. 8-28: Refer to Fig. 8-1.

Fig. 8-29: (B) tries an overhead cudgel strike to (W's) right temple. (W) quickly shifts most weight to the right leg while stepping the left foot forward in a Cat Stance and applies a "White Crane Spreads Its Wings " technique to (B's) cudgel.

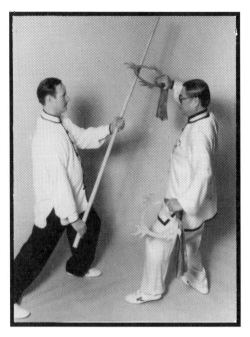 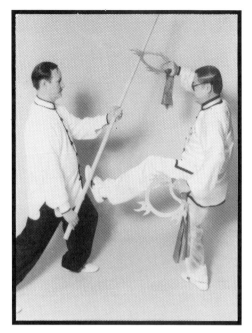

Figure 8-29   **Figure 8-30**

Fig. 8-30: (W) immediately executes a left " Heel Kick" technique to (B).

10. Application Of "Brush Knee And Step Forward"

Fig. 8-31: Refer to Fig. 8-1.

Fig. 8-32: (B) assumes a right Bow Stance and tries a lower straight thrust strike with the cudgel to (W's) knee. (W) quickly steps to the right side and makes a left Cat Stance with a left " Brush Knee" technique to block down (B's) cudgel.

Fig. 8-33: (W) immediately steps into left Bow Stance and strikes (B's) chest with right wheel.

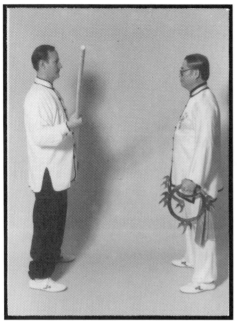

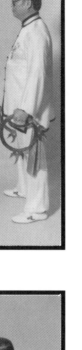

Figure 8-31

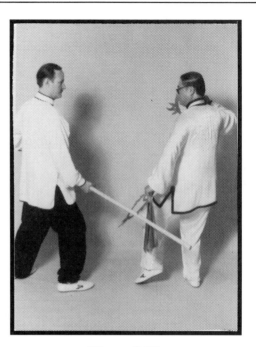

Figure 8-32

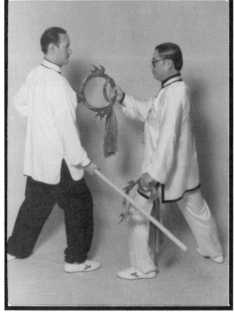

Figure 8-33

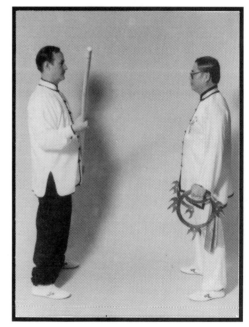

Figure 8-34

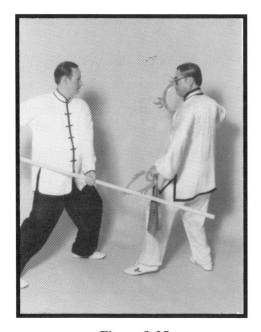

Figure 8-35

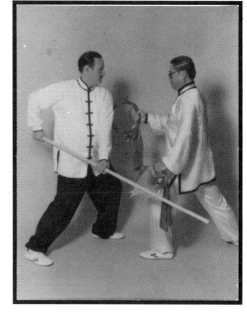

Figure 8-36

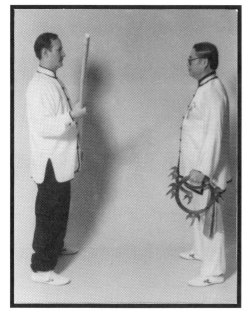

Figure 8-37

11. Application Of "Brush Knee And Step Forward -Alternative Method"

Fig. 8-34: Refer to Fig. 8-1.

Fig. 8-35: (B) makes a left Bow Stance and assumes a lower straight thrust strike with the cudgel to (W's) knee. Then refer to Fig. 8-32.

Fig. 8-36: (W) immediately steps into left Bow Stance and strikes (B's) kidney with right wheel.

297

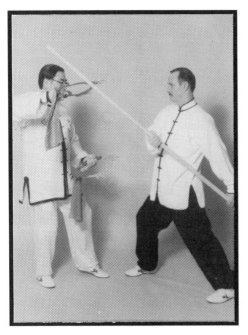

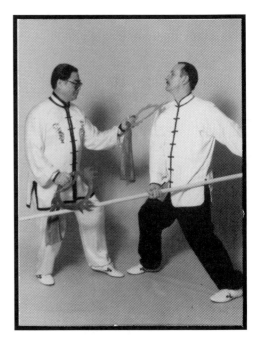

Figure 8-38   Figure 8-39

12. Application Of "Playing The Lute"

Fig. 8-37: Refer to Fig. 8-1.

Fig. 8-38: (B) tries an upward thrust strike with the cudgel pointing directly to (W's) face. (W) quickly steps to left side with a left Cat Stance and blocks the cudgel with the right wheel. (picture shown on other side).

Fig. 8-39: (W) immediately executes a "Playing The Lute" technique striking to (B's) throat with the left wheel while pressing down the cudgel with the right wheel.

13. Application Of "Wind-Fire Protecting The Head And Right Heel Kick"

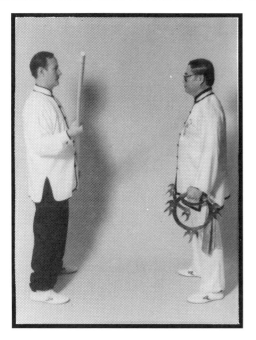

Figure 8-40

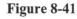

Figure 8-41

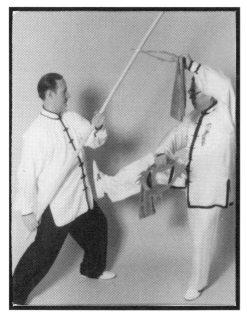

Figure 8-42

Fig. 8-40: Refer to Fig. 8-1.

Fig. 8-41: (B) assumes an overhead attack with the cudgel to (W's) head. (W) quickly steps into a right Cat Stance and uses a "Wind-Fire Protecting The Head" technique with the left wheel blocking and the right wheel slicing to (B's) knee.

Fig. 8-42: (W) immediately executes a " Right Heel Kick" to (B's) left ribs.

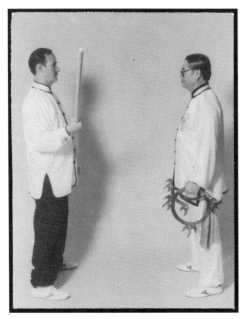

Figure 8-43

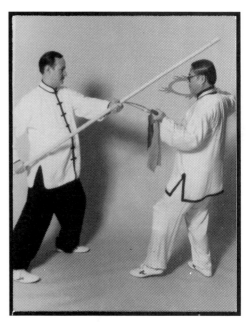

Figure 8-44

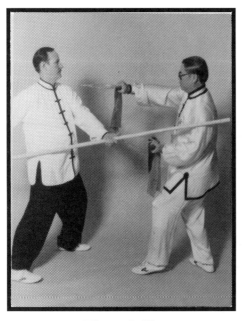

Figure 8-45

14. Application Of "Reverse Reeling Forearm"

Fig. 8-43: Refer to Fig. 8-1.

Fig. 8-44: (B) launches an upward thrust strike with the cudgel to (W's) face. (W) quickly assumes a left Cat Stance and blocks the cudgel with the left wheel using an outward blocking.

Fig. 8-45: (W's) side edge of the left wheel deflects the cudgel down and immediately thrusts the right wheel into (B's) throat.

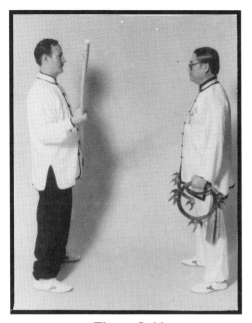

Figure 8-46

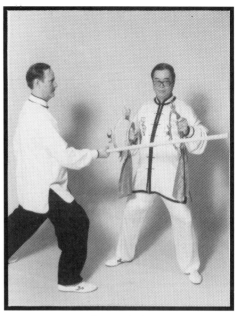

Figure 8-47

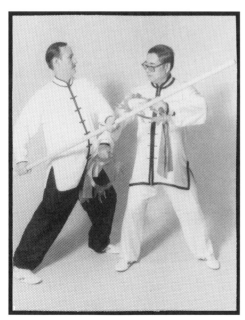

Figure 8-48

15. Application Of "Reverse Reeling Forearm-Alternative Method"

Fig. 8-46: Refer to Fig. 8-1.

Fig. 8-47: (B) launches a straight thrust strike with the cudgel to (W's) chest. (W) quickly steps to the right side into Horse Stance and blocks the cudgel with a "Wind-Fire Commencing" technique.

Fig. 8-48: (W) immediately turns right into a right Bow Stance while deflecting the cudgel with the left wheel and striking (B's) groin with the right wheel. (picture shown on the other side)

301

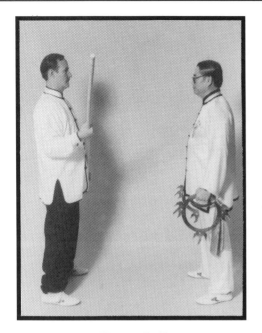

Figure 8-49

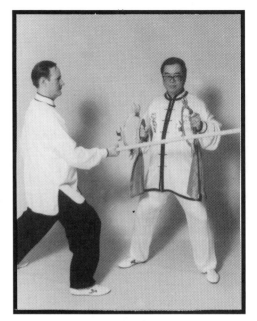

Figure 8-50

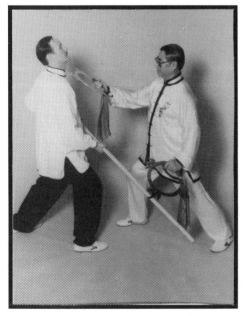

Figure 8-51

16. Application Of "Wind-Fire Commencing" And "Parting Wild Horse's Mane"

Fig. 8-49: Refer to Fig. 8-1.

Fig. 8-50: Refer to Fig. 8-47.

Fig. 8-51: (W) quickly steps right into a right Bow Stance while deflecting the cudgel downward with the left wheel and striking (B's) throat with the right wheel.

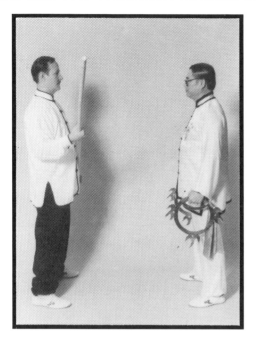

Figure 8-52

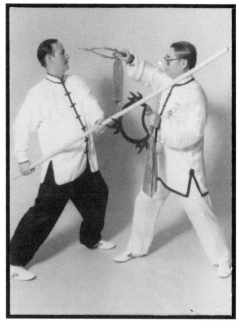

Figure 8-53

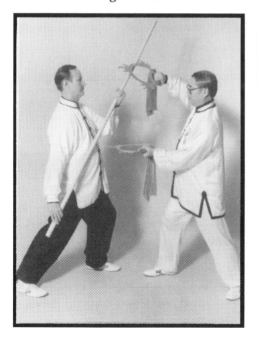

Figure 8-54

17. Application Of "Wave Hands Like Clouds"

Fig. 8-52: Refer to Fig. 8-1.

Fig. 8-53: (B) tries an upward straight thrust strike with the cudgel to (W's) face. (W) quickly deflects the cudgel with the left wheel and strikes to (B's) eyes with the right wheel while shifting into a right Bow Stance.

Fig. 8-54: (W) continues a "Cloud Hand" technique to block and strike (B).

Fig. 8-55: Picture is shown from the other side.

Fig. 8-56 and 8-57: (W) completes the "Wave Hands Like Clouds" technique.

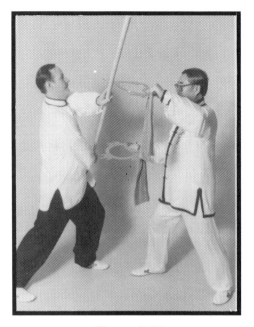

Figure 8-55

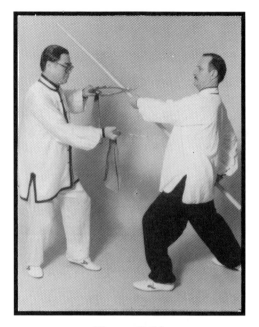

Figure 8-56

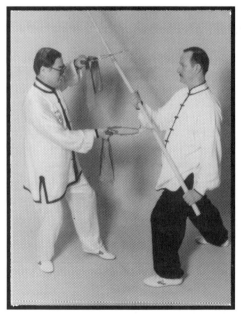

Figure 8-57

18. Application Of "High Pat On Horse"

Fig. 8-58: Refer to Fig. 8-1.

Fig. 8-59: (B) launches a high straight thrust strike with the cudgel to (W's) face. (W) quickly slides to the right into a left Cat Stance while deflecting the cudgel to the left with the outside edge of left wheel.

Fig. 8-60: (W) forcefully presses the cudgel downward with the left wheel and thrusts the front head of the right wheel into (B's) throat completing a " High Pat On Horse" technique.

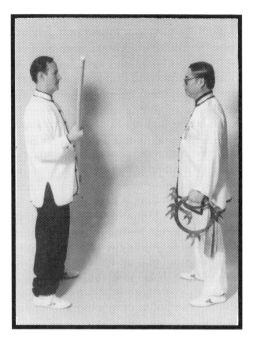

Figure 8-58

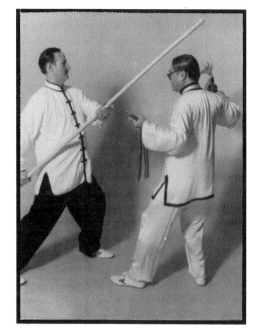

Figure 8-59

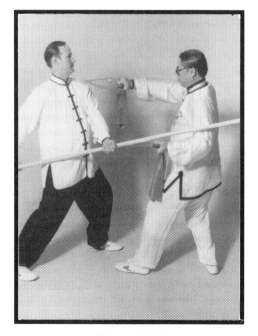

Figure 8-60

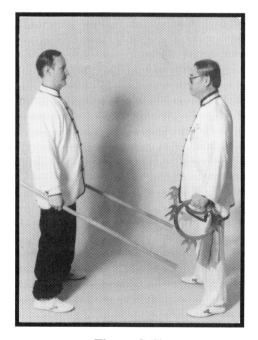

Figure 8-61

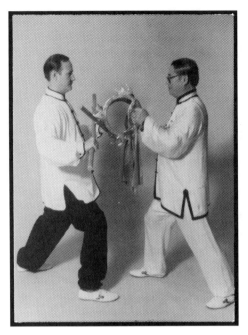
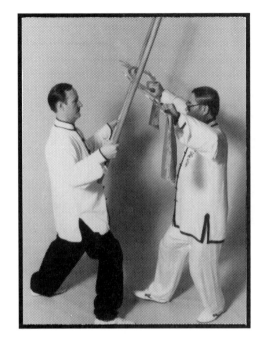

Figure 8-62   Figure 8-63

19. Application Of "Heel Kick And Strikes To Ears"

Fig. 8-61: Refer to Fig. 8-1.

Fig. 8-62: (W) tries a double wheels straight thrust strike to (B's) chest. (B) quickly blocks the wheels with a double cross sticks technique.

Fig. 8-63: (B) launches a double sticks strike to (W's) temples. (W) immediately shifts back the weight to the left leg and tips right heel while upward blocking (B's) sticks with both wheels.

Fig. 8-64: (W) forcefully presses both sticks downward and away with both wheels.

Fig. 8-65: (W) executes a front Heel Kick to (B's) lower section of the body.

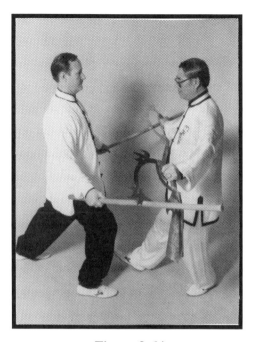

Figure 8-64

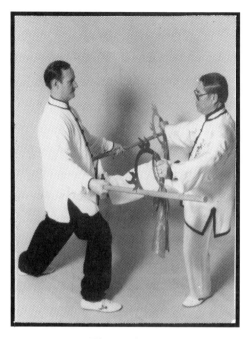

Figure 8-65

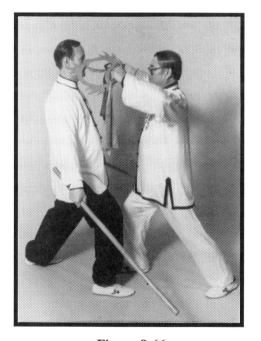

Figure 8-66

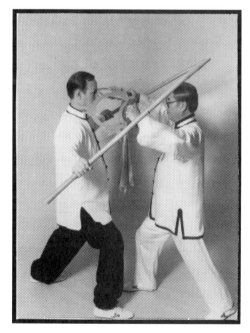

Figure 8-67

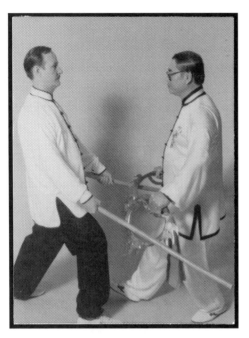

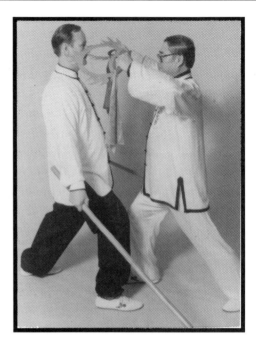

Figure 8-68   Figure 8-69

Fig. 8-66: (W) steps forward with the right foot into a right Bow Stance while striking with both wheels to (B's) temples.

Fig. 8-67: (B) tries a fake double sticks strike to (W's) temples.

Fig. 8-68: (B) suddenly swings both sticks from outside downward to strike both of (W's) knees. (W) immediately blocks both sticks downward and pushes away with both wheels.

Fig. 8-69: (W) once again executes a "Double Wheels Strike Temple" technique.

20. Application Of "Lower Body"

Fig. 8-70: Refer to Fig. 8-1.

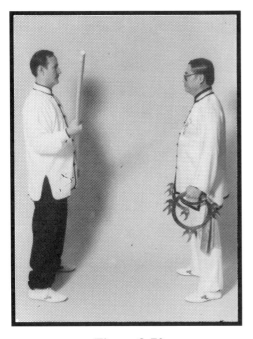

Figure 8-70

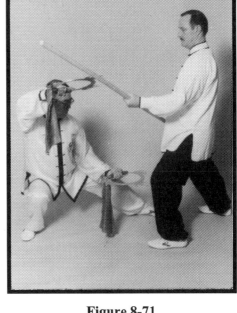

Figure 8-71

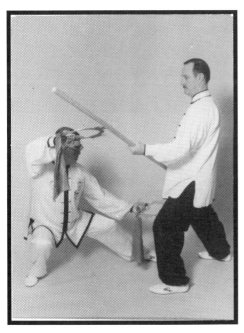

Fig. 8-71: (B) launches a straight thrust strike with the cudgel to (W's) chest. (W) immediately "Lowers Body" into the "Taming The Tiger Stance" while deflecting the cudgel with the right wheel and cutting (B's) knee with the left wheel.

Fig. 8-72: (B) extends the left wheel cutting to (B's) groin.

Figure 8-72

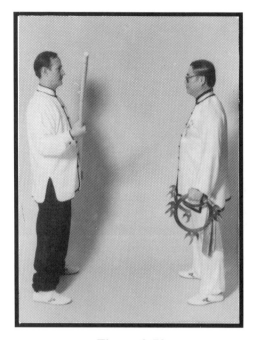

Figure 8-73

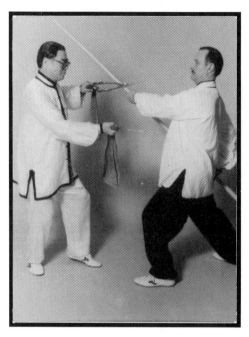

Figure 8-74

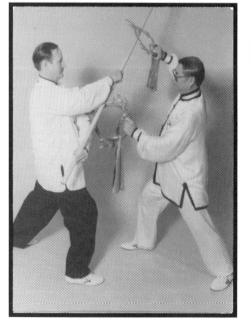

Figure 8-75

21. Application Of "Fair Lady Shuttles Back And Forth"

Fig. 8-73: Refer to Fig. 8-1.

Fig. 8-74: (B) tries a high straight thrust strike to (W's) eyes or face. (W) immediately steps to the right side into left Cat Stance while blocking the cudgel with the left wheel and cutting (B's) arm with the right wheel. (pictures shown on the other side)

Fig. 8-75: (B) quickly uses a reverse striking with the cudgel to (W's) temple. (W) immediately applies a "Fair Lady Shuttles Back And Forth" technique with the right wheel blocking the cudgel and the left wheel striking (B's) chest.

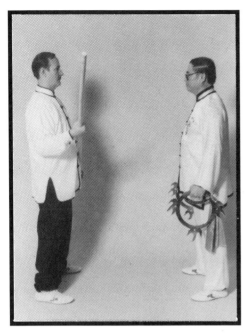

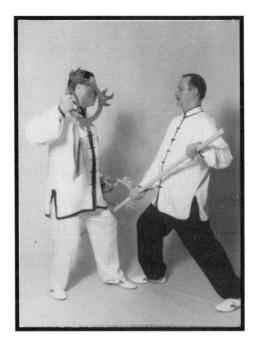

Figure 8-76   **Figure 8-77**

22. Application Of "Needle At Sea Bottom And Fan Through Back"

Fig. 8-76: Refer to Fig. 8-1.

Fig. 8-77: (B) tries a low swing strike with the cudgel to (W's) knee. (W) quickly steps to the right with the left foot into a Cat Stance and blocks the cudgel downward with the left wheel (picture shown on the other side).

Fig. 8-78: (W) forcefully presses the cudgel down with the blocking wheel while cutting (B's) face with the front part of the right wheel.

Fig. 8-79: (W) extends the cutting down to (B's) groin with the same wheel and completes the " Needle At Sea Bottom" technique.

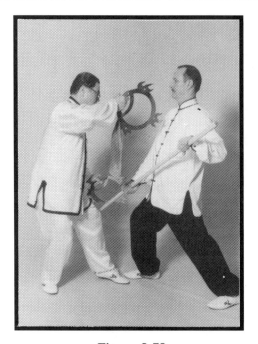

Figure 8-78

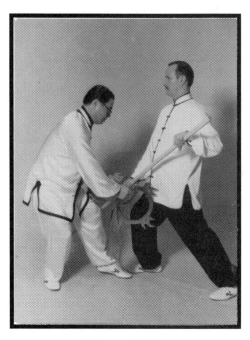

Figure 8-79

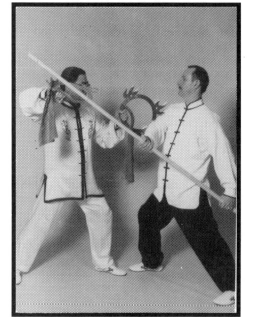

Figure 8-80

Fig. 8-80: (B) assumes a reverse swing strike with the cudgel to (W's) right temple. (W) quickly deflects the cudgel using the right wheel while striking with the left wheel to (B's) arm and completes the " Fan Through Back " technique.

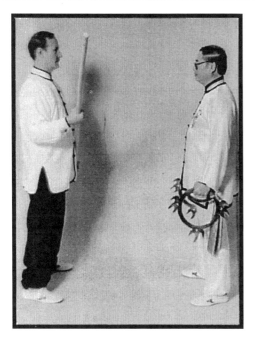

Figure 8-81

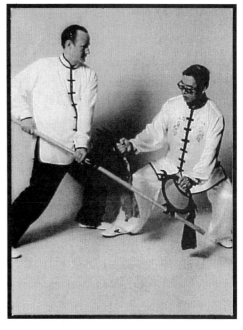

Figure 8-82

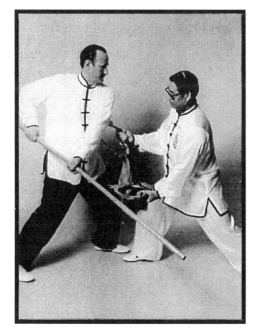

Figure 8-83

23. Application Of "Embrace The Tiger And Return To The Mountain"

Fig. 8-81: Refer to Fig. 8-1.

Fig. 8-82: (B) makes a left Bow Stance and assumes a lower straight thrust strike with the cudgel to (W's) knee. (W) quickly steps to the right side and drops down into a deep Horse Stance while blocking down (B's) cudgel with both wheels.

Fig. 8-83: (W) immediately steps into right Bow Stance and strikes (B's) Kidney with right wheel.

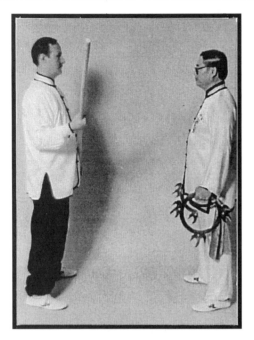

Figure 8-84

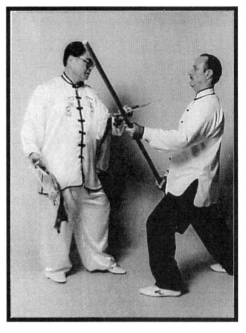

Figure 8-85

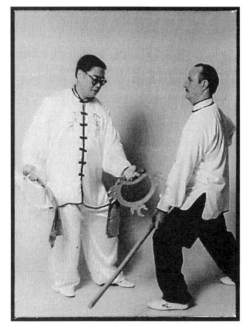

Figure 8-86

24. Application Of "Fist Under The Elbow"

Fig. 8-84: Refer to Fig.8-1.

Fig. 8-85: (B) tries a high straight thrust strike with the cudgel to (W's) face. (W) quickly steps to the left side and assumes a Cat Stance while blocking the cudgel with the left wheel. (Picture shown on the other side.)

Fig. 8-86: (W) maintain same Stance while press down (B's) cudgel with left wheel.

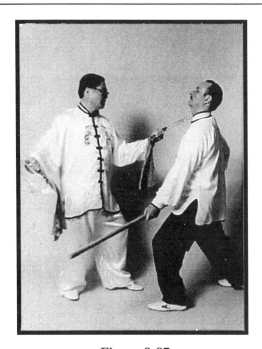

Figure 8-87

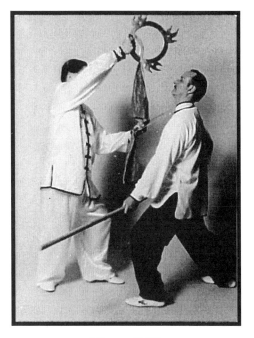

Figure 8-88

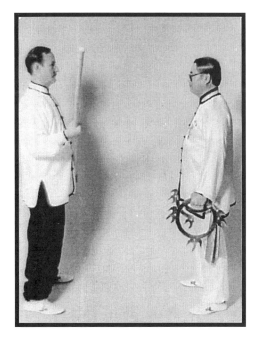

Figure 8-89

Fig. 8-87: (W) quickly uses a left wheel strike to throat height.

Fig. 8-88: (W) executes a right wheel strike, palm to center, in a vertical forward cutting down motion to mid abdomen.

25. Application Of "Diagonal Flying"

Fig. 8-89: Refer to Fig. 8-1.

Fig. 8-90: (B) makes a right Bow Stance and assumes a lower straight thrust strike with the cudgel to (W's) knee. (W) quickly steps to the right side and blocks down (B's) cudgel with both wheels.

315

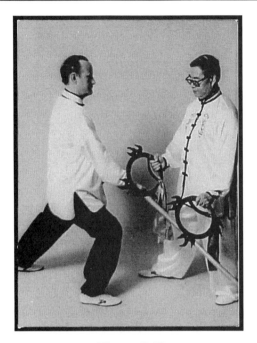

Figure 8-90

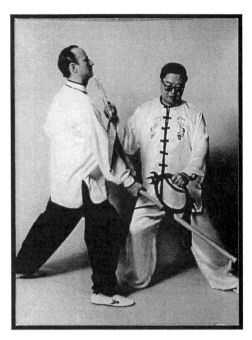

Figure 8-91

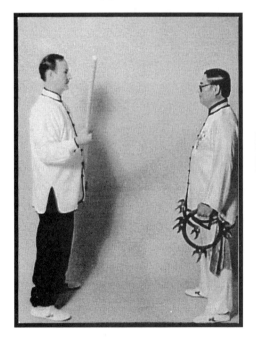

Figure 8-92

Fig. 8-91: (W) immediately steps into right side Bow Stance and strikes (B's) chin with right wheel while blocking and locking the (B's) cudgel with the left wheel.

26. Application Of "Brush Knee And Punch Down"

Fig. 8-92: Refer to Fig. 8-1

Fig. 8-93: (B) makes a right Bow Stance and tries a lower straight thrust strike with the cudgel to (W's) knee. (W) quickly steps to the right side and makes a left Cat Stance with the left "Brush Knee" technique to block down (B's) cudgel.

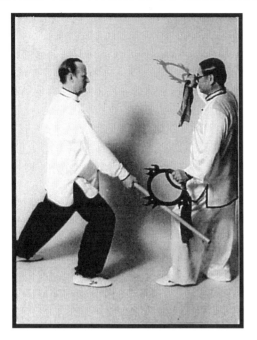

Figure 8-93

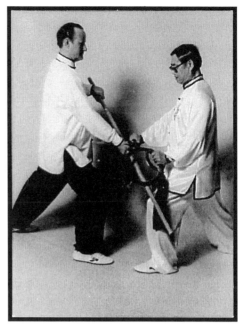

Figure 8-94

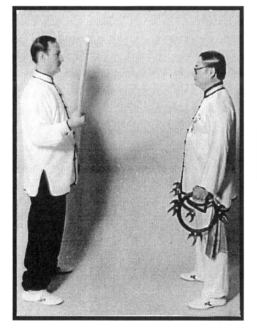

Figure 8-95

Fig. 8-94: (W) immediately steps into left Bow Stance and strikes (B's) groin with a horizontal right wheel.

27. Application Of "Strike The Tiger"

Fig. 8-95: Refer to Fig. 8-1.

Fig. 8-96: (B) tries a low swing strike with the cudgel to (W's) left knee. (W) quickly steps back with the right foot into a left Bow Stance and blocks the cudgel downward with both wheels.

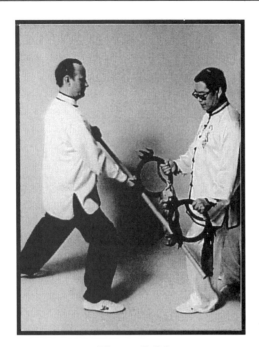

Figure 8-96

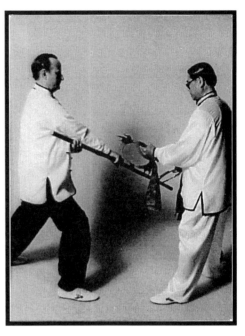

Figure 8-97

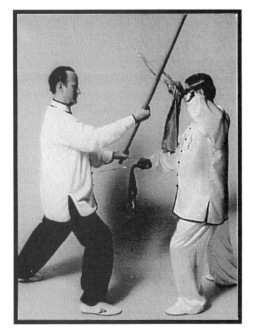

Figure 8-98

Fig. 8-97: (B) assumes a reverse Swing Strike with the cudgel to (W's) right knee. (W) again quickly shifts the weight to the right foot into right Bow Stance while blocking the cudgel downward with both wheels.

Fig. 8-98: (B) makes a high Swing Strike with the cudgel to (W's) temple. (W) immediately shifts the weight to the left foot into left Bow Stance while up blocking the cudgel with the left wheel and cutting from right to left with the horizontal right wheel to (B's) chest.

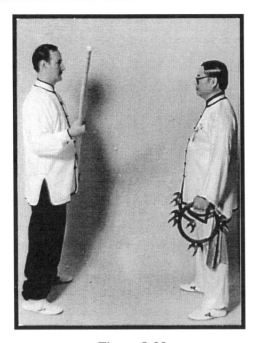

Figure 8-99

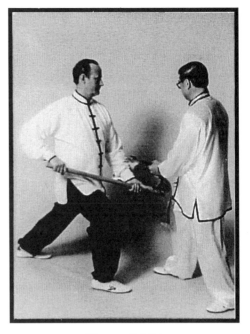

Figure 8-100

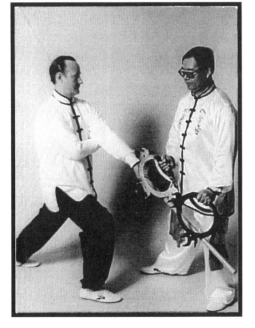

Figure 8-101

28. Application Of "Strike The Tiger-Alternative Method"

Fig. 8-99: Refer to Fig. 8-1.

Fig. 8-100: (B) makes a lower Swing Strike with the cudgel to (W's) right knee. (W) quickly steps back with the left foot into a right Bow Stance and deflects the cudgel downward with both wheels.

Fig. 8-101: (B) assumes a Reverse Swing. Strike with the cudgel to (W's) left knee. (W) immediately shifts the weight to the left foot into a left Bow Stance while blocking the cudgel downward with both wheels.

319

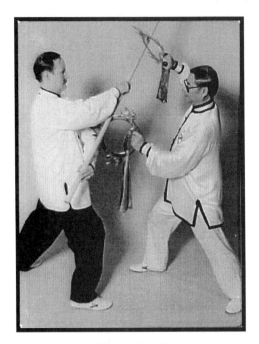

Figure 8-102

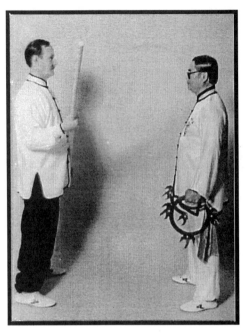

Figure 8-103

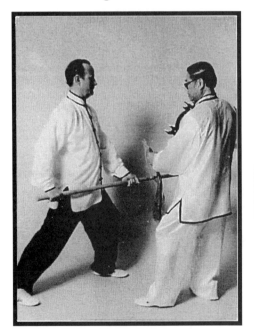

Figure 8-104

Fig. 8-102: (B) tries a high Swing Strike with the cudgel to (W's) right temple. (W) quickly shifts weight to the right foot into right Bow Stance while blocking the cudgel with the right wheel and striking with the vertical left wheel to (B's) chest.

29. Application Of "White Snake Spits The Poison"

Fig. 8-103: Refer to Fig. 8-1.

Fig. 8-104: (B) makes a left Bow Stance and assumes a lower straight thrust strike with the cudgel to (W's) abdomen. (W) quickly steps to the left side into a left Cat Stance and deflect (B's) cudgel with the left wheel.

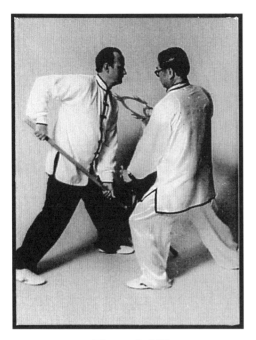

Figure 8-105

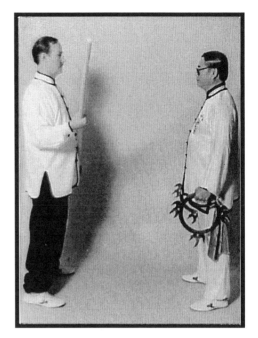

Figure 8-106

Fig. 8-105: (W) presses down (B's) cudgel and executes "White Snake Spits the Poison" technique with the right wheel to (B's) throat.

30. Application Of "Step Back And Ride The Tiger"

Fig. 8-106: Refer to Fig. 8-1.

Fig. 8-107: (W) revolves two wheels with the right wheel down and the left wheel up to strike (B's) mid abdomen. (B) quickly steps right foot out into a right Bow Stance and uses the vertical cudgel to block both (W's) wheels.

Fig. 8-108: (B) makes a high swing strike with the cudgel to (W's) right temple. (W) immediately steps back the right foot into a Cat Stance while bringing the right wheel in an upward arc motion to block the cudgel and bringing the left wheel in a downward arc motion to the left waist of the body.

Fig. 8-109: (W) quickly executes a front kick with the left foot to (B's) groin.

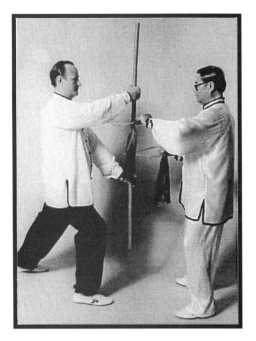

Figure 8-107

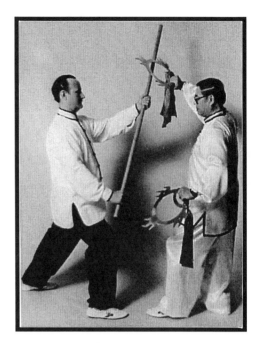

Figure 8-108

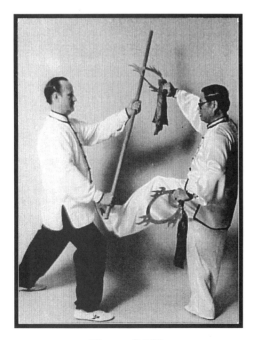

Figure 8-109

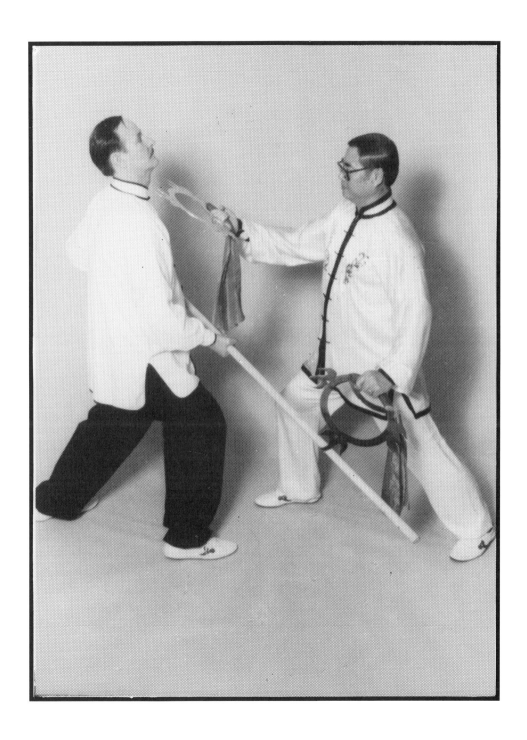

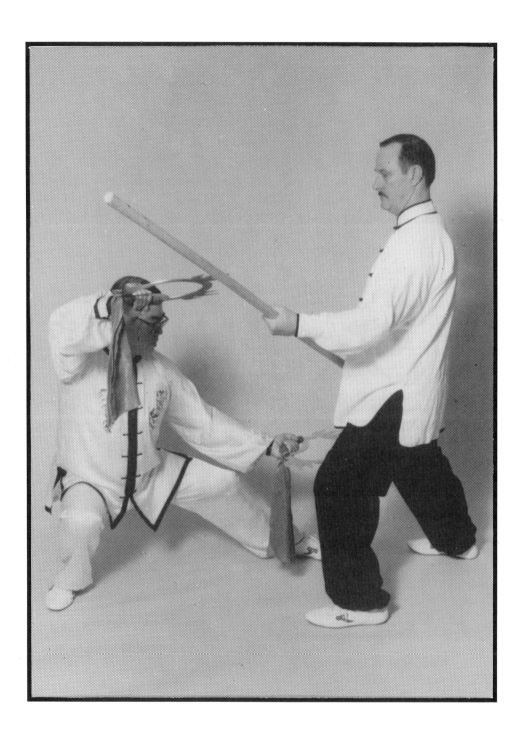

CHAPTER 9

CONCLUSION

This book has defined advanced principles for performing Tai-Chi with Wind-Fire Wheels. Readers have found these principles innovative in that they focus on a weapon that is new to most English speaking Tai-Chi players. However, the book is firmly anchored in the ancient principles of the martial arts and the philosophical underpinnings of Tai-Chi. Those who put those ancient principles to use while using the movements, forms, and applications of this book will be rewarded with new levels of accomplishment in their Tai-Chi and deeper degrees of internal strength and understanding.

It cannot be overemphasized that those who would use the principles of working with the Wind-Fire Wheels need a qualified master to guide them in using the fundamentals of this book in an advanced practice of Tai-Chi Chuan. Without guidance and inspiration from a qualified master, the Wind-Fire Wheels will become a mere novelty. Players who wish to simply brag of prowess with a variety of weapons are advised against practicing the forms and applications in this book for they are dangerous and impossible to appreciate without serious intent and proper guidance.

Serious players with a proper base of skill, internal strength, and loyalty to a qualified master can learn the full sequence of forms presented here in two to

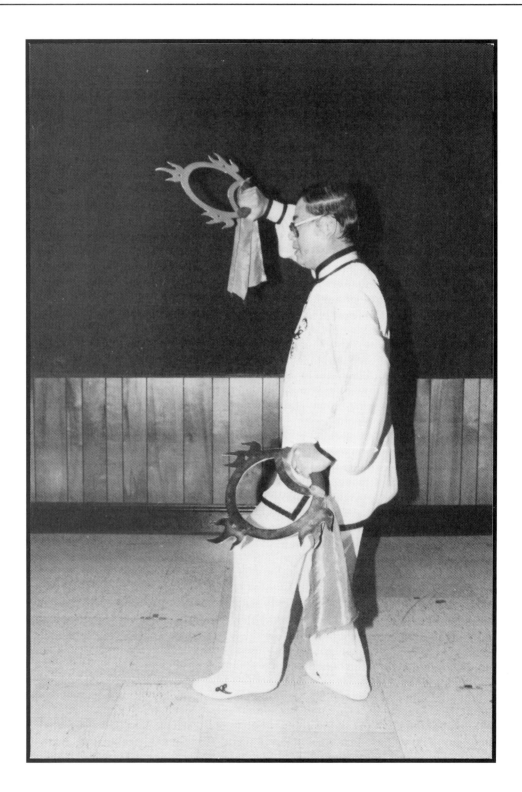

three years. Form Number One was designed to test and extend a players ability in advanced movements in Tai-Chi Chuan. Form Number Two tests and extends a player's internal strength to perform a complex sequence from start to finish with smoothness and intent. Form Number Three was designed to appeal to players who are prepared to advance to the deeper forms of knowledge hidden in the integration of internal flow and external transitions of movement.

The Applications chapter is an especially important part of this book. Indeed, its contents were designed to supplement the players knowledge and ability at each of the stages reached in the forms presented in earlier chapters. Players will find the applications useful after becoming comfortable with the first form in that they will refine the player's knowledge of the structure and purpose of each movement used in the form. Following a command of the second form, players will find themselves able to execute the applications with a confident martial intent. Mastery of the third form prepares players to access the secrets of using the Wind-Fire Wheels in Tai-Chi. That is, for accessing a knowledge of transitions, alterations of emptiness and fullness, and circular transferences that are only being available to those with the competence and openness to experience them. Integration of personal mastery of form with the Wind-Fire Wheel applications will take advanced players an additional three years of study, practice, and consultation.

Players who are legitimately ready to use an advanced book on Tai-Chi know that any form is empty posturing unless it naturally expresses the intent and spirit of the player. Such expression comes only with diligent practice under a master's guidance and with other advanced players. During such development, players may be tempted to modify or otherwise personalize the forms presented here. However, it is essential for players to be true to the contents of this book for to do otherwise is to invite injury to and shallowness in oneself and others. In short, readers of this book should not teach or modify what is presented here until their proficiency has been certified by an accredited Tai-Chi Grand Master. After achieving such certified proficiency, players will experience the deep satisfaction and pleasure I have enjoyed in perfecting and sharing a command of this time-honored weapon.

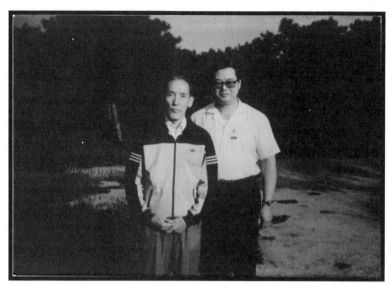

The author posing with Professor Li Tien-Ji (李天驥), world renowned teacher of Tai-Chi Chuan, Beijing, China, 1985.

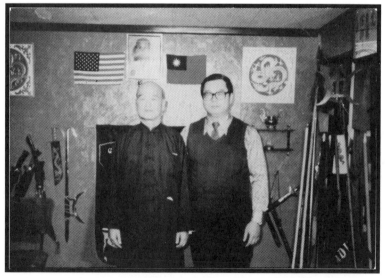

The author posing with Grandmaster Lu Hung-Bin (盧鴻賓), world renowned Pa -Gua Zhang teacher, New Jersey, U.S.A., 1988.

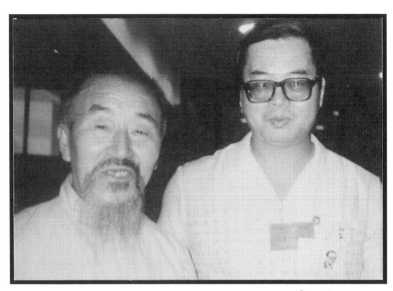

The author posing with Grandmaster Sa Kuo-Zen (沙国政), international renowned Tai-Chi and Chi-Kung teacher, Sian, China, 1985.

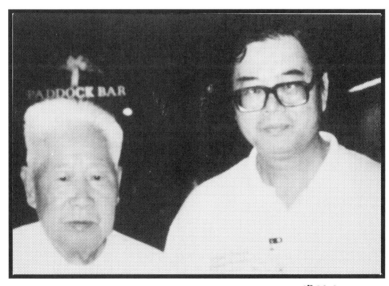

The author posing with Grandmaster Fu Zhong-Wen (傅鍾文), international renowned Tai-Chi Chuan teacher, Baltimore, Maryland, 1994.

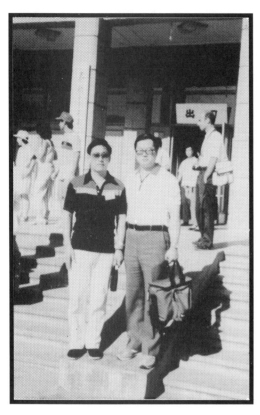

The author posing with Grandmaster
Chen Xiao-Wang (陳曉旺),world
renowned Chen Style Tai-Chi
Chuan teacher, Sian, China, 1985.

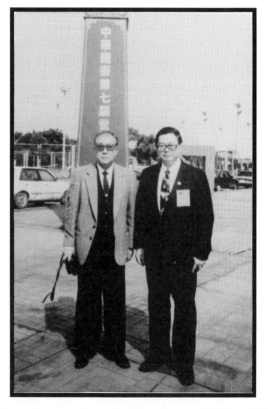

The author posing with Professor Li Mau-Ching
(李茂清), international renowned martial artist,
Taiwan, China, 1992.

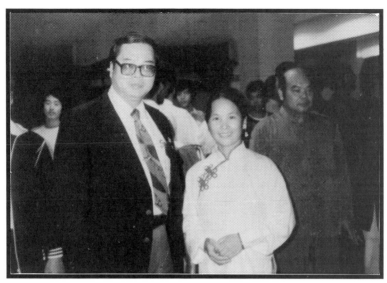

The author posing with Grandmaster Bow Sim Mark (麥寶嬋), Tai-Chi Gold Medalist and world renowned Tai-Chi Chuan teacher, Sian, China, 1985.

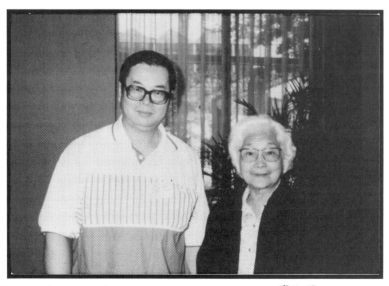

The author posing with Grandmaster Fu Shu-Yun (傅淑雲), international well-known Tai-Chi Chuan teacher, Baltimore, Maryland, 1991.

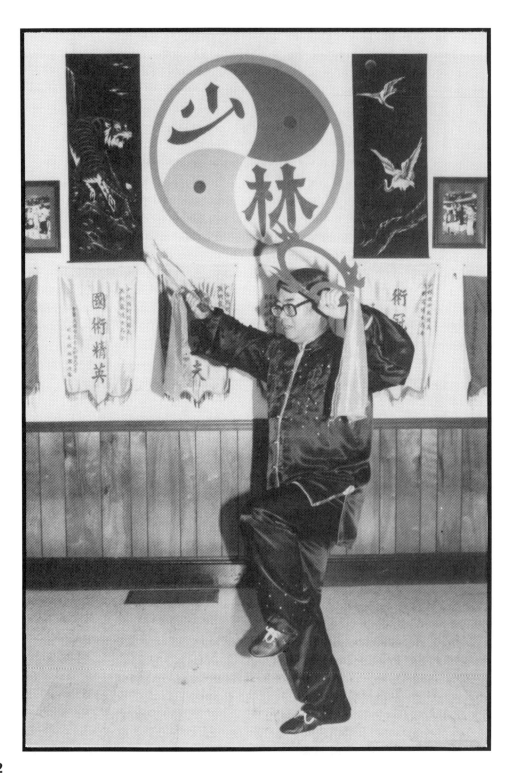

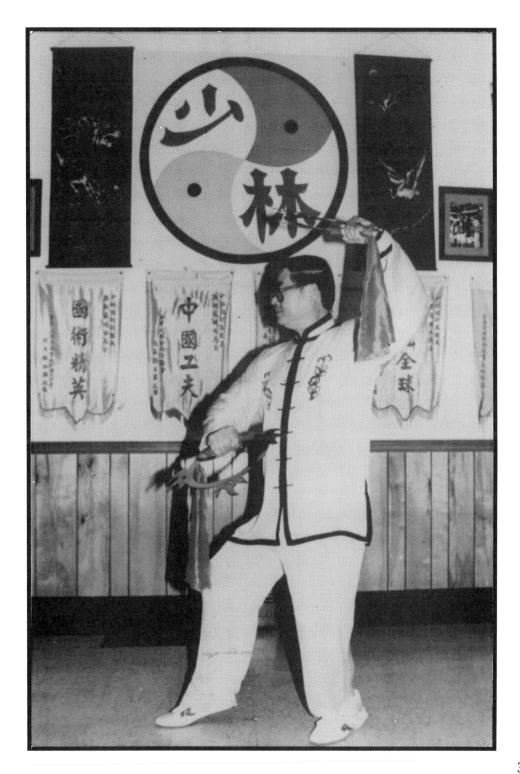

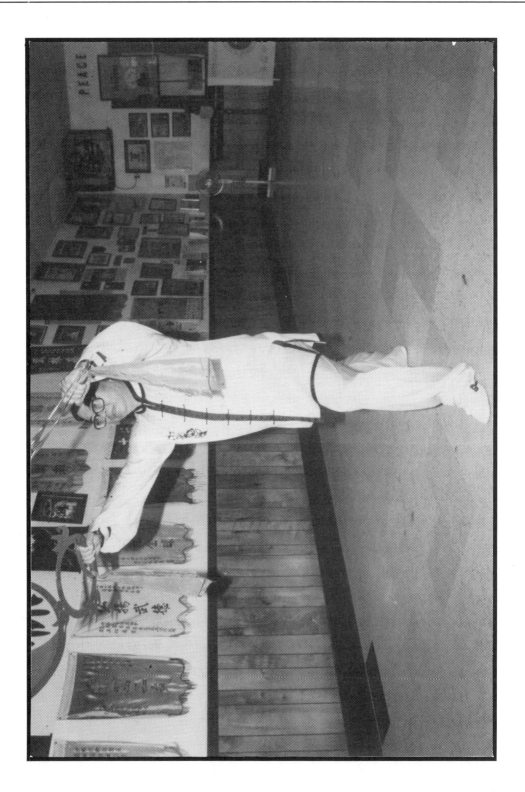

APPENDIX A

TRANSLATIONS IN CHINESE
FOR TAI-CHI WIND-FIRE WHEELS

1. Advanced Form I

2. Advanced Form II

3. Advanced Form III

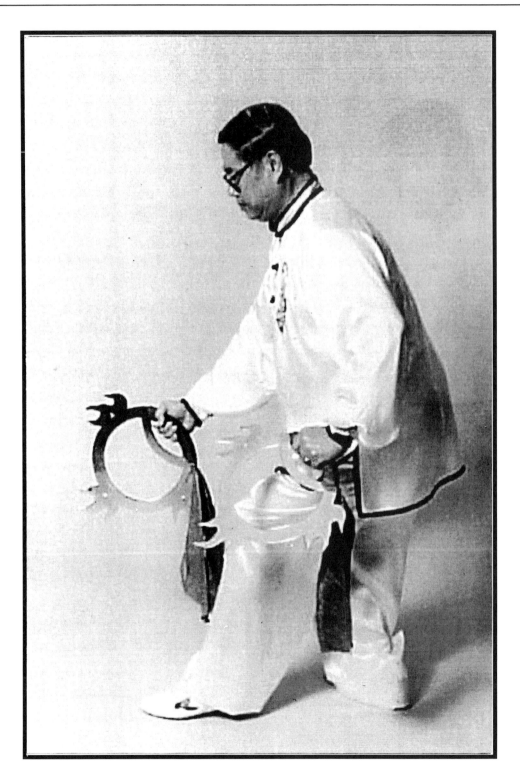

1. Advanced Form I

(1) 預備式　Preparatory Posture

(2) 風火起式　Wind-Fire Commencing

(3) 向前左野馬分鬃　Left Step Forward Part Wild Horse's Mane

(4) 右轉掤,攦,擠,按　Turn Right Ward Off, Roll Back, Press And Push

(5) 左單鞭　Left Single Whip

(6) 右提手上式　Right Lifting Hand

(7) 風火轉輪　Wind-Fire Turning Wheels

(8) 白鶴亮翅與踢腿　White Crane Spreads Its Wings And Left Heel Kick

(9) 左,右,左摟膝拗步　Left, Right, Left Brush Knee And Step Forward

(10) 手揮琵琶式　Playing The Lute

(11) 左掃右沖擊　Left Slicing And Right Striking

(12) 風火上架下腰斬　Wind-Fire Up Blocking And Down Waist Chopping

(13) 抱虎歸山　Embrace The Tiger And Return To The Mountain

(14) 肘底看捶　Fist Under The Elbow

(15) 倒卷肱(三次)　Reverse Reeling Forearm (3 times)

(16) 斜飛式　Diagonal Flying

(17) 海底針　Needle At Sea Bottom

(18) 閃通臂　Fan Through Back

(19) 右轉右野馬分鬃　Right Turn Right Part Wild Horse's Mane

(20) 左單鞭　Left Single Whip

(21) 雲手(三次)　Wave Hands Like Clouds (3 times)

(22) 左單鞭　Left Single Whip

(23) 高探馬　High Pat On Horse

(24) 右蹬腳, 雙峰貫耳   Right Heel Kick And Strike To Ears

(25) 轉身左蹬腳, 雙峰貫耳   Left Turn Body Left Heel Kick And Strike To Ears

(26) 進步栽捶   Brush Knee And Punch Down

(27) 右蹬腳, 雙峰貫耳   Right Heel Kick And Strike To Ears

(28) 左打虎式   Left Strike The Tiger

(29) 雙峰貫耳   Strike To Ears With Both Fists

(30) 右轉左野馬分鬃   Right Turn Left Part Wild Horse's Mane

(31) 右后轉玉女穿梭 (二次)   Right Turn Body Fair Lady Shuttles Back And Forth (right 1 time, left 1 time)

(32) 右下式, 金雞獨立   Right Lower Body And Stand On One Leg

(33) 白蛇吐信   White Snake Spits The Poison

(34) 風火左右斜刺   Wind-Fire High And Low Diagonal Cuts

(35) 進步指擋捶 (左手捶)   Right Step Forward And Left Strike Down

(36) 左下式, 金雞獨立   Left Lower Body And Stand On One Leg

(37) 風火轉輪 (三次)   Wind-Fire Turning Wheels (3 times)

(38) 退步跨虎   Step Back And Ride The Tiger

(39) 轉身風火輪護頂与踢腿   Right Turn Body Wind-Fire Protecting The Head And Right Heel Kick

(40) 左掃右沖擊   Left Slicing And Right Striking

(41) 上步兩沖擊   Step Forward Left And Right Strikings

(42) 如封似閉   Appears Closed

(43) 風火收勢   Wind-Fire Closing

(44) 還原   Return To Origin

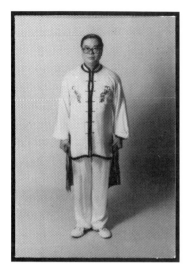

Figure A1-1

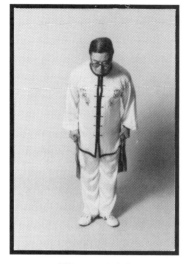

Figure A1-2

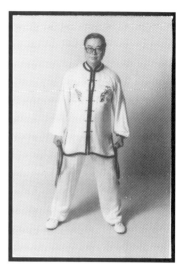

Figure A1-3

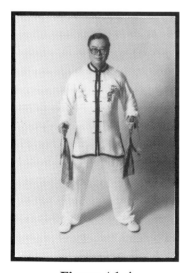

Figure A1-4

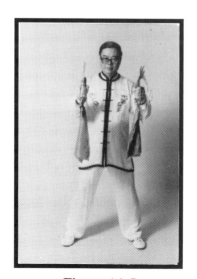

Figure A1-5

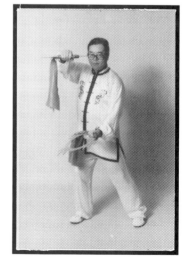

Figure A1-6

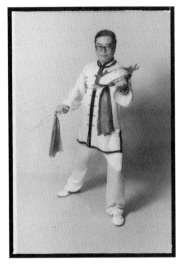

Figure A1-7

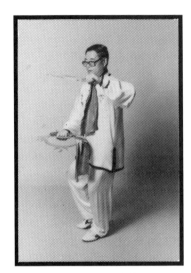

Figure A1-8

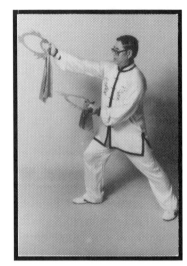

Figure A1-9

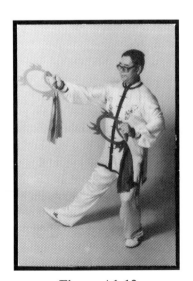

Figure A1-10

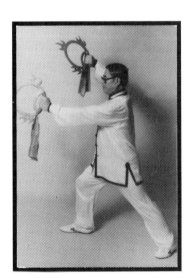

Figure A1-11

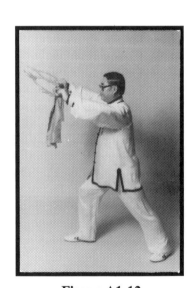

Figure A1-12

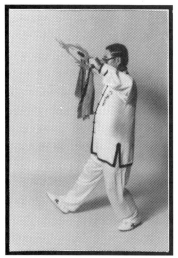

Figure A1-13

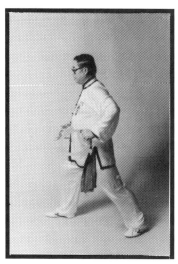

Figure A1-14

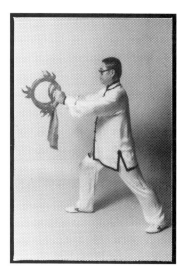

Figure A1-15

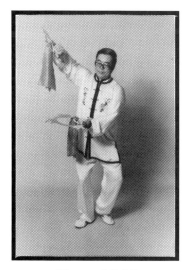

Figure A1-16

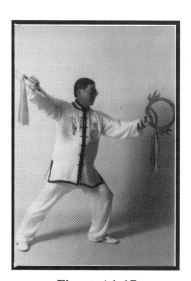

Figure A1-17

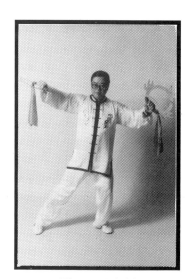

Figure A1-18

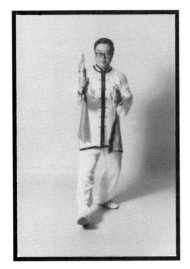

Figure A1-19

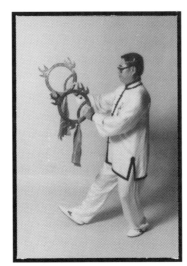

Figure A1-20

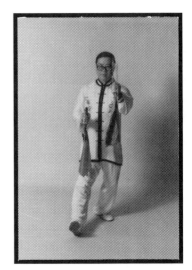

Figure A1-21

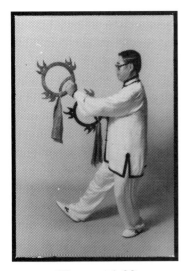

Figure A1-22

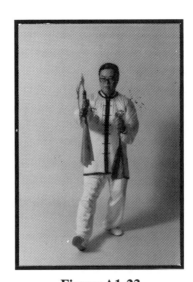

Figure A1-23

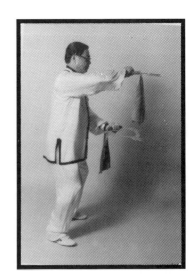

Figure A1-24

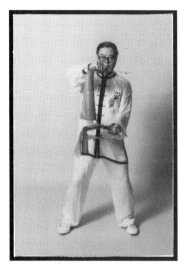

Figure A1-25

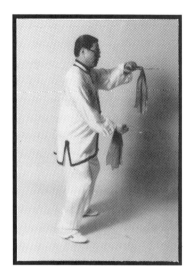

Figure A1-26

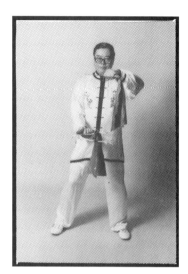

Figure A1-27

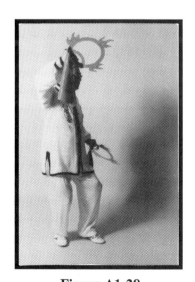

Figure A1-28

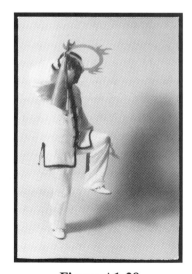

Figure A1-29

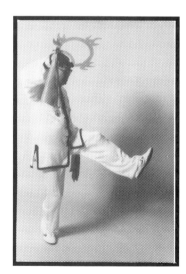

Figure A1-30

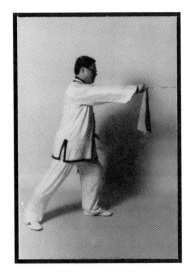
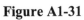

Figure A1-31

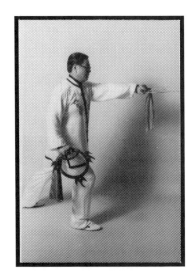

Figure A1-32

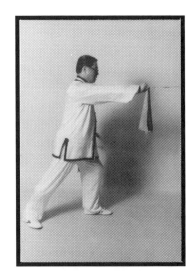

Figure A1-33

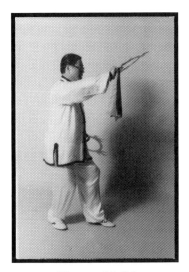

Figure A1-34

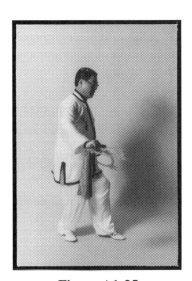

Figure A1-35

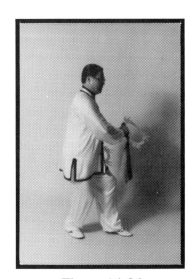

Figure A1-36

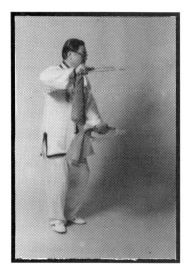

Figure A1-37

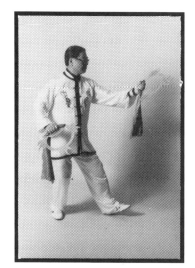

Figure A1-38

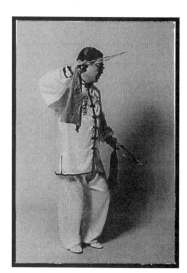

Figure A1-39

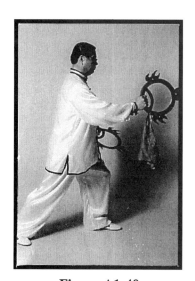

Figure A1-40

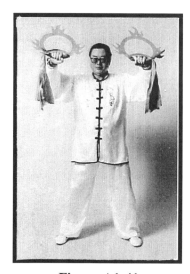

Figure A1-41

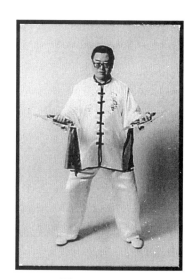

Figure A1-42

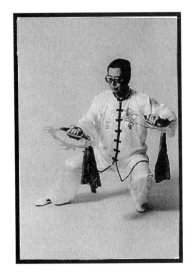

Figure A1-43

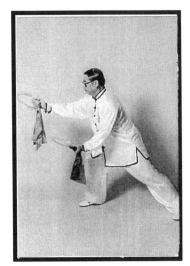

Figure A1-44

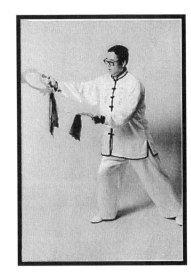

Figure A1-45

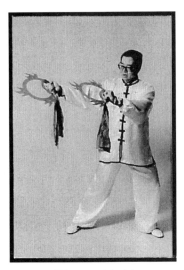

Figure A1-46

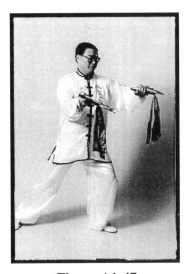

Figure A1-47

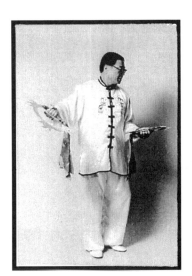

Figure A1-48

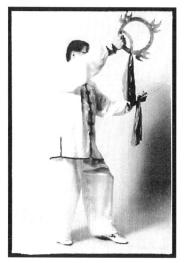

Figure A1-49

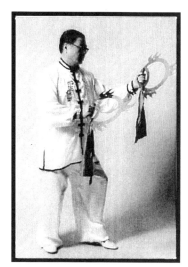

Figure A1-50

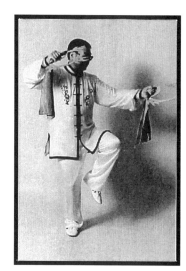

Figure A1-51

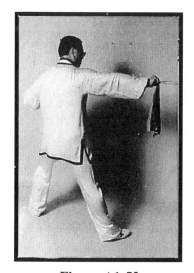

Figure A1-52

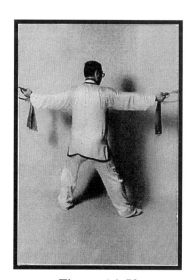

Figure A1-53

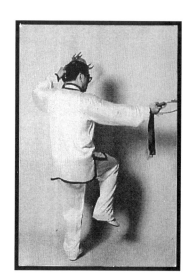

Figure A1-54

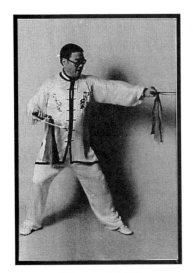
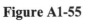

Figure A1-55

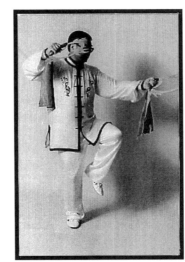

Figure A1-56

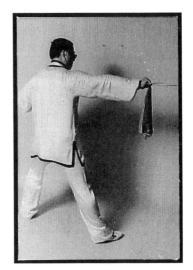

Figure A1-57

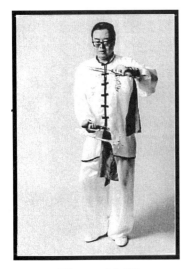

Figure A1-58

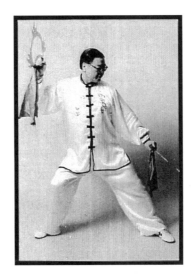

Figure A1-59

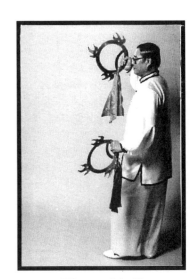

Figure A1-60

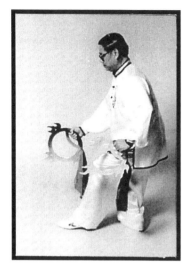

Figure A1-61

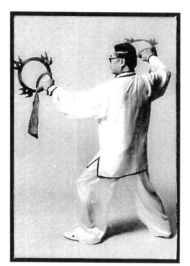

Figure A1-62

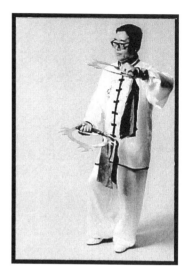

Figure A1-63

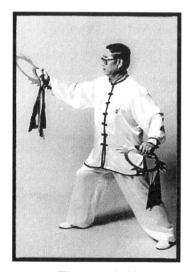

Figure A1-64

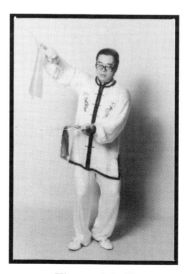

Figure A1-65

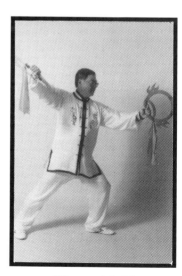

Figure A1-66

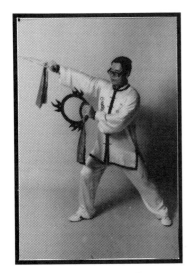
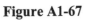

Figure A1-67

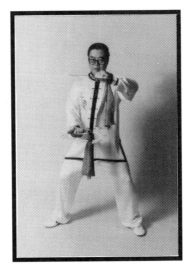

Figure A1-68

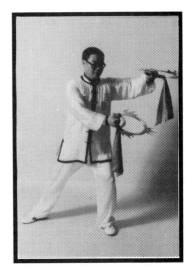

Figure A1-69

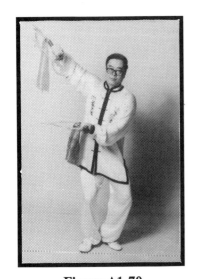

Figure A1-70

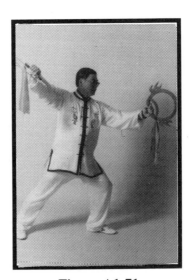

Figure A1-71

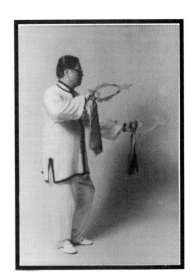

Figure A1-72

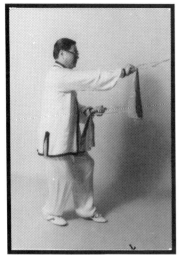

Figure A1-73

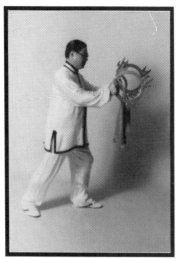

Figure A1-74

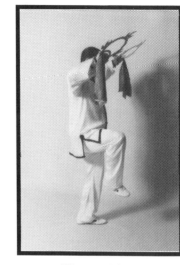

Figure A1-75

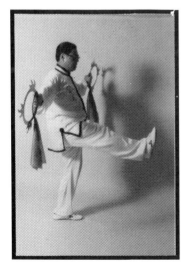

Figure A1-76

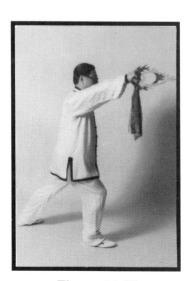

Figure A1-77

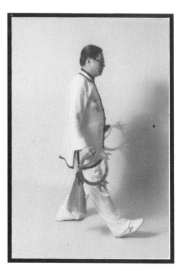

Figure A1-78

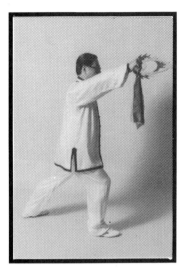

Figure A1-79

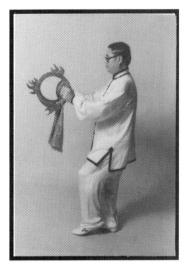

Figure A1-80

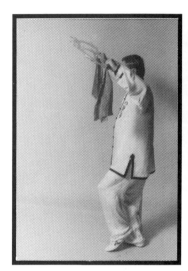

Figure A1-81

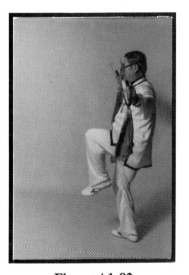

Figure A1-82

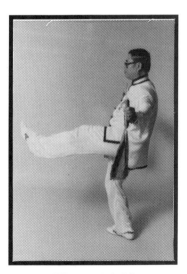

Figure A1-83

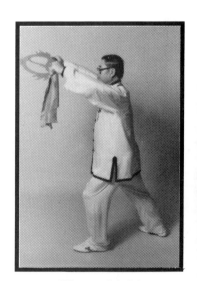

Figure A1-84

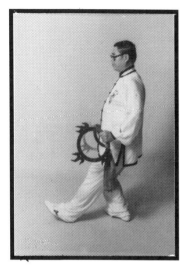

Figure A1-85

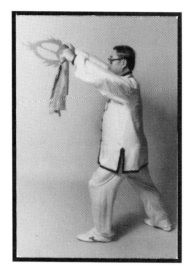

Figure A1-86

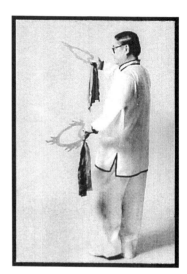

Figure A1-87

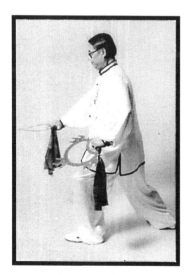

Figure A1-88

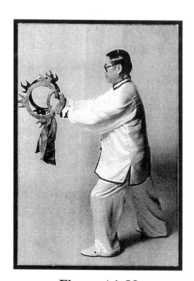

Figure A1-89

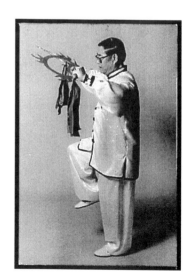

Figure A1-90

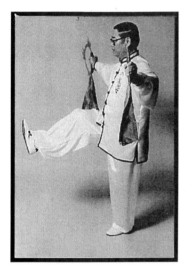

Figure A1-91

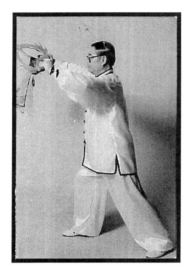

Figure A1-92

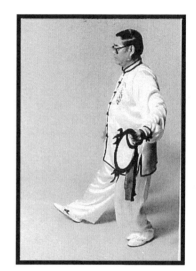

Figure A1-93

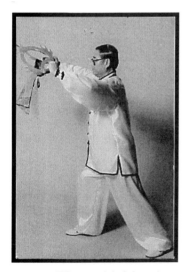

Figure A1-94

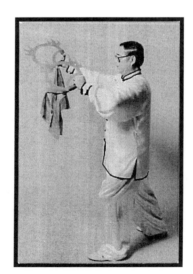

Figure A1-95

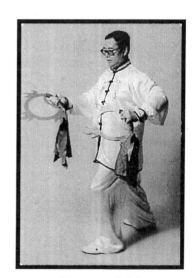

Figure A1-96

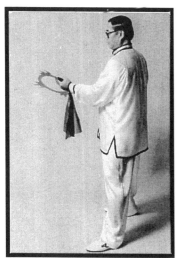

Figure A1-97

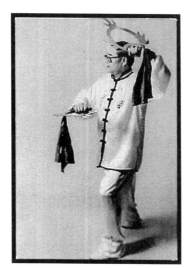

Figure A1-98

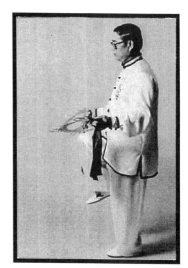

Figure A1-99

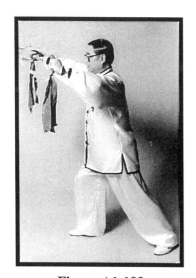

Figure A1-100

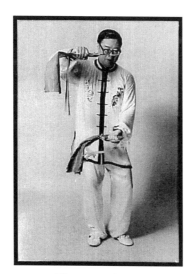

Figure A1-101

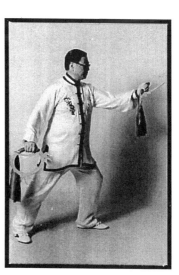

Figure A1-102

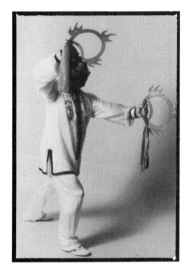

Figure A1-103

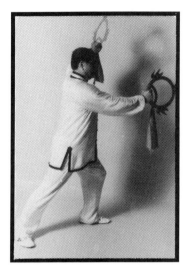

Figure A1-104

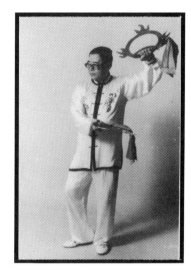

Figure A1-105

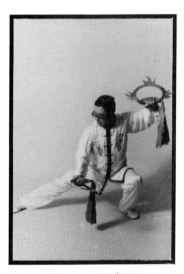

Figure A1-106

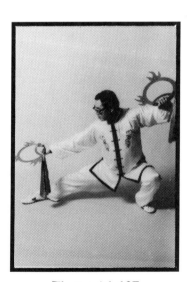

Figure A1-107

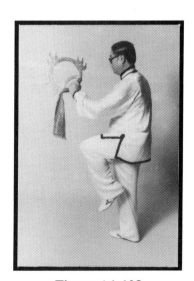

Figure A1-108

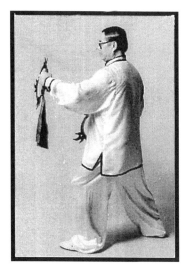

Figure A1-109

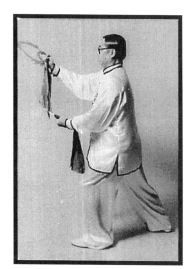

Figure A1-110

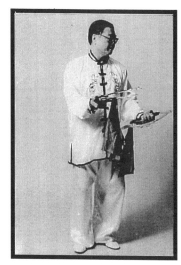

Figure A1-111

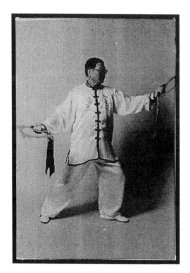

Figure A1-112

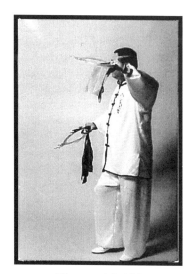

Figure A1-113

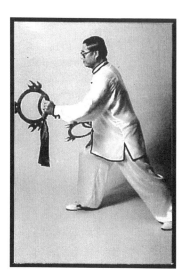

Figure A1-114

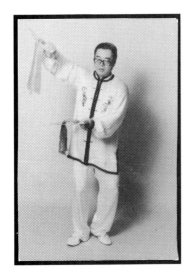

Figure A1-115

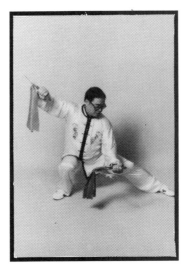

Figure A1-116

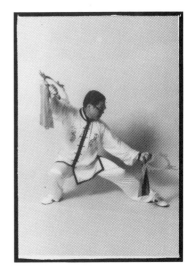

Figure A1-117

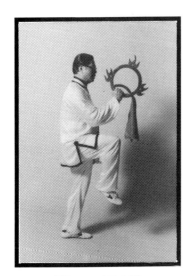

Figure A1-118

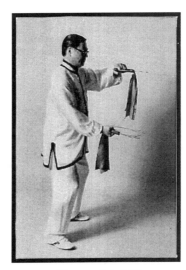

Figure A1-119

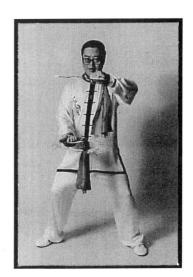

Figure A1-120

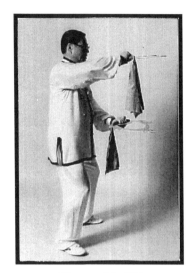

Figure A1-121

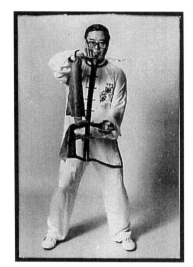

Figure A1-122

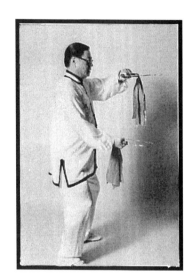

Figure A1-123

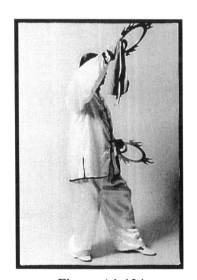

Figure A1-124

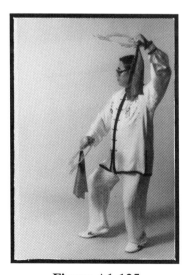

Figure A1-125

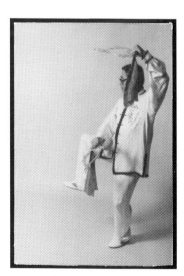

Figure A1-126

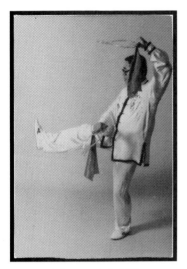

Figure A1-127

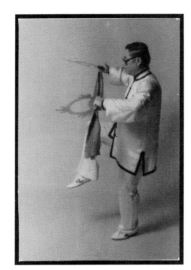

Figure A1-128

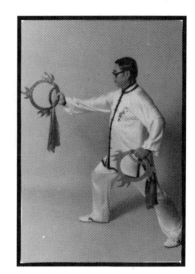

Figure A1-129

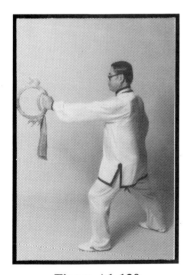

Figure A1-130

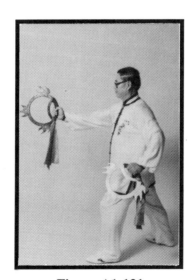

Figure A1-131

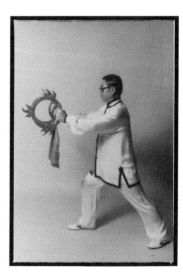

Figure A1-132

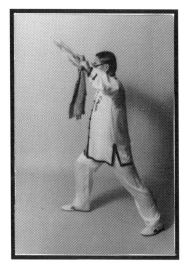

Figure A1-133

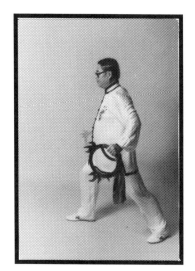

Figure A1-134

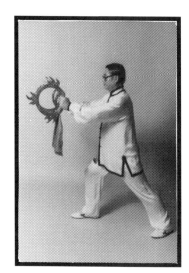

Figure A1-135

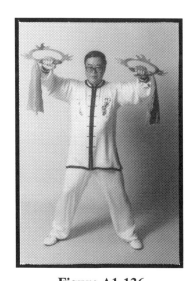

Figure A1-136

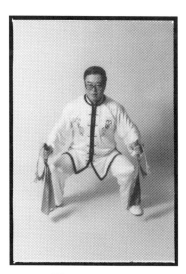

Figure A1-137

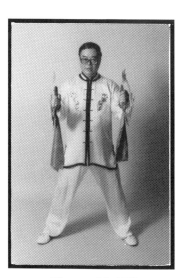

Figure A1-138

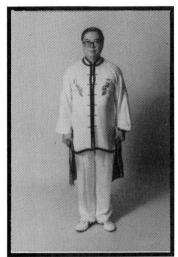

Figure A1-139

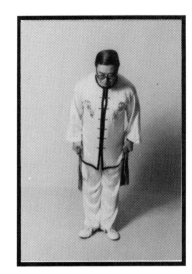

Figure A1-140

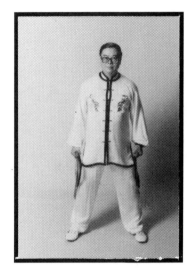

Figure A1-141

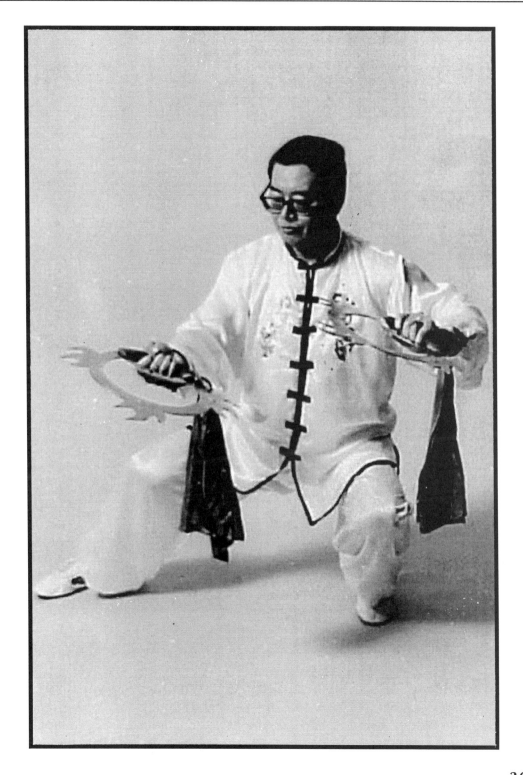

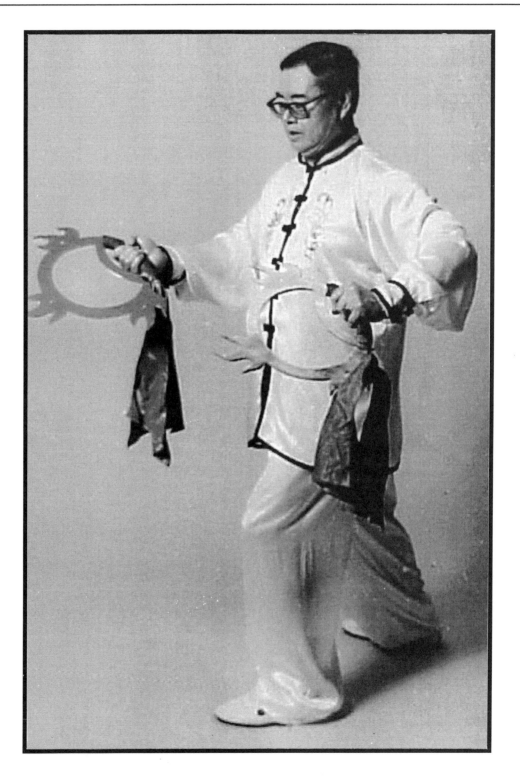

2. Advanced Form II

(1)   預備式   Preparatory Posture

(2)   風火起勢   Wind-Fire Commencing

(3)   向前左野馬分鬃   Left Step Forward Part Wild Horse's Mane

(4)   右轉掤,攦,擠,按   Turn Right Ward Off, Roll Back, Press And Push

(5)   左單鞭   Left Single Whip

(6)   右提手上式   Right Lifting Hand

(7)   風火轉輪   Wind-Fire Turning Wheels

(8)   白鶴亮翅与踢腿   White Crane Spreads Its Wings And Left Heel Kick

(9)   左,右,左摟膝拗步   Left, Right, Left Brush Knee And Step Forward

(10)   手揮琵琶   Playing The Lute

(11)   左掃右沖擊   Left Slicing And Right Striking

(12)   斜飛式   Diagonal Flying

(13)   肘底看捶   Fist Under The Elbow

(14)   倒卷肱(四次)   Reverse Reeling Forearm (4 times)

(15)   右后轉玉女穿梭(二次)   Right Turn Body Fair Lady Shuttles Back And Forth (left 1 time, right 1 time)

(16)   左野馬分鬃   Left Part Wild Horse's Mane

(17)   右野馬分鬃   Right Part Wild Horse's Mane

(18)   左單鞭   Left Single Whip

(19)   雲手(三次)   Wave Hands Like Clouds (3 times)

(20)   左單鞭   Left Single Whip

(21)   高探馬   High Pat On Horse

(22)   右蹬腳,雙峰貫耳   Right Heel Kick And Strike To Ears

(23)   轉身左蹬腳,雙峰貫耳   Left Turn Body Left Heel Kick And Strike To Ears

(24) 海底針　Needle At Sea Bottom

(25) 扇通背　Fan Through Back

(26) 白蛇吐信　White Snake Spits The Poison

(27) 風火左右斜刺　Wind-Fire High And Low Diagonal Cuts

(28) 左野馬分鬃　Left Part Wild Horse's Mane

(29) 右蹬腳,雙峰貫耳　Right Heel Kick And Strike To Ears

(30) 左打虎式　Left Strike The Tiger

(31) 右打虎式　Right Strike The Tiger

(32) 左野馬分鬃　Left Part Wild Horse's Mane

(33) 右單鞭下式,金雞獨立　Right Lower Body And Stand On One Leg

(34) 進步指擋捶　Left Step Forward And Right Strike Down

(35) 上步掤,攦,擠,按　Step Forward Ward Off, Roll Back, Press And Push

(36) 左單鞭下式,金雞獨立　Left Lower Body And Stand On One Leg

(37) 風火轉輪(三次)　Wind-Fire Turning Wheels (3 times)

(38) 退步跨虎　Step Back And Ride The Tiger

(39) 風火輪護頂与踢腿　Right Turn Body Wind-Fire Protecting The Head And Right Heel Kick

(40) 左掃右沖擊　Left Slicing And Right Striking

(41) 上步兩沖擊　Step Forward Left And Right Strikings

(42) 如封似閉　Appears Closed

(43) 風火收勢　Wind-Fire Closing

(44) 還原　Return To Origin

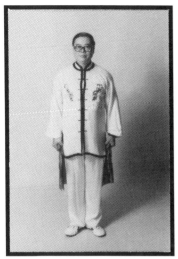

Figure A2-1

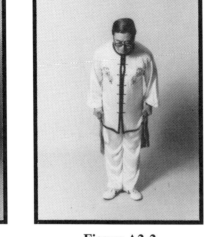

Figure A2-2

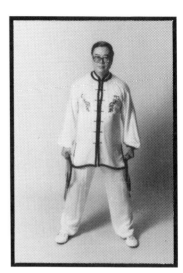

Figure A2-3

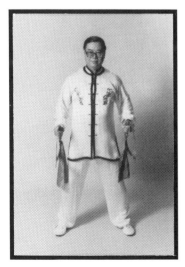

Figure A2-4

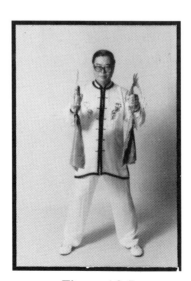

Figure A2-5

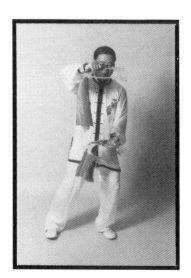

Figure A2-6

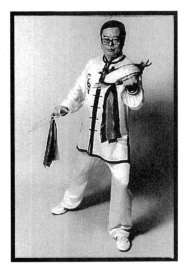

Figure A2-7

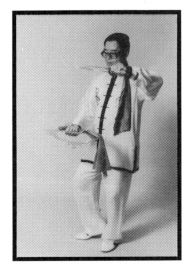

Figure A2-8

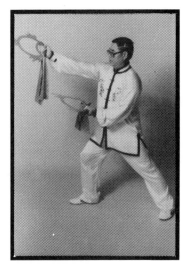

Figure A2-9

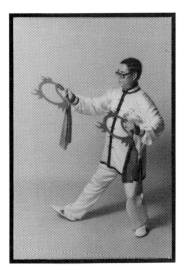

Figure A2-10

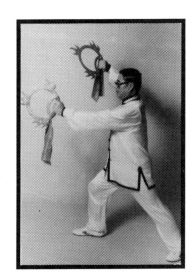

Figure A2-11

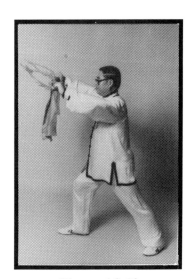

Figure A2-12

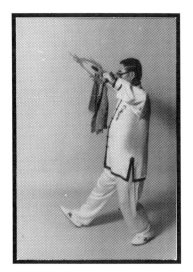

Figure A2-13

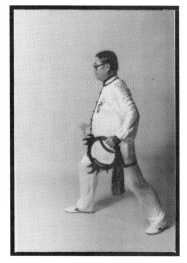

Figure A2-14

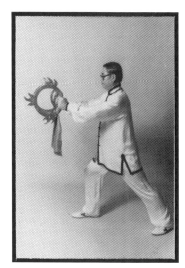

Figure A2-15

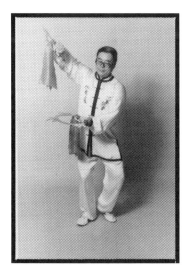

Figure A2-16

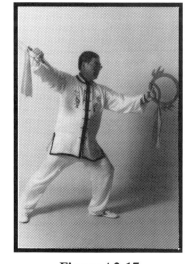

Figure A2-17

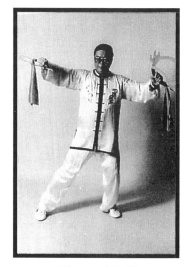

Figure A2-18

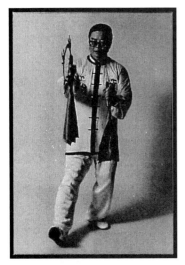

Figure A2-19

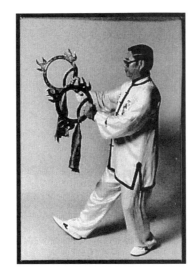

Figure A2-20

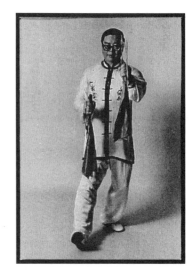

Figure A2-21

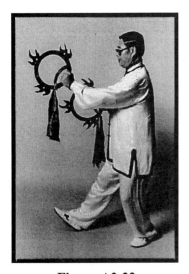

Figure A2-22

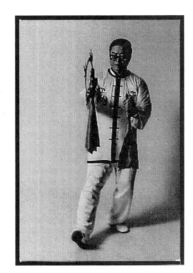

Figure A2-23

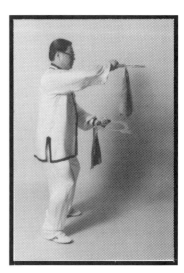

Figure A2-24

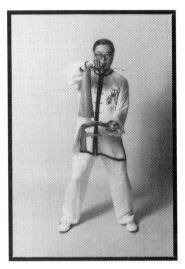

Figure A2-25

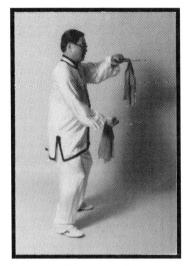

Figure A2-26

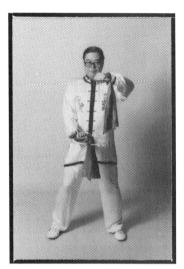

Figure A2-27

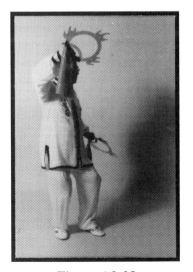

Figure A2-28

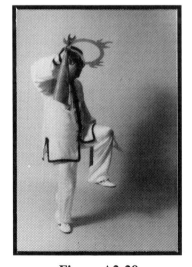

Figure A2-29

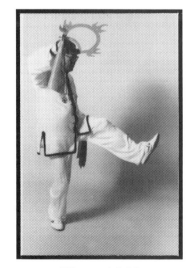

Figure A2-30

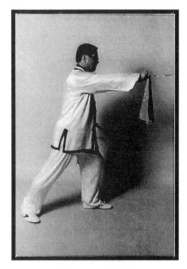

Figure A2-31

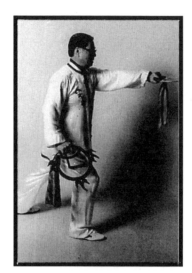

Figure A2-32

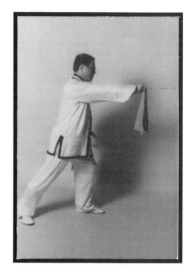

Figure A2-33

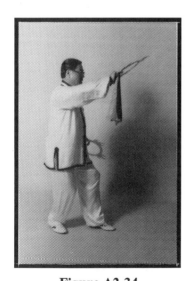

Figure A2-34

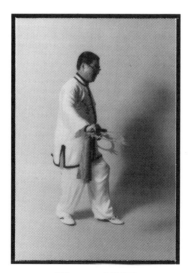

Figure A2-35

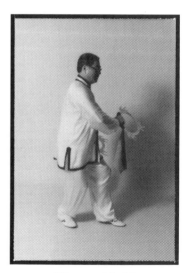

Figure A2-36

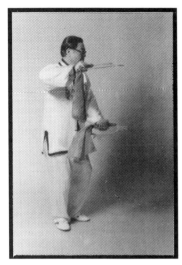

Figure A2-37

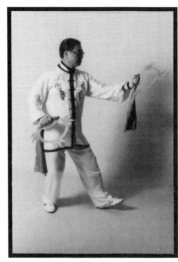

Figure A2-38

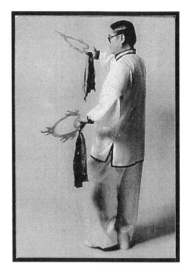

Figure A2-39

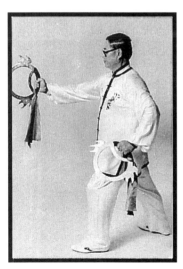

Figure A2-40

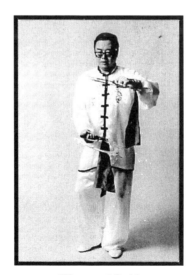

Figure A2-41

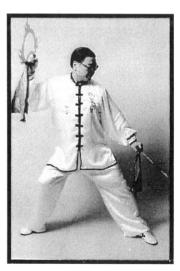

Figure A2-42

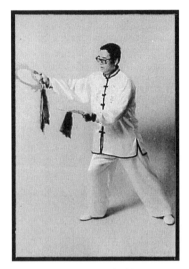

Figure A2-43

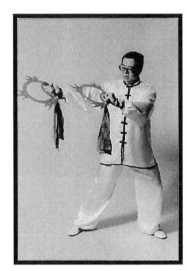

Figure A2-44

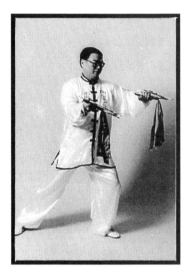

Figure A2-45

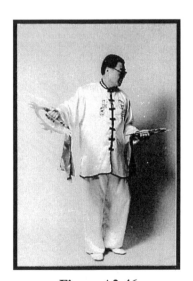

Figure A2-46

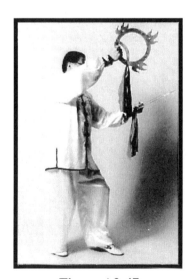

Figure A2-47

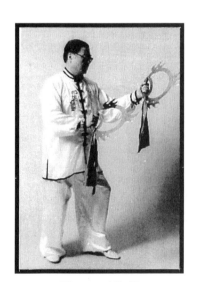

Figure A2-48

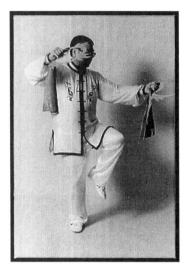

Figure A2-49

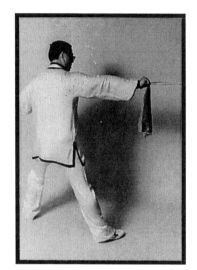

Figure A2-50

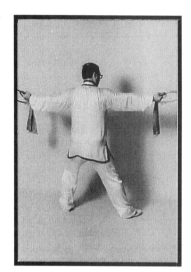

Figure A2-51

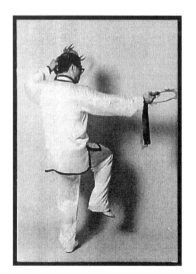

Figure A2-52

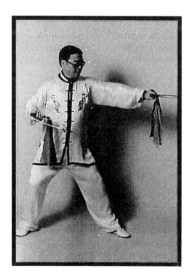

Figure A2-53

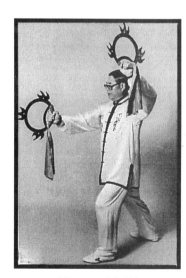

Figure A2-54

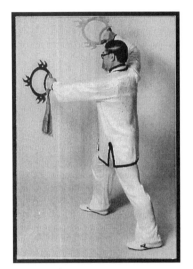

Figure A2-55

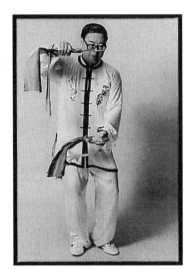

Figure A2-56

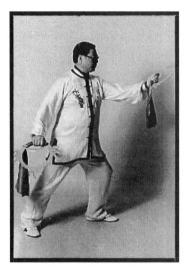

Figure A2-57

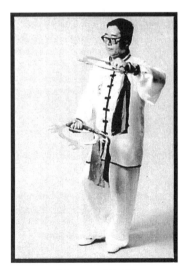

Figure A2-58

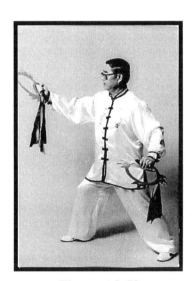

Figure A2-59

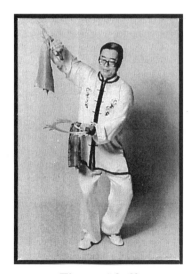

Figure A2-60

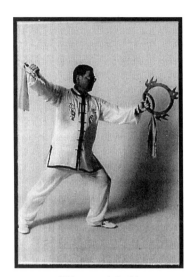

Figure A2-61

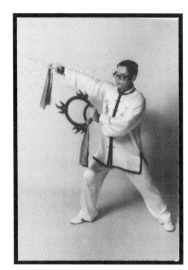

Figure A2-62

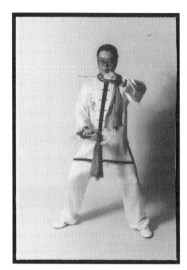

Figure A2-63

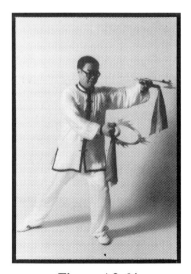

Figure A2-64

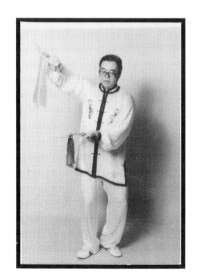

Figure A2-65

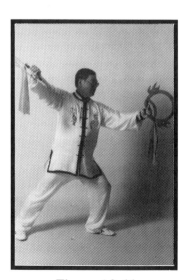

Figure A2-66

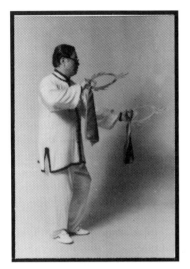

Figure A2-67

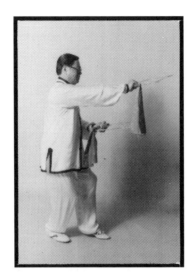

Figure A2-68

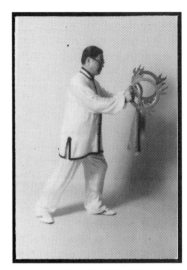

Figure A2-69

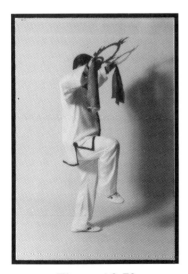

Figure A2-70

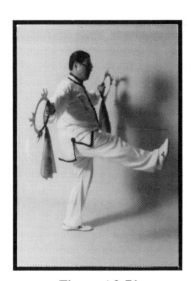

Figure A2-71

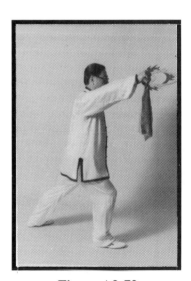

Figure A2-72

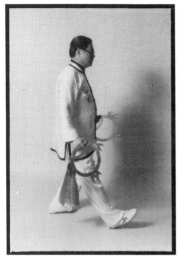

Figure A2-73

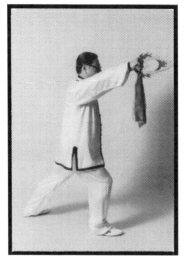

Figure A2-74

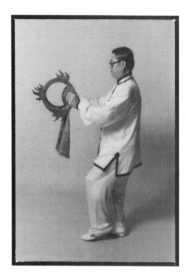

Figure A2-75

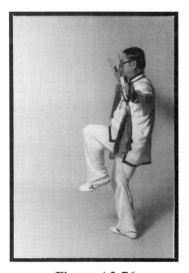

Figure A2-76

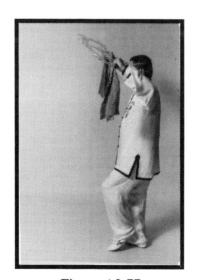

Figure A2-77

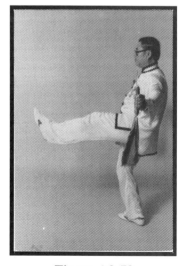

Figure A2-78

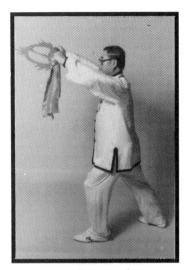

Figure A2-79

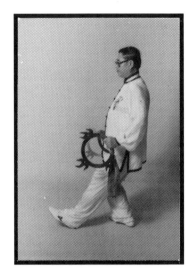

Figure A2-80

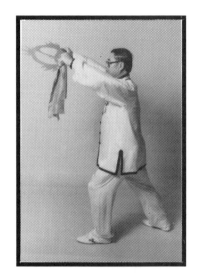

Figure A2-81

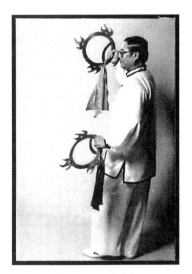

Figure A2-82

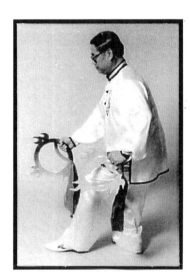

Figure A2-83

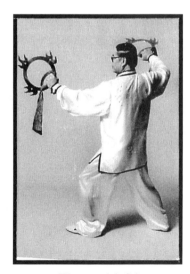

Figure A2-84

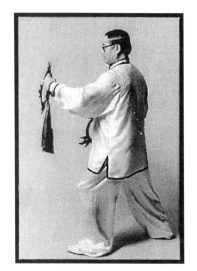

Figure A2-85

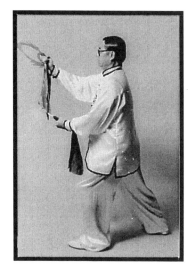

Figure A2-86

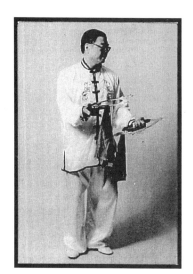

Figure A2-87

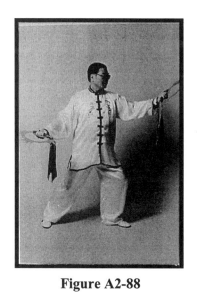

Figure A2-88

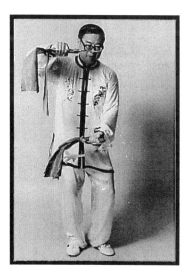

Figure A2-89

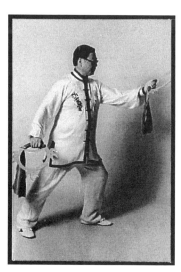

Figure A2-90

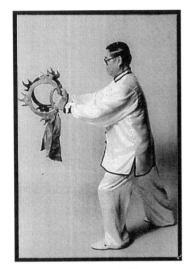

Figure A2-91

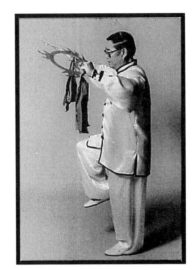

Figure A2-92

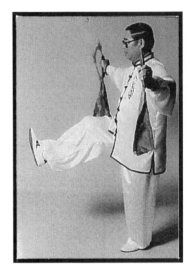

Figure A2-93

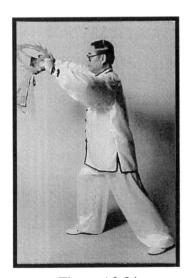

Figure A2-94

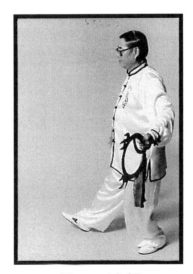

Figure A2-95

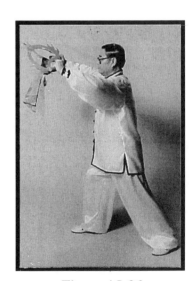

Figure A2-96

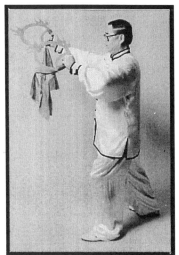
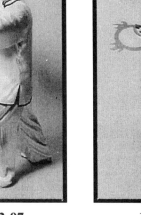

Figure A2-97

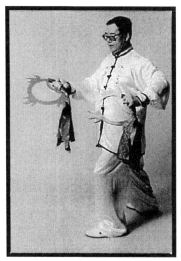

Figure A2-98

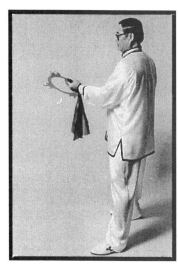

Figure A2-99

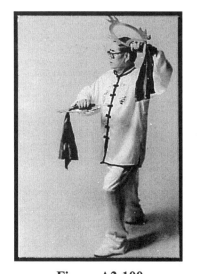

Figure A2-100

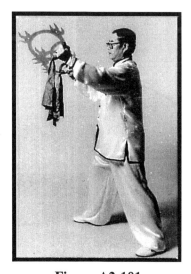

Figure A2-101

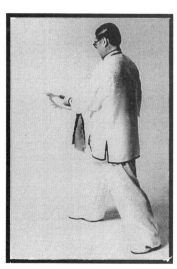

Figure A2-102

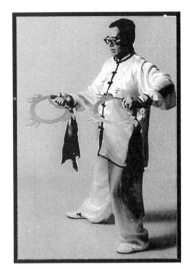

Figure A2-103

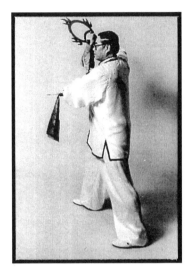

Figure A2-104

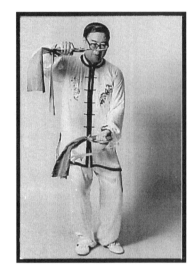

Figure A2-105

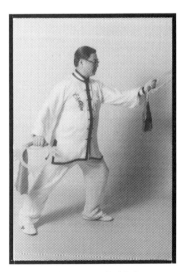

Figure A2-106

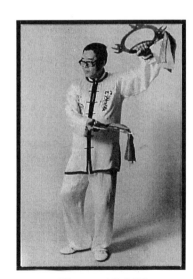

Figure A2-107

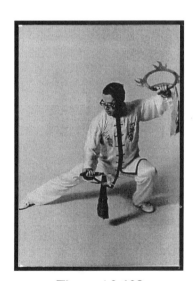

Figure A2-108

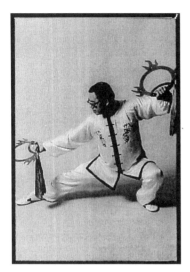

Figure A2-109

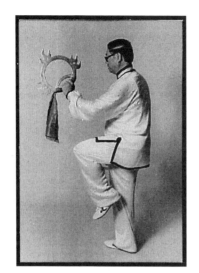

Figure A2-110

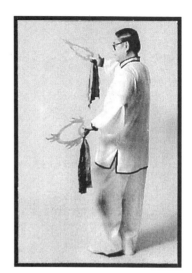

Figure A2-111

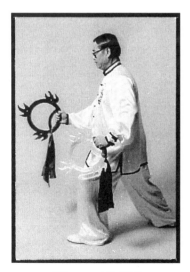

Figure A2-112

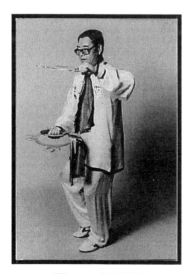

Figure A2-113

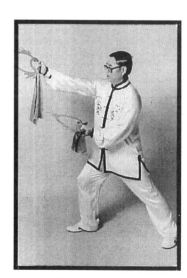

Figure A2-114

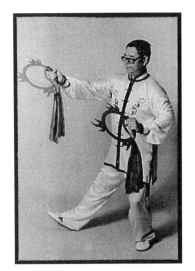

Figure A2-115

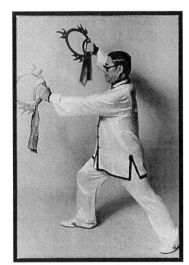

Figure A2-116

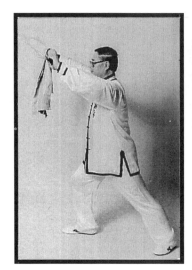

Figure A2-117

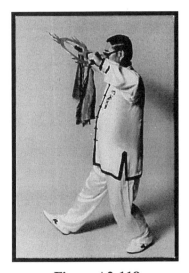

Figure A2-118

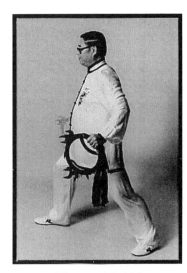

Figure A2-119

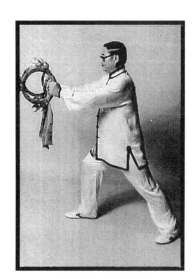

Figure A2-120

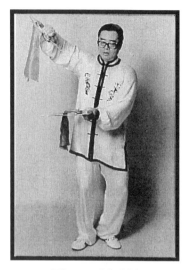

Figure A2-121

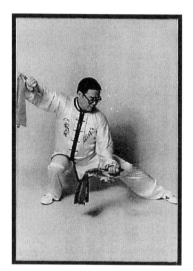

Figure A2-122

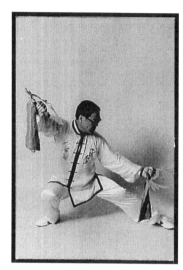

Figure A2-123

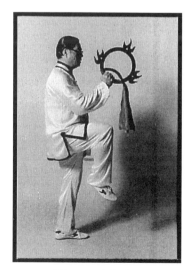

Figure A2-124

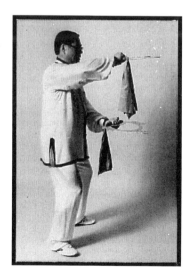

Figure A2-125

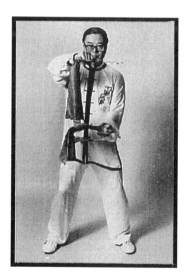

Figure A2-126

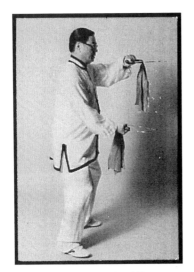

Figure A2-127

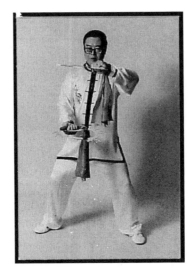

Figure A2-128

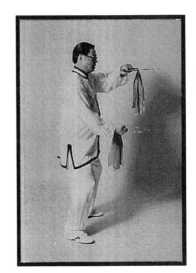

Figure A2-129

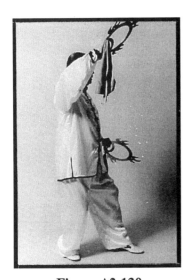

Figure A2-130

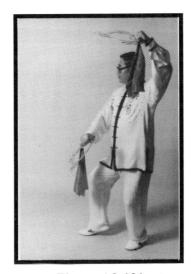

Figure A2-131

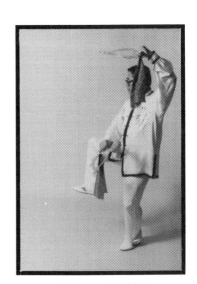

Figure A2-132

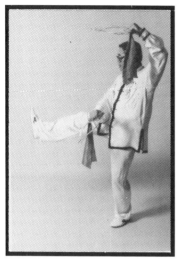

Figure A2-133

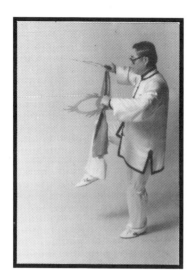

Figure A2-134

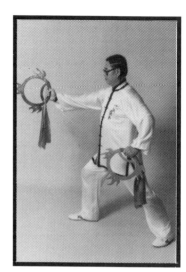

Figure A2-135

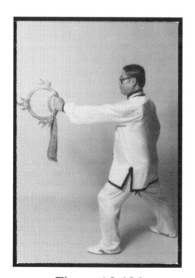

Figure A2-136

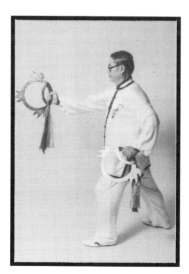

Figure A2-137

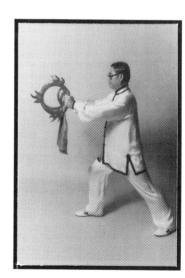

Figure A2-138

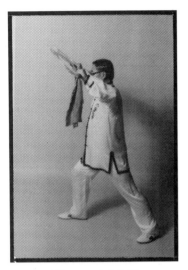

Figure A2-139

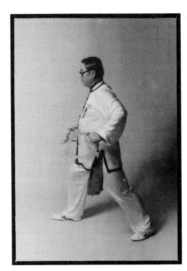

Figure A2-140

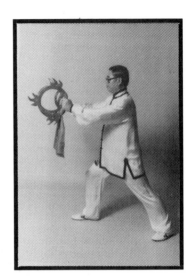

Figure A2-141

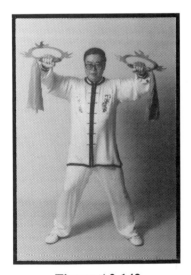

Figure A2-142

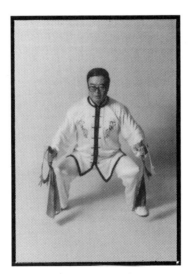

Figure A2-143

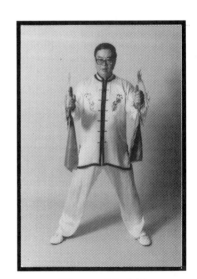

Figure A2-144

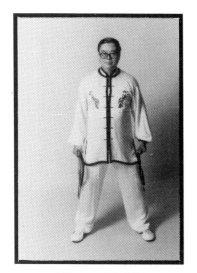

Figure A2-145

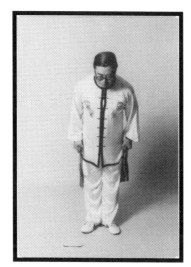

Figure A2-146

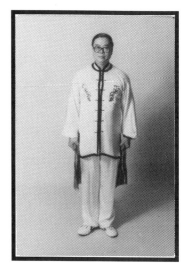

Figure A2-147

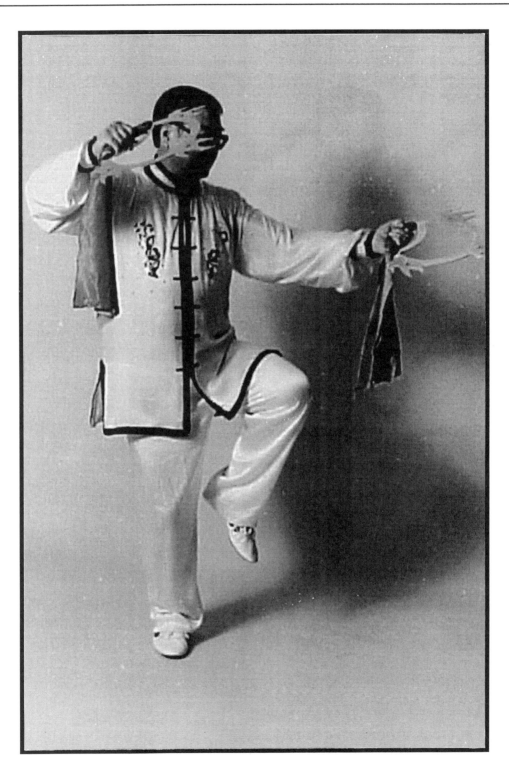

3. Advanced Form III

(1) 預備式 Preparatory Posture

(2) 風火起勢 Wind-Fire Commencing

(3) 向前左野馬分鬃 Left Step Forward Part Wild Horse's Mane

(4) 右轉掤,擺,擠,按 Turn Right Ward Off, Roll Back, Press And Push

(5) 左單鞭 Left Single Whip

(6) 雲手(三次) Wave Hands Like Clouds (3 times)

(7) 左單鞭 Left Single Whip

(8) 蛇身下式 Left Lower Body

(9) 左金雞獨立 Left Golden Rooster Stands By One Leg

(10) 右金雞獨立 Right Golden Rooster Stands By One Leg

(11) 倒卷肱(三次) Reverse Reeling Forearm (3 times)

(12) 斜飛式 Diagonal Flying

(13) 右提手上式 Right Lifting Hand

(14) 風火轉輪 Wind-Fire Turning Wheels

(15) 白鶴亮翅与踢腿 White Crane Spreads Its Wings And Left Heel Kick

(16) 左摟膝拗步 Left Brush Knee And Step Forward

(17) 海底針 Needle At Sea Bottom

(18) 扇通背 Fan Through Back

(19) 高探馬 High Pat On Horse

(20) 右蹬腳,雙峰貫耳 Right Heel Kick And Strike To Ears

(21) 轉身左蹬腳,雙峰貫耳 Left Turn Body Left Heel Kick And Strike To Ears

(22) 左摟膝拗步 Left Brush Knee And Step Forward

(23) 手揮琵琶 Playing The Lute

(24)　摟膝栽捶　Brush Knee And Punch Down

(25)　右轉右野馬分鬃　Right Turn Right Part Wild Horse's Mane

(26)　左蹬腳, 雙峰貫耳　Left Heel Kick And Strike To Ears

(27)　右打虎式　Right Strike The Tiger

(28)　左打虎式　Left Strike The Tiger

(29)　右打虎式　Right Strike The Tiger

(30)　右單鞭下式, 金雞獨立　Right Lower Body And Stand On One Leg

(31)　白蛇吐信　White Snake Spits The Poison

(32)　風火左右斜剌　Wind-Fire High And Low Diagonal Cuts

(33)　左野馬分鬃　Left Part Wild Horse's Mane

(34)　右蹬腳, 雙峰貫耳　Right Heel Kick And Strike To Ears

(35)　左轉玉女穿梭　Left Turn Body Fair Lady Shuttles Back And Forth
　　　　　　　(forward 1 time, backward 1 time)

(36)　左轉右野馬分鬃　Left Turn Right Part Wild Horse's Mane

(37)　轉左, 肘底看捶　Left Turn Body Fist Under The Elbow

(38)　指擋捶　Step Forward And Strike Down

(39)　風火轉輪(三次)　Wind-Fire Turning Wheels (3 times)

(40)　退步跨虎　Step Back And Ride The Tiger

(41)　轉身風火輪護頂与踢腿　Right Turn Body Wind-Fire Protecting The Head
　　　　　　　And Right Heel Kick

(42)　左掃右沖擊　Left Slicing And Right Striking

(43)　上步兩沖擊　Step Forward Left And Right Strikings

(44)　如封似閉　Appears Closed

(45)　風火收勢　Wind-Fire Closing

(46)　還原　Return To Origin

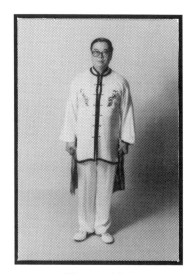

Figure A3-1

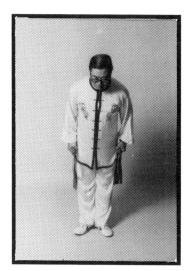

Figure A3-2

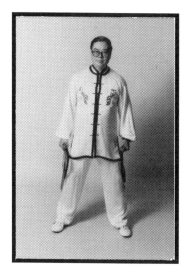

Figure A3-3

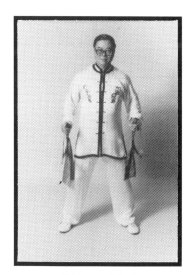

Figure A3-4

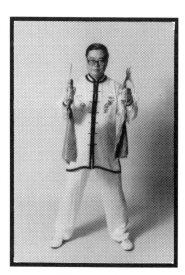

Figure A3-5

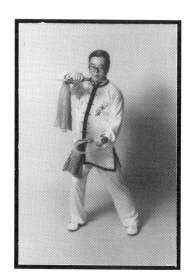

Figure A3-6

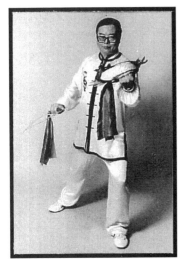

Figure A3-7

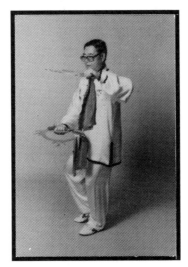

Figure A3-8

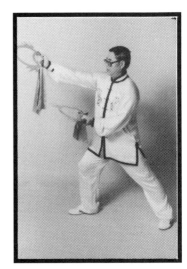

Figure A3-9

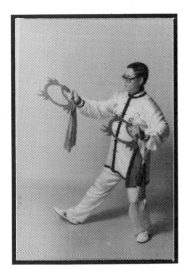

Figure A3-10

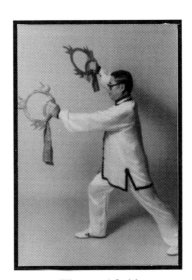

Figure A3-11

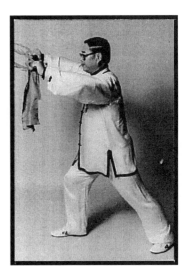

Figure A3-12

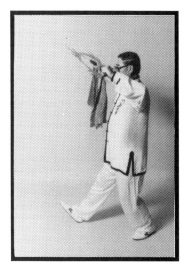

Figure A3-13

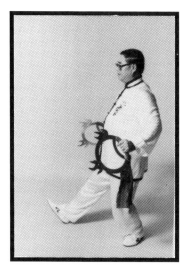

Figure A3-14

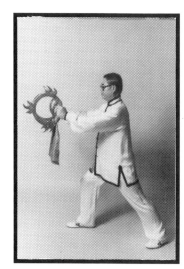

Figure A3-15

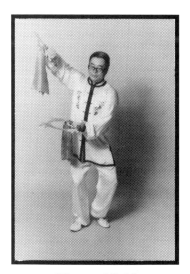

Figure A3-16

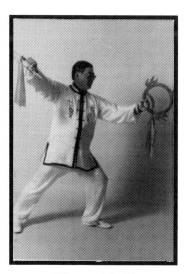

Figure A3-17

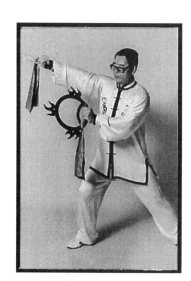

Figure A3-18

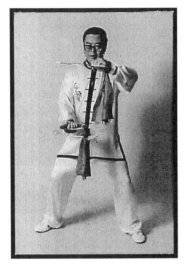

Figure A3-19

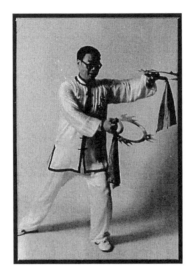

Figure A3-20

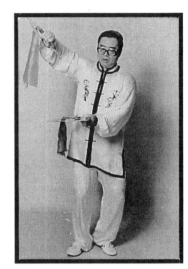

Figure A3-21

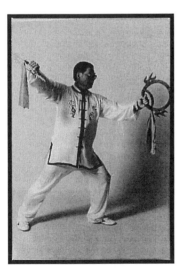

Figure A3-22

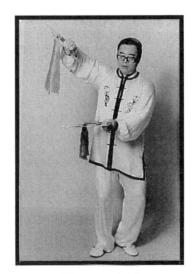

Figure A3-23

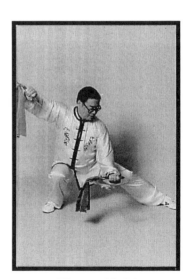

Figure A3-24

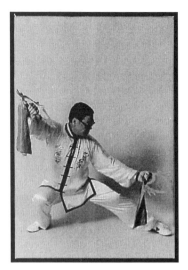

Figure A3-25

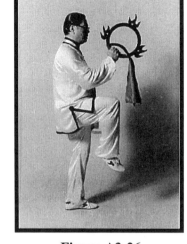

Figure A3-26

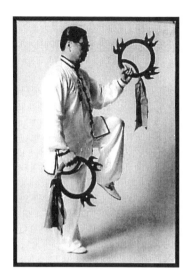

Figure A3-27

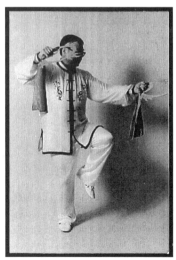

Figure A3-28

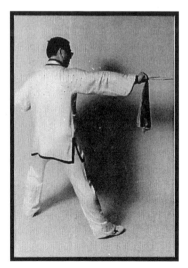

Figure A3-29

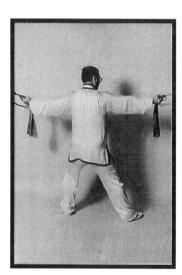

Figure A3-30

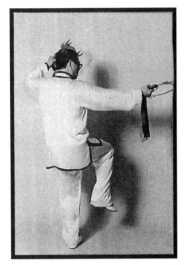

Figure A3-31

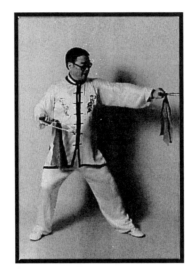

Figure A3-32

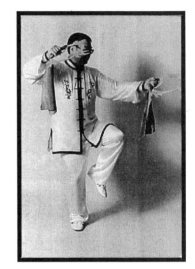

Figure A3-33

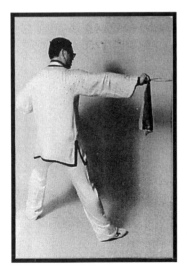

Figure A3-34

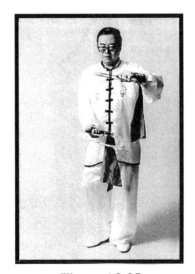

Figure A3-35

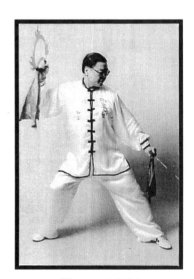

Figure A3-36

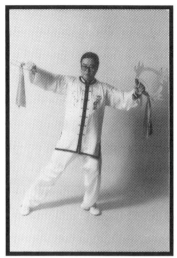

Figure A3-37

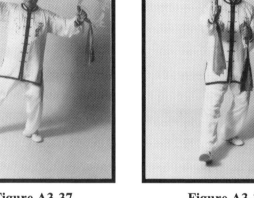

Figure A3-38

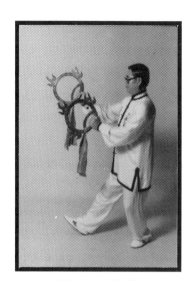

Figure A3-39

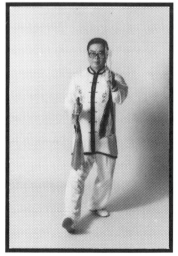

Figure A3-40

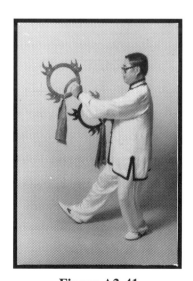

Figure A3-41

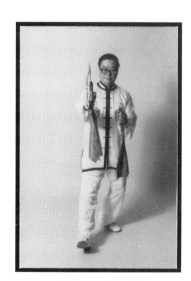

Figure A3-42

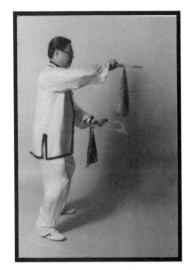

Figure A3-43

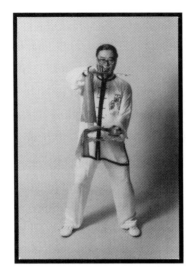

Figure A3-44

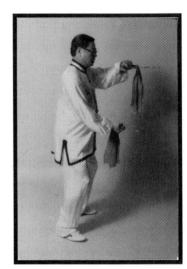

Figure A3-45

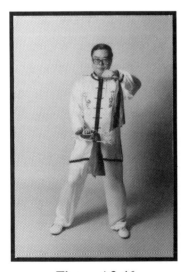

Figure A3-46

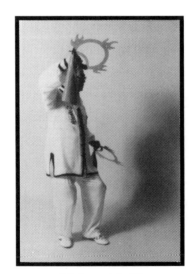

Figure A3-47

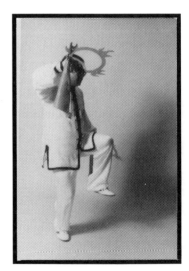

Figure A3-48

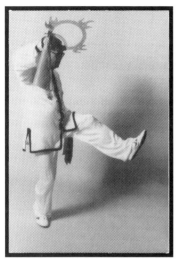

Figure A3-49

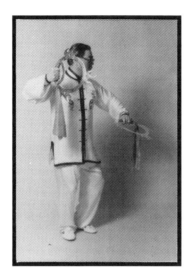

Figure A3-50

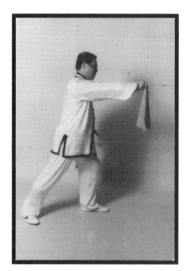

Figure A3-51

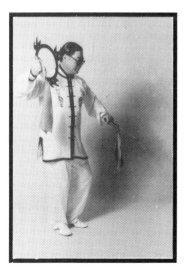

Figure A3-52

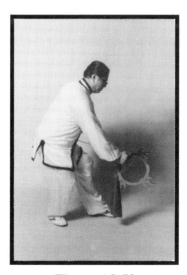

Figure A3-53

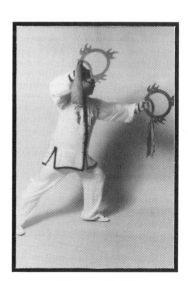

Figure A3-54

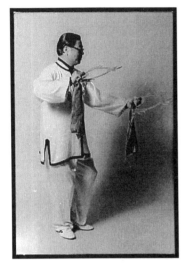

Figure A3-55

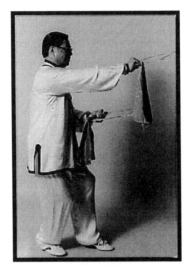

Figure A3-56

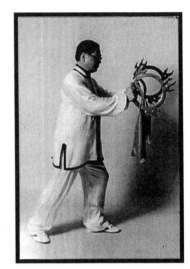

Figure A3-57

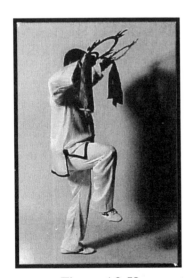

Figure A3-58

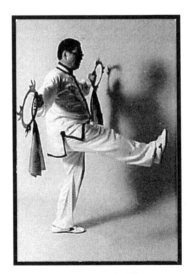

Figure A3-59

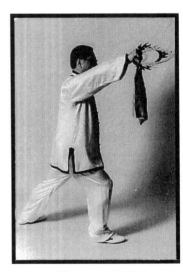

Figure A3-60

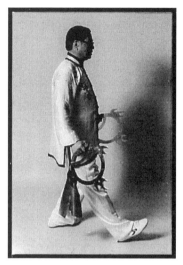

Figure A3-61

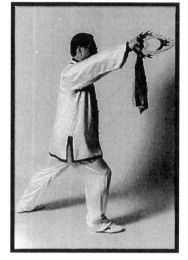

Figure A3-62

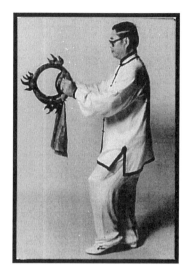

Figure A3-63

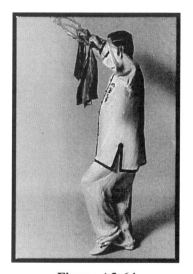

Figure A3-64

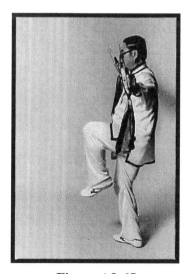

Figure A3-65

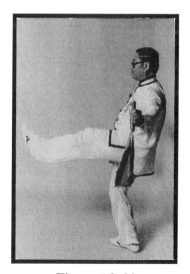

Figure A3-66

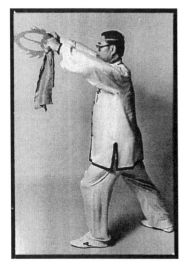

Figure A3-67

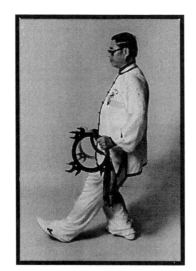

Figure A3-68

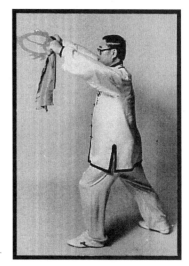

Figure A3-69

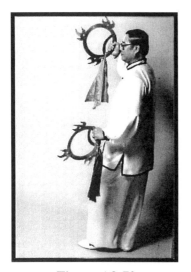

Figure A3-70

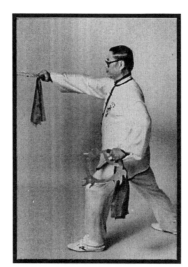

Figure A3-71

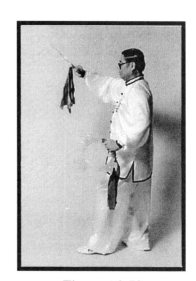

Figure A3-72

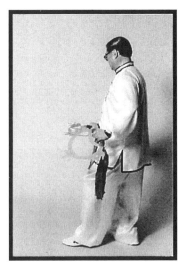

Figure A3-73

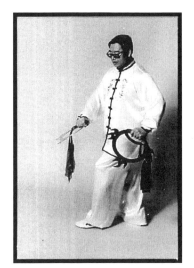

Figure A3-74

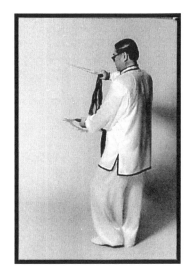

Figure A3-75

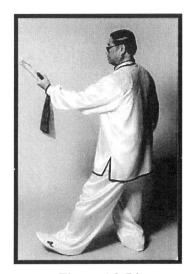

Figure A3-76

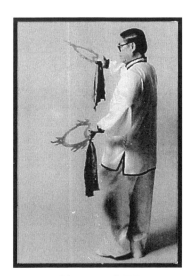

Figure A3-77

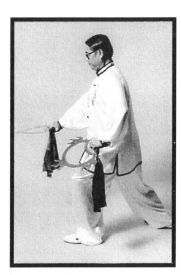

Figure A3-78

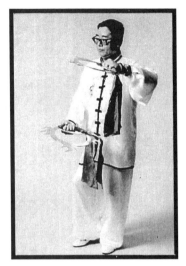
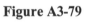

Figure A3-79

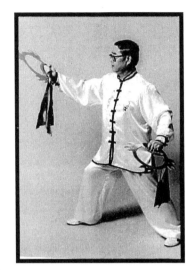

Figure A3-80

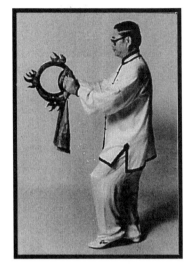

Figure A3-81

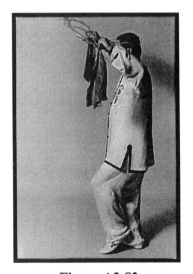

Figure A3-82

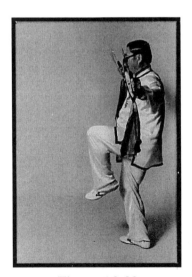

Figure A3-83

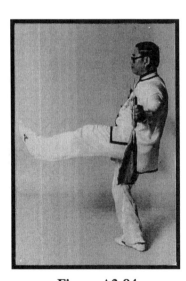

Figure A3-84

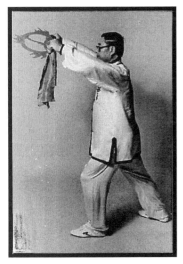

Figure A3-85

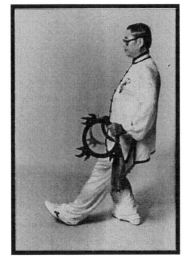

Figure A3-86

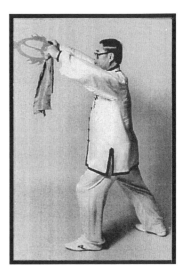

Figure A3-87

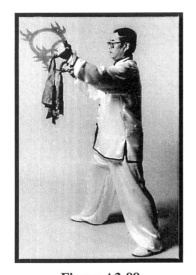

Figure A3-88

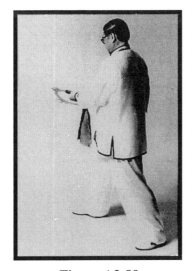

Figure A3-89

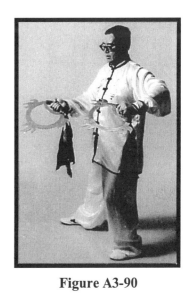

Figure A3-90

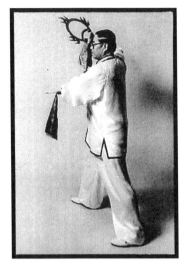

Figure A3-91

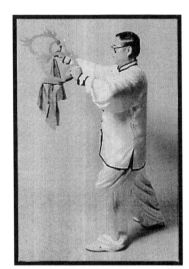

Figure A3-92

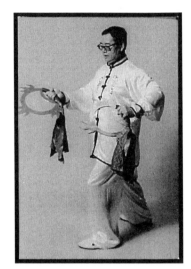

Figure A3-93

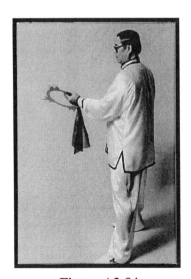

Figure A3-94

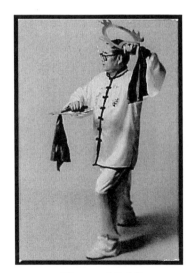

Figure A3-95

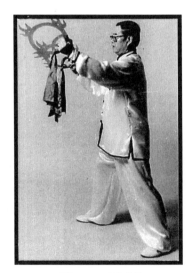

Figure A3-96

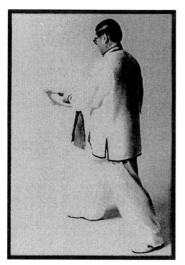

Figure A3-97

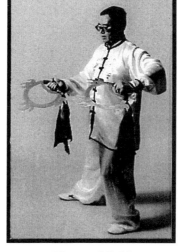

Figure A3-98

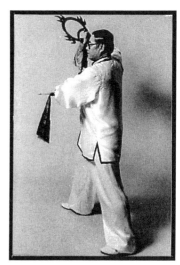

Figure A3-99

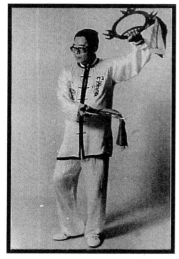

Figure A3-100

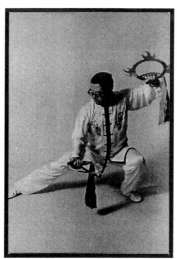

Figure A3-101

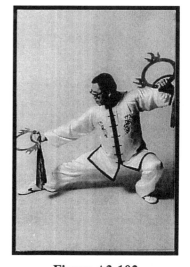

Figure A3-102

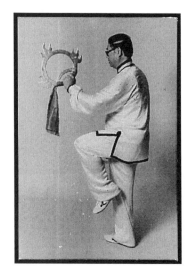

Figure A3-103

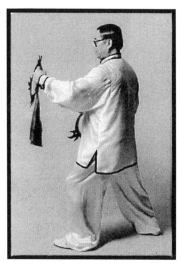

Figure A3-104

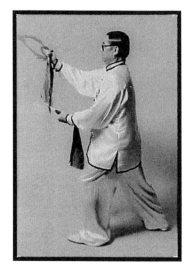

Figure A3-105

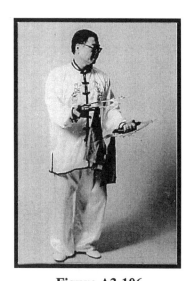

Figure A3-106

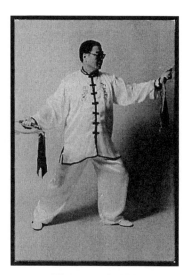

Figure A3-107

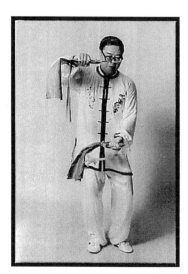

Figure A3-108

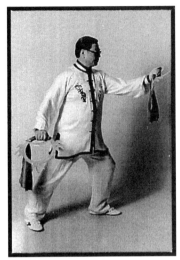

Figure A3-109

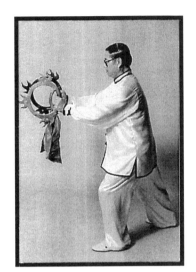

Figure A3-110

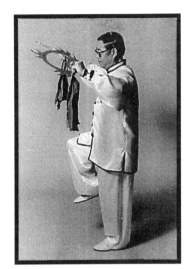

Figure A3-111

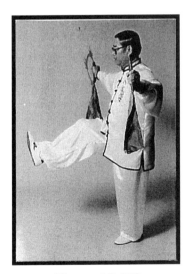

Figure A3-112

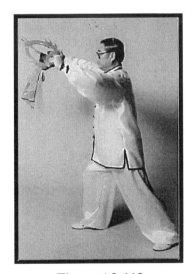

Figure A3-113

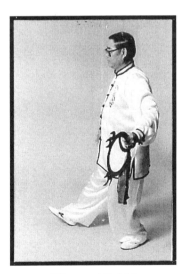

Figure A3-114

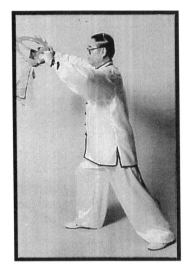

Figure A3-115

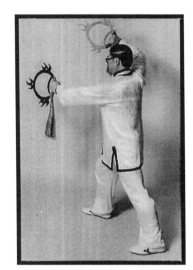

Figure A3-116

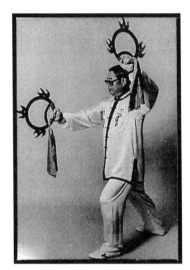

Figure A3-117

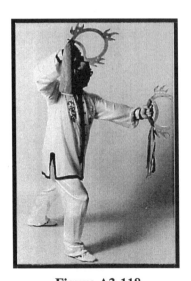

Figure A3-118

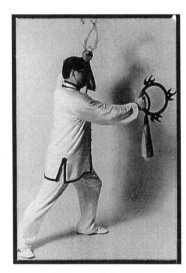

Figure A3-119

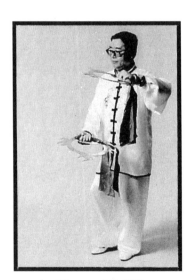

Figure A3-120

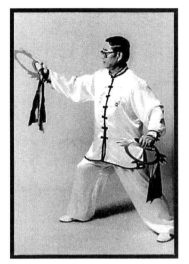

Figure A3-121

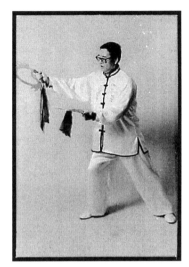

Figure A3-122

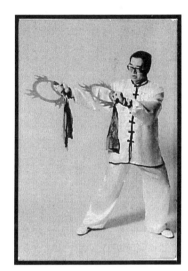

Figure A3-123

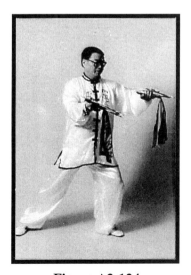

Figure A3-124

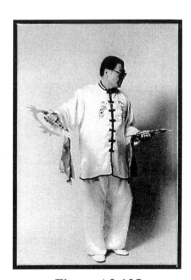

Figure A3-125

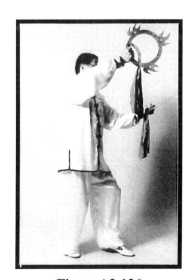

Figure A3-126

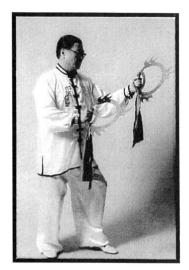

Figure A3-127

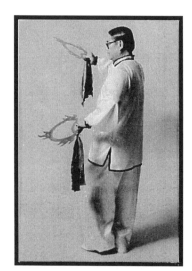

Figure A3-128

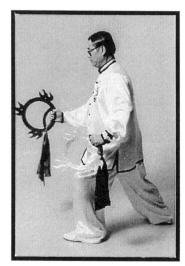

Figure A3-129

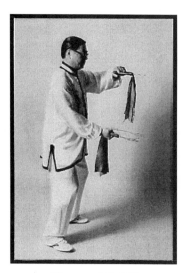

Figure A3-130

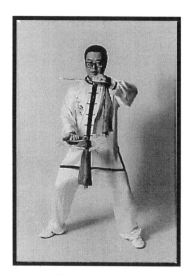

Figure A3-131

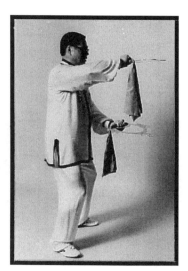

Figure A3-132

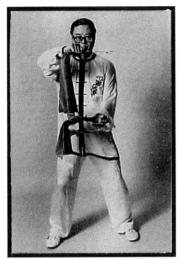

Figure A3-133

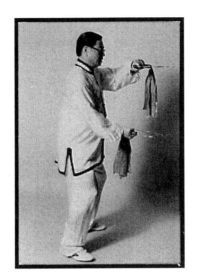

Figure A3-134

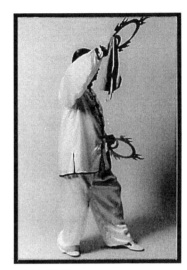

Figure A3-135

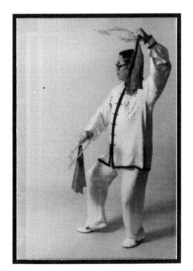

Figure A3-136

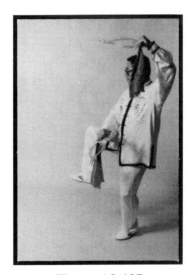

Figure A3-137

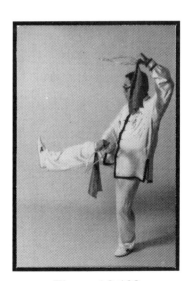

Figure A3-138

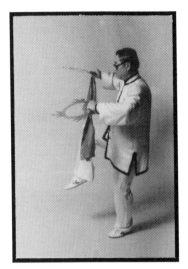

Figure A3-139

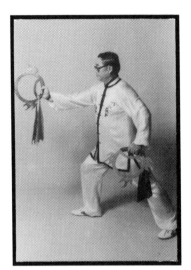

Figure A3-140

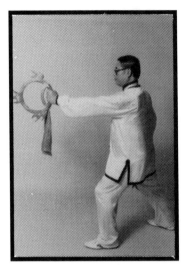

Figure A3-141

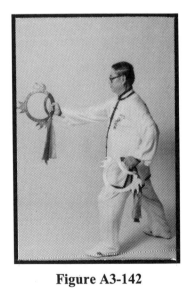

Figure A3-142

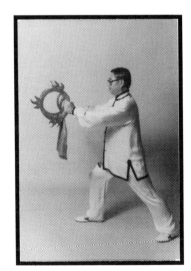

Figure A3-143

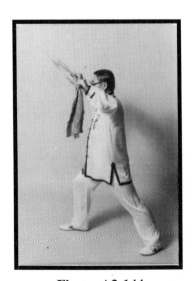

Figure A3-144

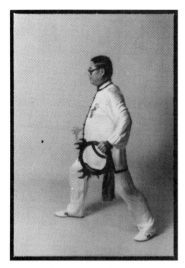

Figure A3-145

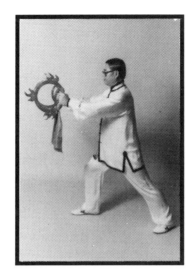

Figure A3-146

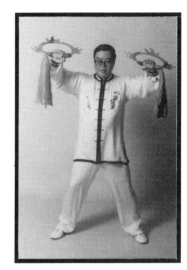

Figure A3-147

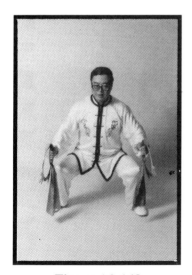

Figure A3-148

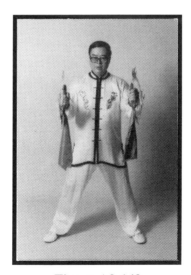

Figure A3-149

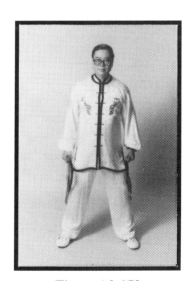

Figure A3-150

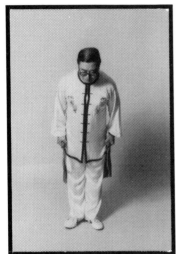
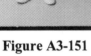
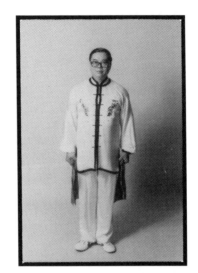

Figure A3-151   **Figure A3-152**

APPENDIX B

LIST OF PUBLISHED WIND-FIRE WHEELS ARTICLES IN MARTIAL ARTS MAGAZINE

1. <u>Inside Kung-Fu</u> , July, 1996
   Topics: " The (Wind) Fire Inside Your Tai-Chi "
        By Harriet Ellen Thompson

2. <u>Tai Chi & Alternative Health,</u> Vol. 1-Issue 12, 1997
   Topics: " Rebirth Of An Ancient Tai Chi Weapon "
        By Shahab S. Minassian, M.D.

3. <u>Wu Gong Journal Of Chinese Martial Arts,</u>
   Vol. 4, #20, 1999
   Topics: " A Book Review "
        By Harriet Thompson-Laurin

4. <u>Inside Kung-Fu,</u> October, 1999
   Topics: " The Wind Beneath Your Wheels "
        By Shahab S. Minassian

APPENDIX B

LIST OF PUBLISHED WIND-FIRE WHEELS ARTICLES IN MARTIAL ARTS MAGAZINE

5. <u>Qigong & Wushu Kung-Fu, November, 1999</u>
    Topics:"The Tai Chi Chuan Wind-Fire Wheels—
        A Nearly Lost Chinese Weapon Returns To
        The Scene"
    By Shahab S. Minassian, M.D. And
    Maryann Leonard, M.R.S.

APPENDIX C

LIST OF SPECIAL LETTER
AND GOLDEN AWARDS

(1) Grandmaster Jou Tsung Hwa's Letter to the Author

(2) Certificate of Seven Most Outstanding Golden
     Awards for "Tai Chi Chuan Wind & Fire Wheels"
     from the "World Chinese Medicine And Herbs
     United Association", November, 1998

(3) One of Seven Most Outstanding Golden Awards

(4) 1999 USA WKF Hall Of Fame
     "Outstanding Master Award"

Dear **Grandmaster Jou :** **May 18, 1998**

As has been requested by a number of people, mainly students of Tai Chi, I have recently completed writing a book on the use of the Tai Chi Wind Fire Wheels. As you know, I began teaching some of my students these unique weapons just a few years ago. The form has been seen in demonstrations and in competitions.

I have enclosed a prototype of the book. I would greatly appreciate it if you would review the transcript and provide a letter expressing your positive thoughts regarding the contents. As a recognized authority in the Tai Chi community, your feedback would greatly assist in helping the book become available in the community.

I look forward to your comments and to seeing you personally in the near future.
Thank you for your time and assistance.

Yours,

Steve L. Sun

Dr. Steve L. Sun, Ph.D.

树森老弟：书收到了，非常精采，但没有
"Foreword"之份，我想打电话给您，您的
电话，电话局不肯告诉我，你能签名在
纸上，多谢，祝好！

Jou, Tsung Hwa   Jou, Tsung Hwa
周宗桦

Sponsored by World Chinese Medicine
and Herbs United Association
A Non-Profit Organization
世界中醫藥聯合總會主辦

The Third World And Asian
Traditional Medicine Conference
第三屆世界亞裔傳統醫學大會

世界最佳
優秀醫學論文著作
OUTSTANDING MEDICAL THESIS

著作內容____太極拳風火輪____
Thesis Title
Tai Chi Chuan Wind & Fire Wheels

作者:____孫樹霖____醫師

NAME: DR. **Steve L. Sun Ph.D.**____

世界中醫藥聯合總會
評鑑委員會評鑑通過
**Approved by the Evaluation
Committee of W.C.M.U.A.**

總會主席: 江志成
President: Che Cheng Chiang

審委主委: 劉家駿
Chief Referee: George C. Liu

評 委: 黃 雷
Referee: Huang Lei

世界中醫藥聯合總會
WORLD CHINESE MEDICINE AND HERBS UNITED ASSOCIATION
987 N. BROADWAY, LOS ANGELES, CA 90012
Tel: (213)625-2112, (888)625-2112   Fax: (213)625-0001

425

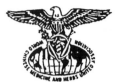 # WORLD CHINESE MEDICINE & HERBS UNITED ASSOCIATION

a non-profit corporation (非營利社團)

財團法人 世界中醫藥聯合總會

This is to certify that: **November 28, 1998**

Grandmaster Dr. Steve L. Sun's Latest work. "Tai Chi Chuan Wind & Fire Wheels", recovers a lost art that is over one hundred years old. Dr. Sun has not only brought new glory to Tai Chi Chuan, he has also discussed it with great depth in a very profound, logical and scientific fashion. This historic work has earned seven outstanding awards from the World Chinese Medicine and Herbs United Association in 1998. It is widely acclaimed as one of the few masterpieces, that is on Martial Arts and Chi Kung that will last beyond the next millennium.

Wind & Fire Wheels can be used as a special implement in Martial Arts which promotes health. They also contribute to a significant increase of inner strength. Many people have testified that Wind and Fire Wheels have brought glory to people of Asian descent and made special contributions to human health and the training in Chi Kung.

The Board of Referees of the World Chinese Medicine and Herbs United Association bestows to Grandmaster Dr. Steve L. Sun the following seven awards:

(1) 學術論文金牌獎   *Outstanding Medical Thesis Golden Award*
(2) 傑出成就金牌獎   *Outstanding Medical Achievement Golden Award*
(3) 診療專家金牌獎   *Outstanding Medical Treatment Golden ward*
(4) 健康器材金牌獎   *Outstanding Health Equipment Golden Award*
(5) 亞裔領袖金牌獎   *Asian American Outstanding Leadership Golden Award*
(6) 亞裔終身成就獎   *Asian American Outstanding Lifetime Achievement Award*
(7) 亞裔服務貢獻獎   *Asian American Outstanding Service & Contribution Award*

Dr. Che Cheng Chiang
Chairman of A.A.F.

Dr. Chia Chua Liu
Chief Referee

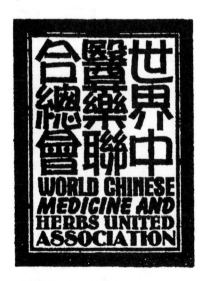

---

987 N. Broadway, Los Angeles, CA 90012, USA. TEL: (213) 625-2112, **(888)** 625-2112. FAX: (213) 625-0001

兹證明　　　　　　　　　　　　　November 28, 1998

　孫樹森　博士的巨著　"太極拳風火輪"(*Tai Chi Chuan Wind & Fire Wheels*)為最新出版的一本新書．已有百年以上失傳，現被孫樹森　博士重新發揚光大，內容深奧，合乎邏輯，並且非常科學化的偉大著作．經本聯盟總會評審為 1998 年七項大獎的歷史性大傑作，被譽為純屬壹本跨世紀的不可多得的武術與氣功結合的華麗名著．

　風火輪 (*Wind & Fire Wheels*) 可作為特殊健康用的武術器材，對增進內氣的功用非常顯著，並得到不少使用者的印證，對人類健康及氣功鍛鍊有特殊貢獻，可造福社會，為亞裔民族爭光．

　經本聯盟總會大會評審通過，特頒發世界最佳七項大獎：

(1) 學術論文金牌獎　*Outstanding Medical Thesis Golden Award*
(2) 傑出成就金牌獎　*Outstanding Medical Achievement Golden Award*
(3) 診療專家金牌獎　*Outstanding Medical Treatment Golden Award*
(4) 健康器材金牌獎　*Outstanding Health Equipment Golden Award*
(5) 亞裔領袖金牌獎　*Asian American Outstanding Leadership Golden Award*
(6) 亞裔終身成就獎　*Asian American Outstanding Lifetime Achievement Award*
(7) 亞裔服務貢獻獎　*Asian American Outstanding Service & Contribution Award*

　以資鼓勵，並向社會推廣．

Dr. *Che Cheng Chiang*
Chairman of A.A.F.　總會主席

Dr. *Chia Chun Liu*
Chief Referee　審委會主委

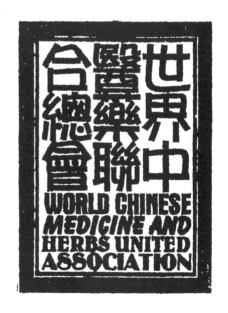

WORLD CHINESE MEDICINE AND HERBS UNITED ASSOCIATION

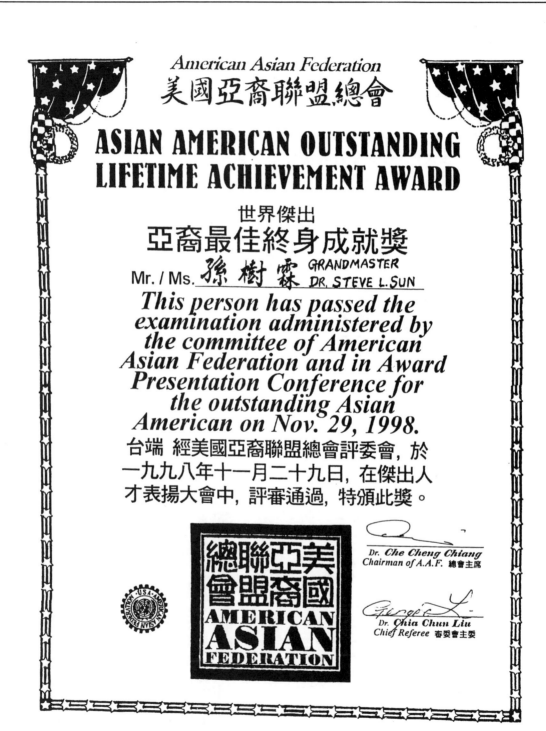

1999 USAWKF
Hall of Fame

Outstanding Master

presented to

Dr. Steven L. Sun

In recognition of the depth of your achievements in the art, in your teaching, and in your profound ability to inspire the many people around you.

August 8, 1999
_____
Date

_____
President

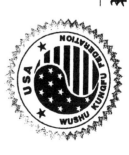

Special Comments

★ <u>Inside Kung-Fu</u>: 1996

" Rare Weapon Makes Triumphant Return"

★ <u>Tai Chi & Alternative Health:</u> 1997

"Rebirth Of An Ancient Tai Chi Weapon"

★ <u>Inside Kung-Fu</u>: 1999

" The Wind-Fire Wheels Bring Tai-Chi Forms To Life With A Beauty And Grace That Belie The Deadliness"

Special Comments

★ <u>Qigong & Wushu Kung-Fu:</u> 1999

"A Nearly Lost Chinese Weapon Returns To The Scene"

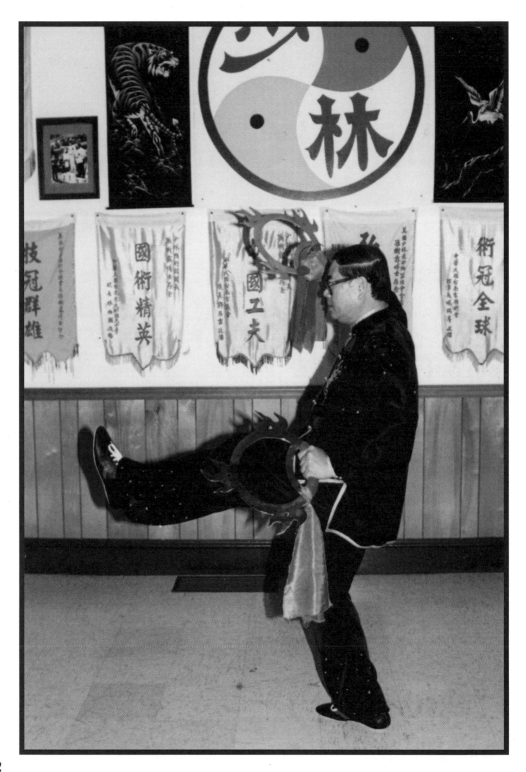

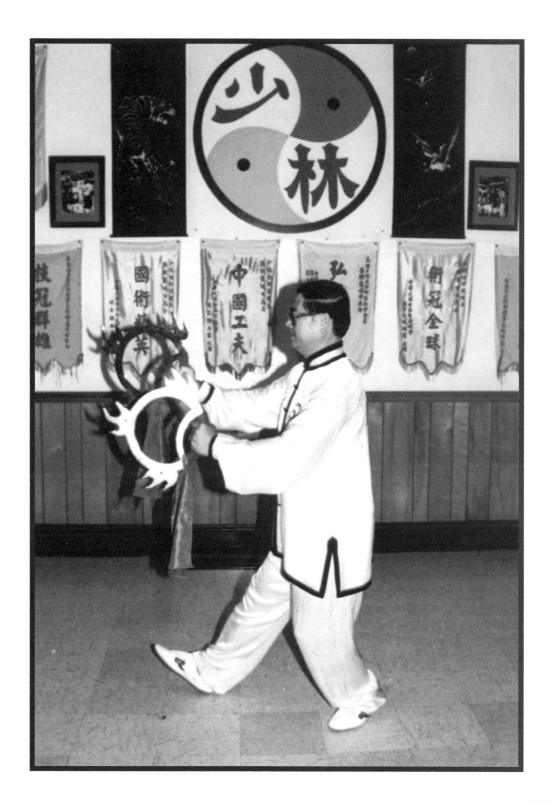

433

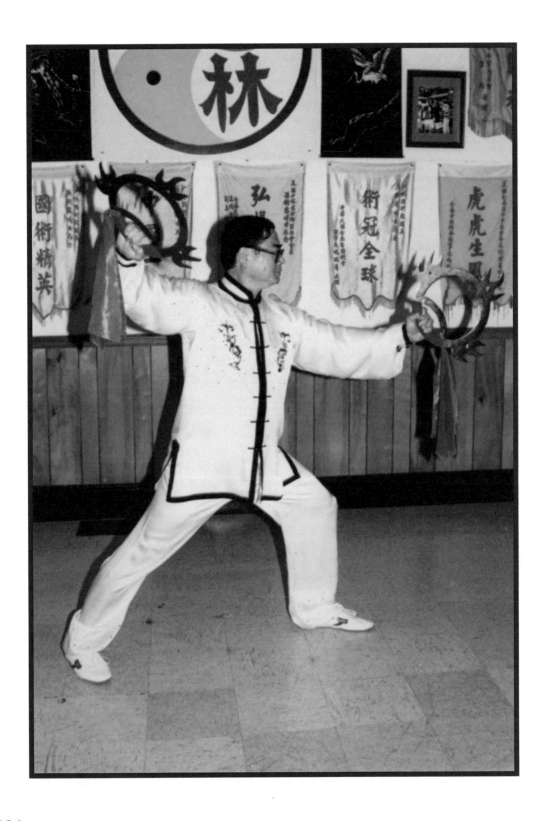

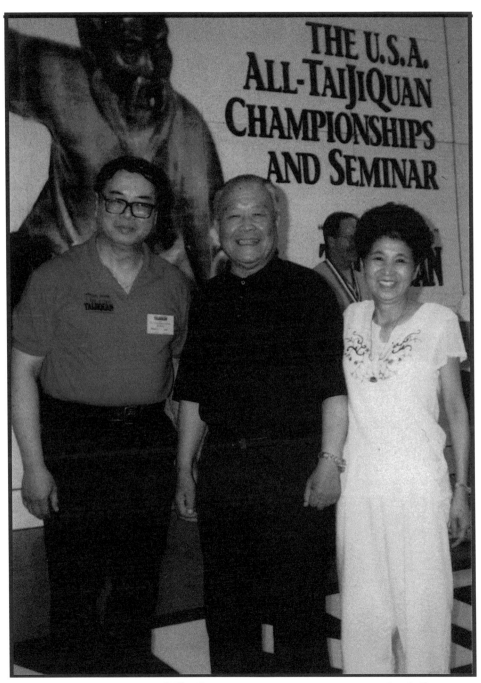

**The author(孫樹霖) and his wife, Emilia(吳碧霞),
with Grandmaster Yang Zhen-Duo(楊振鐸)
at "A Taste of China", Winchester, Virginia, 1998.**

Notes

Notes